This book is dedicated to our dear and inspiring friend Dr. Tom Ferguson (DocTom), a radical physician who championed healthcare consumers and encouraged them to use communication as a tool to get the most out of health care. Tom recently died after a long and courageous battle with myeloma. He worked tirelessly to empower the public to use relevant health information, gathered from many sources, especially the Internet, to confront and overcome health threats. Tom coined the term "e-patients" to describe the new generation of informed and assertive health care consumers who use health information to promote their health and the health of their loved ones. He leaves a large legacy of e-patients who are transforming and improving the modern healthcare system. Thank you DocTom!

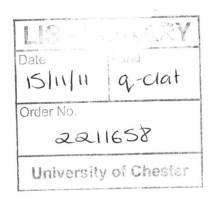
Handbook of Communication and Cancer Care

edited by

Dan O'Hair
University of Oklahoma

Gary L. Kreps
George Mason University

Lisa Sparks
Chapman University

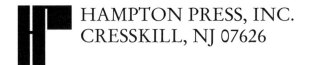

HAMPTON PRESS, INC.
CRESSKILL, NJ 07626

Libarary of Congress Cataloging-in-Publication Data

Handbook of communication and cancer care / edited by Dan O'Hair, Gary L. Kreps, Lisa Sparks.
    p. cm. -- (The Hampton Press communication series)
  Includes bibliographical references and index.
  ISBN 1-57273-682-8 (cloth) -- ISBN 1-57273-683-6 (pbk.)
    1. Cancer--Social aspects. 2. Cancer--Psychological aspects. 3. Communication in medicine. I. O'Hair, Dan. II.Kreps, Gary L. III. Sparks, Lisa Daniel. IV. Series.

RC262.H277 2006
362.196'994--dc22   2005058904

Hampton Press, Inc.
23 Broadway
Cresskill, NJ 07626

362
196
994
OHA

Handbook of Communication
and Cancer Care

HEALTH COMMUNICATION
Gary L. Kreps, series editor

Communication in Recovery: Perspectives on Twelve-Step Groups
  Lynette S. Eastland, Sandra L. Herndon, and *Jeanine R. Barr (eds.)*

Communicating in the Clinic: Negotiating Frontstage and Backstage Teamwork
  Laura L. Ellingson

Media-Mediated Aids
  Linda K. Fuller (ed.)

Cancer-Related Information Seeking
  J. David Johnson

Changing the Culture of College Drinking: A Socially Situated
    Health Communication Campaign
  Linda C. Lederman and *Lea P. Stewart*

Handbook of Communication and Cancer Care
  Dan O'Hair, Gary L. Kreps, and *Lisa Sparks, (eds.)*

forthcoming

A Natural History of Family Cancer
  Wayne Beach

Crisis Communication and the Public Health
  Matthew Seeger and *Timothy Sellnow (eds.)*

Cancer Communication and Aging
  Lisa Sparks, Dan O'Hair, and *Gary L. Kreps (eds.)*

Communicating Spirituality in Health Care
  Maggie Wills (ed.)

Contents

1 | Conceptualizing Cancer Care and Communication

H. Dan O'Hair
University of Oklahoma

Gary L. Kreps
George Mason University

Lisa Sparks
Chapman University

Great strides have been made in cancer care over the last two decades based in large part on the efforts of biomedical scientists, physician-researchers, and other medical personnel in the cancer research community. With each new discovery, individuals who are diagnosed with cancer find hope and encouragement for overcoming what was once considered to be a certain fatal disease. Due to advances in early detection and treatment of cancer, many people are living with cancer, rather than dying from cancer. A recent report released by the Centers for Disease Control and Prevention, (CDC) based on research at the National Cancer Institute (NCI), announced that more than 9.8 million people in the United States are cancer survivors, and this number is growing (CDC, 2004). Many cancers have become curable diseases for some people and chronic illnesses for others. Cancer care for those confronting cancer has never been more important than it is now because effective care can help cancer patients live longer, healthier, and higher quality of lives.

Yet cancer is still a serious health problem in the United States. More than 25% of all deaths in the United States are attributable to cancer (Wallace, 2001) and only cardiovascular disease accounts for more deaths in adults 65 years of age and older. Twenty-five percent of all deaths are attributable to cancer for adults between the ages of 65 and 74. Further, about 20% of all deaths are caused by cancer for those aged between 74 and 84. After the age of 85, the percentage of adults dying of cancer decreases to about 12% (Solomon, 1999). Males over the age of 65 are most likely to contract cancers of the lung, prostate, colon, rectum, urinary system, and bladder. Females of that age cohort are most vulnerable to cancers of the breast, colon, rectum, lung, and pancreas (Solomon, 1999).

Perhaps the one aspect of cancer care that has lagged behind until recently is communication. Compelling, empirically based research in cancer communication did not emerge until the last decade when funding for communication research began to find its way into the hands of communication scholars and research-practitioners. A major impetus for this funding was the development of the Health Communication and Informatics Research Branch of the National Cancer Institute, and the development of cancer communications research as a significant area of investment (Kreps, 2005). Through various programs and funding mechanisms, cancer communication research has been elevated to unprecedented levels (Kreps, 2003a). The accompanying "translation" of that research has begun to reach the level of the patients, although many important advancements will only be realized over the next several years.

Cancer care is a multifaceted process involving scores of medical personnel, numerous teams of care delivery, and a large investment on the part of the patient and her or his family. Cancer is not just a physical challenge to patients, family members, and health care providers, but also poses significant psychological challenges. Being diagnosed with cancer is often frightening for all involved and treatments can often be quite complex and uncomfortable. Some types of cancer are more easily managed than others. For example, although breast, colon, and skin cancers are still quite dangerous, especially when diagnosed at advanced stages of development, many patients with these diseases are living full lives for long periods of time, but this generally does not occur without concerted cancer care. The critical issue we want to stress is that although being diagnosed with cancer is not necessarily a death sentence, it is also not a disease that is effortlessly managed. It is a health problem that demands attention, examination, and decision making. An extraordinary number of issues must be considered in the conduct of cancer care, not the least of which are critical communication factors, including gathering and interpreting relevant health information; eliciting coordination among interdependent patients, providers, and family members, and/or caregivers; and providing social support and promoting psychosocial adjustment (O'Hair, Villagran, Wittenberg, Brown, Hall, Ferguson, & Doty, 2003). The contributors to this volume make compelling cases that communication is an inherent component of cancer care, and although we understand communication processes much better than we did even 10 years ago, there is still much work to do before we arrive at levels of excellence in cancer care and communication. It is important that we gain a deeper understanding of the complexities involved in effective and appropriate communication with cancer patients across the continuum of cancer care from diagnosis to survivorship. Effective health communication is the crucial link that can provide and encourage cancer prevention, inform cancer detection and diagnosis, guide cancer treatment, support successful cancer survivorship, and, finally promote the best end-of-life care in unique ways (Kreps, 2003b). To influence entrenched health behaviors, communicative messages of all types need to be relevant and compelling, with appropriate and pertinent health information that provides direction and rationale for making the best health-related decisions and adopting health-preserving behaviors. By gaining this knowledge, researchers and health care providers can give better cancer care to patients, and partners and family members can more easily acquire health information that will help them to help themselves in more productive and efficient ways.

We have organized the volume into sections in which conceptual connections among the chapters seemed to make the most sense. The sections are arranged into the following six parts: Providers, Patients, Communication, and Outcomes; Contextual Issues; Self, Identity, and Support; Special Patient Populations; Treatment Issues; and Patient Skills, Control, and Decision Making.

PROVIDERS, PATIENTS, COMMUNICATION, AND OUTCOMES

The first part begins with a selection of chapters that focus on some aspect of communication and medical outcomes. In the first chapter, "Importance of Physicians' Communication Behavior across the Cancer Care Continuum," Rutten and Arora review previous research on physician and patient communication specific to cancer prevention, control, treatment, and post-treatment care. Their discussion includes models of physician-patient interaction and important content goals for this type of interaction. The authors offer a summary of the various elements of physician communication across the continuum of cancer care from primary prevention, early detection, diagnosis and treatment, and survivorship, to end of life. The authors propose a number of limitations of the existing literature and suggest that future research efforts should address the limitations identified in past research by conducting longitudinal evaluations of physician and patient interaction episodes utilizing large, representative, and diverse samples.

The following chapter, "Health Care Partnership Model of Doctor-Patient Communication in Cancer Prevention and Care Among the Aged" by Kahana and Kahana, proposes a comprehensive and testable model of health communication termed the Health Care Partnership (HCP) model. The model was developed based on an understanding of the influence of communication among health care partners on patient outcomes in both cancer prevention and cancer care. Their model emphasizes content and relational aspects of doctor-patient communication but also positive patient behaviors in information-gathering and communication. Kahana and Kahana also emphasize the critical role played by health significant others (HSOs) in providing advocacy and support. The HCP model is a shift in thinking about how patients and HSOs can take a greater proactive role in cancer prevention and care and improved patient outcomes.

In the chapter by Harris, Kreps, and Dresser entitled "Coordinating Cancer Communication through Technology," technology takes center stage in the consideration of cancer care. The authors examine the uses of health communication technologies, often referred to as e-health, to support cancer care. Based on the argument that communication demands in cancer care are very complex, including the gathering, interpreting, and sharing of complicated and emotionally laden information, it is suggested that the time is ripe for the widespread implementation of communication technologies (such as interactive computer systems, advanced telecommunications programs, and multimedia educational programs) to help individuals confronting cancer meet the unique communication demands of cancer care. The chapter describes two approaches from IOM and NCI that can be used to enhance the use of health communication technologies in cancer care.

The focus of DiMatteo's chapter "Communication, Adherence, and Outcomes of Cancer Prevention and Treatment: Recommendations for Future Research" is on consumer-provider communication and patient adherence. DiMatteo noted a relative lack of adherence research in the area of cancer care (five studies in 30 years). A number of recommendations were offered for future work, including research on various regimens using a variety of measure-

ment strategies, and research on cancer prevention and treatment that includes effective
assessments of patient adherence for understanding the possible attenuating role of nonadherence. Because data are limited on variations in adherence among different cancers and levels
of cancer care, DiMatteo urges researchers to pursue empirical research that addresses those
issues as well.

CONTEXTUAL ISSUES

The second part shifts attention to some of the more salient contextual issues inherent in cancer communication research. The part opens with the chapter, "Communication in Context:
New Directions in Communication Research," by Bensing, van Dulmen, and Tates, who
argue that it is now time to direct communication research toward the study of specific contextual conditions that promise to broaden the base of knowledge in cancer communication
research. They suggest four areas of research, each informed by different theories. First, context should be determined by the goals or targets pursued by both parties in the medical
encounter. The second area takes up the issue of time, referring to the influence of previous
and future medical encounters. The third area involves the influence of the organizational
context in which an interaction takes place. Finally, context is construed by looking at a medical encounter as a meeting between two multifaceted parties. The authors contend that
studying medical communication in its broader context provides insight into issues that have
been neglected in previous research.

Taking a slightly different but complementary perspective, Ledlow, Moore, and
O'Hair's chapter, "Systemic Influences on Cancer Care," contends that environmental influences on cancer care emanate from a host of sources, including professional or institutional
pressures that have some impact, either direct or indirect, on the quality or duration of the
delivery of cancer care. In sections to follow, the authors briefly describe some of the more
prominent environmental influences: (a) the disease context, which include types of cancer,
pain management, and standards of cancer care; (b) sociocultural, with a focus on cultural
competence of cancer care delivery systems along with poverty's sociolinguistic influence;
(c) institutional/regulatory with, related discussions on HIPPA and FMLA; (d) paying for
care, with directed attention on insurance and managed care; and (e) cancer care delivery systems, including provider privileging, cancer care teams, and clinical trials programs. Moore
et al. suggest a number of implications for future work in the area of environmental influences on cancer care and communication.

In the final contribution of the section, Kim focuses exclusively on advocacy efforts in
her chapter entitled, "Public Advocacy for Cancer Care." Kim explores the world of advocacy with a specific focus on cancer research. She sets up her treatise with the axiom, "Science
follows money, money creates opportunity, opportunity brings discovery and discovery
brings money." Her chapter charts a historical view of advocacy efforts and lays bare the
political issues involved with funding cancer research. Many of the private, nonprofit, and
governmental advocacy organizations are described, and she offers some interesting detail for
how her own advocacy work began as a personal quest, quickly turning into one of the more
successful advocacy stories of its kind in cancer research.

SELF, IDENTITY, AND SUPPORT

Cancer is a formidable disease in its effects on the psyche and persona of patients. Patients experience deep psychological and emotional turmoil as they come to grips with the fact that they now have cancer and many of their significant others do not. This section raises a number of issues that seek to identify issues of self, identity, and the support offered to help patients cope with their internal strife. In the first chapter, "Patient Communication Processes: An Agency-Identity Model for Cancer Care," Villagran, Jones, and O'Hair put forward the notion that identity plays an indispensable role in the health care of cancer patients, and after a cancer diagnosis, the identity of a patient undergoes significant changes based on perceptions of powerfulness/powerlessness to participate in subsequent processes of decision making, reconstitution of relationships, and survivorship. The authors argue that communication is not merely a vehicle for the implementation for agency, but rather the basis of co-creation of an agentic identity after a cancer diagnosis. Agentic patients have the opportunity and responsibility to analyze the context and available options for care and make decisions that best serve their own heath care needs. According to this perspective, agency, then, opens the door of opportunity for choice within the patient-health care context.

In the next chapter, "Cancer, Communication, and the Social Construction of Self: Modeling the Construction of Self in Survivorship," by Richey and Brown propose a model of the social construction of self with the goal of understanding the relationship between a patient's interpretation of self and the lived experience of cancer diagnosis and resultant care. The model of the emergent self intends to conceptualize the process of social self-construction by suggesting that the development of self and the restructuring of self are inherent within the ongoing, shared locus of lived communicative experience. The model consists of three interrelated systems of self: (a) the experiential or existential self, (b) the relational self, and (c) the cultural self. The authors present a number of implications for future work in the area.

Babers, McWherter, and Brown expand our thinking about identity and support by redirecting attention to caregiving processes by nonmedical advocates. Their chapter, "Advocate/Caregiver Process in Cancer Care," begins with some interesting statistics about caregivers. It is estimated that as many as 75% of cancer patients bring a caregiver with them to medical appointments and that they do so to help with the communication aspect of the therapeutic episode. More specific reasons for the large number of advocate/caregivers who accompany patients include assistance with language or cultural barriers, and these instances more frequently involve frail or infirmed elderly people. Often, family members and caregivers put in many hours toward the care of patients in what is referred to as the "third shift"; an addition to the caregiver's "first shift" of paid work and the "second shift" of ordinary housework and childcare. The authors report a study demonstrating a number of dialectics operating in this context that illustrate the difficulty of this cancer care context.

Wright and Frey explore the communicative reasons that influence patients' decisions to join a cancer support group in their chapter, "Support Groups for Cancer Patients." In addition to an exploration of characteristics of cancer support group participants, their chapter delineates those communication processes that characterize cancer support groups as well as potential outcomes that result from participating in these groups. Other issues that are analyzed include how stigma, social isolation, and communication difficulties result in patients seeking support groups. Demographics are reported for those who participate in groups, and other issues include the topics discussed, types of messages, and narratives. The chapter concludes with an extensive discussion of the outcomes of support groups (e.g., coping, empowerment, and activism).

Brown and Bakos take up a little-studied cancer phenomenon, but one that is highly salient for many cancer patients, "Spiritual Care." Brown and Bakos position their chapter through a spiritual lens, arguing that spirituality is a powerful resource for coping with health-related problems. For the purpose of this chapter spirituality is conceived as a multifaceted, fundamental part of each person that drives a search for one's purpose in life. This search is often facilitated through religious practice and involves relationships with self, others, and a transcendent being. Issues discussed include diagnosis, emotions, coping, pain, and family adjustment. Brown and Bakos recommend that researchers studying health communication should incorporate spirituality in the health care setting and attempt to learn the influence of spirituality on health status and recovery issues as well as what effects spirituality has on the processing of messages in the health care realm.

SPECIAL PATIENT POPULATIONS

Cancer can strike anyone at anytime; however, special groups or populations susceptible to cancer are important to emphasize for a variety of reasons. This section targets aging cancer patients, ethnic groups, and children as cancer victims. In the first chapter, "Cancer Care for the Aging Patient," Sparks focuses exclusively on the aging cancer patient. Taking a perspective grounded in life-span development, Sparks analyzes the communicative characteristics of the aging patient in the context of a complex and overwhelming cancer care environment. Sparks proposes that cancer communication messages must match the specific communication skills, needs, and predispositions of the older adult population. She goes on to suggest that messages and interventions should focus on encouraging aging patients to be active participants in cancer care by focusing on message strategies that have proven their effectiveness. Toward that end, Sparks proposes the Selection, Optimization, and Compensation Model, which is intended to overcome age-related communication barriers. Through application of the model researchers, practitioners, and family members can construct interpersonal and mediated messages in a systematic, understandable way that will have a greater likelihood of reaching the aging patient diagnosed with cancer.

Ramirez's chapter, "Consumer-Provider Communication Research with Special Populations," shifts the reader's thinking toward ethnic groups as special cancer populations. Ramirez cites a number of statistics that convincingly report that special populations (African Americans, Appalachians, Asian and Pacific Islanders, Hispanic/Latinos, and Native Americans) suffer from a disproportionate cancer burden, often experiencing higher morbidity and mortality rates than the general population. Special populations also suffer unequally from specific cancers, such as prostate and breast cancers among African Americans, lung cancer among Appalachians, stomach and liver cancers among Asian Americans, and cervical cancer among Hispanic/Latinos. The chapter focuses on a number of barriers to cancer care specific to special populations including ethnic/racial, cultural, and linguistic challenges, and it concludes with a discussion on efforts and strategies to reduce the cancer burden for special populations.

In one of the more heartfelt chapters, Husain and Moore focus on "Communication and Childhood Cancer." Husain's daughter died from cancer as a child, and the authors make it poignantly clear that childhood cancer is a particularly distressing situation for children as well patients and their families. Husain and Moore point out that despite the importance of understanding communication processes in childhood cancer care, there has been an absence of literature in the area. Perhaps this lack of research is due to methodological challenges, not the least of which is access to the children and their families, and the emotional nature of the topic itself. The authors discuss several topics believed to be unique to childhood cancer, including developmental identity and emotion/cognition issues, family relational issues, and specialized communication issues. Major sections in the chapter focus on the child's perspective, the family's perspective, and the special communicative circumstances of childhood cancer.

TREATMENT ISSUES

In this section, several of the chapters delve deeply into the communication implications of treatment issues. The first chapter, "Palliative Care," by Wittenberg-Lyles and Ragan, contends that the dying process requires a paradigm shift from the perspective of health care providers and patients—a shift "that moves the focus from curing to healing and is characterized by a loss of control by all involved; that is, neither doctors nor other caregivers nor the patients themselves are able to keep the patient from an inevitable demise." The authors put forward the notion that narrative research can make meaningful contributions in three main areas of palliative care: the coping needs of terminally ill patients, their families, and their health care staff; as a pedagogical tool in teaching health care staff about patients' needs in the dying process; and as a means to evaluating current palliative care practices. The authors conclude that narrative research could create awareness of palliative care as a practice throughout the course of life-threatening illness and not just at its end stages.

The next chapter by Query, Wright, and Gilchrist takes up the issues of "Hospice Communication and Its Roles in Cancer Contexts." Increasingly, hospice is an option that a larger number of cancer patients are selecting for themselves. Query, Wright, and Gilchrist note the lack of systematic research in the area of communication and hospice care and recommend a systematic examination of interpersonal communication in providing cancer patients and their loved ones with social support in hospice contexts. Their chapter focuses on Western views of death and dying, examination of decision-making and referral processes, explanations of key definitions, a summary of the history of hospice care, and an assessment of communication issues surrounding the caregiver-patient relationship and their implications for individuals with cancer and their caregivers. End-of-life issues are discussed with an eye toward communication features. The chapter concludes with recommendations and directions for future research.

Gordon's chapter, "Care Not Cure: Dialogues at the Transition," draws attention to some of the challenges preventing effective communication in the context of palliative care. As a review of communication skills training for cancer physicians, the chapter raises questions for further research studies in the area of palliative care. Gordon argues that training programs can be effective in improving the communication skills of cancer clinicians at various levels of training. Training initiatives are supported by medical communication education programs that are competency-based assessments with optional certification of individuals and training programs. Health care organizations are also taking a careful look at communication as an essential element of patient safety and quality of care. These initiatives should offer opportunities for research on "patient-centered and systems-based teaching and practice," including communication and the management of cancer.

PATIENT SKILLS, CONTROL, AND DECISION MAKING

The concluding section of the volume includes chapters that focus squarely on patients, their skills in dealing with cancer treatment, and issues of decision making. The first chapter, "Cancer Patients as Active Participants in their Care," is authored by Krupat and Irish and centers on the communication process exclusively from the patient's perspective. Initially the authors ask about patient preferences for communication and the extent to which they express their needs and desires. In the second part of the chapter, Krupat and Irish explore research on strategies intended to induce patient activation interventions. Because much of this research has been conducted in health care contexts other than cancer, they extrapolate these findings to the care of patients with cancer. At the end of the chapter, the authors propose directions in which future programs of research and intervention might proceed to create better patient-provider communication, increased quality of life, and more positive health outcomes.

How patients come to an agreement with their cancer care provider is the subject of the next chapter by Chewning, "Concordance and Communication in Cancer Management" This chapter explores the concept of concordance and its potential for enhancing the communication between health care providers and individuals who have cancer. *Concordance* refers to the agreement between an individual and health care provider around a range of issues such as visit agendas, approaches to diagnosis and treatment, calibration of ongoing regimens, and even how actively an individual wishes to participate in a particular decision or visit. The nature and quality of the communication process influences their quality of life immeasurably. The authors review cancer literature related to individuals' preference for involvement, their visit agendas, their symptom monitoring and pain management between visits, and patients' interactions with multiple providers related to pharmaceutical decisions regarding chemotherapy and palliative therapy. To guide the discussion of possible approaches, the authors trace the experience of one individual with cancer who was a colleague.

Kerr redirects attention to an issue that is increasingly challenging for both cancer patients and providers—information seeking through information technology. In his chapter, "Health Informatics and Decision Technologies in Cancer Care Communication," Kerr delves into an area of patient communication with which most people are now familiar— using information technology for accessing health information. Kerr identifies and analyzes numerous Web sites pertaining to cancer care, and he cites a number of statistics related to information technology and cancer information. The core of his position is that patients and caregivers must become facile in evaluating a burgeoning pool of cancer information. One method of facilitating this goal is the application of criteria for evaluating health information. These criteria include credibility, content, disclosure, links, design, interactivity, and caveats.

In the chapter "Patient Participation, Health Information, and Communication Skills Training: Implications for Cancer Patients," Cegala presents the Integrated Patient Participation Model (IPPM). This model integrates health information with patient communication skills training. The basic premise of the model is that information about cancer alone is insufficient to prepare most patients to communicate effectively with physicians about their illness. It is suggested that communication skills training will enhance patients' use of information and promote more informed, adaptive decision making. The IPPM may be applied to several illnesses, including cancer; however, it is illustrated here with respect to prostate cancer. The integration of tailored information with communication skills training is the key feature of the IPPM. As patients are presented with tailored information about their illness, they are exposed to prompts and models of communication skills illustrating what they can do with the information during their appointment with a physician.

In the final chapter of the volume, O'Hair draws attention to several previous lines of health communication research that peer into patients' perceptions of communication quality, preferences for provider communication style, and relational messages that attempt communication control. O'Hair suggests a number of implications these lines of research have for cancer communication research and poses several limitations of their utility for health communication scholars.

PROLOGUE TO THE VOLUME

The goal of this chapter was to introduce the major communication approaches to cancer care that are covered in the chapters. It is the editors' hope that the chapters in this book encourage concerted investigation into the important functions and strategies for effective communication in cancer care. Researchers have the potential to conduct important studies that inform health communication practice, providing health care consumers and providers with evidence-based strategies for using communication to build meaningful collaborative relationships in cancer care that can help reduce cancer risks, incidence, morbidity, and mortality, while enhancing quality of life across the continuum of cancer care. Health communication scholars have a plethora of theoretical, methodological, and pragmatic communication-based approaches that can greatly contribute to enhancing the understanding of the many complex yet unique communicative contexts of cancer care (O'Hair, 2003). Health communication scholars must engage the health care community in cancer care research and actively translate research findings into strategies for effective cancer care. It is the editors' sincere hope that the chapters in this book begin this important process of applying communication research and theory to enhancing cancer care.

ACKNOWLEDGEMENTS

A volume such as this is impossible to produce without the expertise of many talented individuals. The editors extend deep appreciation to the contributors who shared their scholarly prowess and infinite wisdom in each of the chapters contained here. The assemblage of authors is a virtual Who's Who among noted health communication scientists. We are also deeply grateful to Barbara Bernstein, Publisher of Hampton Press, for having the faith, and especially the patience, in this project. Finally, we thank our families who gave us the time to bring this collection together: Mary John, Erica, Jonathan, Stephanie, Becky, David, Daniele, Elena, Arianna, and John O. We also deeply appreciate the inspiration from our parents (living and dead), many of whom have confronted cancer. This book is dedicated to you and to all the cancer patients, providers, and their families.

Proceeds from this volume are being dedicated to the Association for Cancer Online Resources, which provides a very important and powerful communication forum for tens of thousands of cancer survivors and their loved ones.

REFERENCES

Centers for Disease Control and Prevention (CBC). (2004). Cancer survivorship—United States, 1971–2001. *Morbidity and Mortality Weekly Report, 53(24), 526-529.*

Kreps, G. L. (2003a). Opportunities for health communication scholarship to shape public health policy and practice: Examples from the National Cancer Institute. In T. Thompson, R. Parrott, K. Miller, & A. Dorsey (Eds.), *The handbook of health communication* (pp. 609-624), Hillsdale, NJ: Erlbaum.

Kreps, G.L. (2003b). The impact of communication on cancer risk, incidence, morbidity, mortality, and quality of life. *Health Communication, 15*(2), 163-171.

Kreps, G. L. (2005). Cancer communication research at the National Cancer Institute. In M. Haider (Ed.), *Public health communications utility, values, and challenges* (pp. 379-390). Sudbury, MA: Jones & Bartlett.

O'Hair, D. (2003). Research traditions in provider-consumer interaction: Implications for cancer care. *Patient Education and Counseling, 50*, 5-8.

O'Hair, D., Villagran, M., Wittenberg, E., Brown, K., Hall, T., Ferguson, M., & Doty, T. (2003). Cancer survivorship and agency model (CSAM): Implications for patient choice, decision making, and influence. *Health Communication, 15*, 193-202.

Solomon, D. H. (1999). The role of aging processes in aging-dependent diseases. In V. L. Bengsten & K. W. Schaie (Eds.), *Handbook of theories of aging* (pp. 133-150). New York: Springer.

Wallace, R. B. (2001). *Prevention of cancer in the elderly.* In E. Swanson, T. Tripp Reimer, & K. Buckwalter (Eds.), *Health promotion and disease prevention in the older adult: Interventions and recommendations* (pp. 146–155). New York: Springer.

I

PROVIDERS, PATIENTS, COMMUNICATION, AND OUTCOMES

2 | Importance of Physicians' Communication Behavior Across the Cancer Care Continuum

Lila J. Finney Rutten, Ph.D., MPH
National Cancer Institute, SAIC-Frederick, Inc.

Neeraj K. Arora, Ph.D.
National Cancer Institute

The manner in which physicians communicate with their patients has a significant impact on patient health behaviors and health outcomes. Physicians' communication skills are fundamental to the effective delivery of clinical services across the continuum of cancer care from risk assessment, primary prevention, early detection, diagnosis and treatment, and survivorship, to end of life. Patients view physicians as expected sources of preventive health information (Kottke, Edwards, & Hagen, 1999), and physicians generally value their role in health promotion (Levine, 1987; Valente, Sobal, Muncie, Levine, & Antlitz, 1986). Physician-patient communication is vital in assessing cancer risk, motivating cancer prevention measures, and increasing patient adherence to cancer screening recommendations. The physician-patient interaction is also significant within the context of providing care to cancer patients. Cancer patients rely on their physician for support at the time of diagnosis, assistance with decisions about treatment, and follow-up care during cancer survivorship (Arora, 2003). Physician communication is also important to patients and their families as they struggle with the physical and emotional challenges of end-of-life care (Kreps, 2003).

In this chapter, the authors examine the literature on physician-patient communication relevant to cancer prevention, control, treatment, and post-treatment care. The discussion begins with a description of proposed models of physician-patient interaction and important content goals for this interaction. Then, the relevant literature is summarized to highlight the significance of various elements of physician communication across the continuum of cancer care from primary prevention, early detection, diagnosis and treatment, and survivorship, to end of life. Finally, the authors discuss some of the key limitations of the existing literature, and offer directions for future research.

MODELS OF THE PHYSICIAN-PATIENT INTERACTION

Three distinct models (paternalism, consumerism, and shared decision making) that differ in their relative emphasis on physician authority and patient autonomy have typically described the physician-patient interaction. In reality, physician-patient interactions fall along a continuum of these models; however, these conceptual frameworks provide an understanding of the range of, and distinctions between, various behaviors that may occur during the medical consultation (Charles, Gafni, & Whelan, 1999; Chewning & Sleath, 1996).

On one end of the continuum lies the *paternalistic approach,* also known as the *biomedical model,* which has traditionally dominated the physician-patient interaction. It casts the patient in a passive, dependent role and the physician in a position of dominance and authority (Parsons, 1951). This model emphasizes physician control over medical decisions and assumes that the physician can discern what is in the best interest of the patient independent of the patient's values and preferences (Ballard-Reisch, 1990; Emanuel & Emanuel, 1992). Patient autonomy is largely ignored as the patient is expected to accept and comply with the decisions made by the physician.

On the other end of the continuum lies the *consumeristic approach,* also referred to as the *informed* or *independent choice model.* According to this model, the physician's primary role is to inform the patient about the various diagnostic and therapeutic options, their risks and benefits, and their odds of success (Emanuel & Emanuel, 1992). Equipped with this information, the patient is free to make an independent decision, which is then implemented by the physician. This model emphasizes complete patient autonomy and control over medical decisions and excludes the physician from the decision-making process (Balint & Shelton, 1996; Ballard-Reisch, 1990; Quill & Brody, 1996).

Interactions between physicians and their cancer patients that are based on the paternalistic approach require physicians to make treatment decisions that are likely to have a significant impact on the physical, emotional, and social aspects of their patients' lives with minimal input from the patients themselves; the consumeristic approach, on the other hand, requires patients to make often complex decisions regarding cancer prevention, detection, or treatment without adequate physician guidance. Both of these approaches could lead to suboptimal decisions with far-reaching implications for the well being of patients (Butler, Campion, & Cox, 1992; Quill & Brody, 1996).

The limitations of the paternalistic and consumeristic approaches to the physician-patient interaction have led to the rise of the shared decision-making model, which is increasingly being advocated as the "ideal/preferred" model of interaction between physicians and their chronically ill patients (Charles et al., 1999; Golin, DiMatteo, & Gelberg, 1996). This model requires mutual participation by physicians and patients in the decision-making process. Patients and physicians are required to actively exchange information and ideas, negotiate differences, and share power and influence to arrive at decisions that would be most beneficial to the patient (Ballard-Reisch, 1990; Charles et al., 1997; Lazare, Eisenthal, & Wasserman,

1975). Also referred to as the *"relationship-centered" model* (Quill & Brody, 1996; Roter, 2000), it emphasizes patient autonomy without sacrificing physician authority. Although the final decisions may belong to the patient, these decisions (such as deciding whether to engage in prostate specific antigen screening or choosing between a lumpectomy or a mastectomy for breast cancer patients) are informed by both the physician's medical expertise and by the patient's personal values and thus have the potential to result in optimal patient health outcomes (Quill & Brody, 1996; Szasz & Hollender, 1956).

CONTENT OF THE PHYSICIAN-PATIENT INTERACTION: THE THREE "I"S OF PHYSICIAN BEHAVIOR

Consistent with the shared decision-making model, three important goals have been identified for physicians to accomplish during interactions with their patients: establish a good interpersonal relationship, facilitate information exchange, and facilitate patient involvement in decision making (Beisecker, 1996; Keller & Carroll, 1994; Ong, de Haes, Hoos, & Lammes, 1995). The authors have discussed these tasks in detail elsewhere (see Arora, 2003) and summarize them next.

Establish Interpersonal Relationship

Although critical in cancer, it is recommended that, in general, a physician should create a warm and trusting atmosphere in which the patient is treated as a "person" and feels that the physician shows interest in, and is sensitive to, his or her problems and feelings (Bakker, Fitch, Gray, Reed, & Bennett, 2001; Bensing & Dronkers, 1992; DiMatteo, 1994). Several researchers consider such interpersonal communication by physicians to be a prerequisite for successful information exchange and collaborative decision making to take place (e.g., Bakker et al., 2001; Ballard-Reisch, 1990; Finset, Smedstad, & Ogar, 1997; Golin et al., 1996). The Kalamazoo consensus statement (Makoul, 2001) concludes that establishing an interpersonal relationship with a patient is an ongoing task within and across encounters, and it undergirds the relatively more sequential tasks of information exchange and decision making.

Facilitate Information Exchange

A large proportion of time during clinical visits is typically spent in information exchange (Cegala, 1997; Ong et al., 1995). Information exchange encompasses three key subtasks for the physician: listening to the patient's story, giving information to the patient, and ensuring that the patient understands the imparted information.

Active Listening

Prior to imparting information, physicians have been recommended to actively listen to the patients' story without interruption (Rosenblum, 1994; Simpson et al., 1991). Physicians who provide their patients with the opportunity to establish their identity with uninterrupted talk often generate greater rapport and a feeling of openness with their patients (Rosenblum, 1994). Attentive, uninterrupted listening also helps physicians to get a better understanding of patients' subjective experiences, which is likely to result in clinical decisions that minimize disruption in patients' quality of life (QOL).

Information Giving

As a rapidly expanding area of inquiry, cancer prevention and control has produced multiple and occasionally conflicting recommendations regarding cancer prevention and early detection through diet, exercise, and cancer screening. Patients often rely on their physicians to distill this large body of knowledge and to make tailored recommendations. Furthermore, studies have consistently reported that a majority of cancer patients desire detailed information on a variety of topics such as prognosis, treatment options, associated side effects, risks, benefits, and so on (Blanchard, Labrecque, Ruckdeschel, & Blanchard, 1988; Cassileth, Zupkis, Sutton-Smith, & March, 1980; Jenkins, Fallowfield, & Saul, 2001). Moreover, they consider physicians to be one of the most important sources of such information (Bakker et al., 2001; Finney Rutten, Arora, Bakos, Rowland, & Aziz, 2004; Silliman, Dukes, Sullivan, & Kaplan, 1998). However, research in cancer as well as primary care suggests that physicians often underestimate patients' desire for information and overestimate their own informativeness (Cegala, 1997; Chaitchik, Kreitler, Shaked, Schwartz, & Rosin, 1992; Strull, Lo, & Charles, 1984).

Ensure Patient Understanding

While imparting information, physicians often use medical terms that cancer patients may not understand (Lerman et al., 1993; Lobb, Butow, Kenny, & Tattersall, 1999). At the same time, physicians tend to overestimate cancer patients' understanding of information given to them (Chaitchik et al., 1992; Gattellari, Butow, Tattersall, Dunn, & MacLeod, 1999). Even though physicians have been recommended to minimize the use of medical jargon during visits and to explicitly assess patients' understanding of the information imparted, such assessment is one of the least conducted communication activities in both oncology and primary care (Braddock, Edwards, Hasenberg, Laidley, & Levinson, 1999; Gattellari, Voigt, Butow, & Tattersall, 2002).

Facilitate Patient Involvement in Decision Making

Successful information exchange between physicians and patients ensures that patient concerns are elicited and explanations about prevention, screening, and treatment options are understood, thus laying the foundation for shared decision making (Richards et al., 1995). As Charles et al. (1999) explain, on the basis of this information exchange, a patient's options can be evaluated "within the context of the patient's specific situation and needs rather than as a standard menu of options whose impact and outcomes are assumed to be similar for clinically similar patients" (p. 654). This process of evaluating options and arriving at the final decision requires physicians to elicit patient preferences for outcomes and opinions about their preferred course of action. Physicians also need to explain the rationale for their recommendations. When difference in opinion and preference exists, physicians are required to facilitate discussion and negotiation with patients and arrive at a mutually acceptable decision (Charles et al., 1999; DiMatteo & Lepper, 1998).

This shared decision-making approach requires physicians to involve patients at various stages of the process; however, studies show that cancer patients who prefer greater involvement often fail to achieve their desired role during consultations (Degner et al., 1997; Gattellari, Butow, & Tattersall, 2001). Kaplan, Greenfield, Gandek, Rogers, and Ware (1996) suggest that in order to facilitate shared decision making, physicians have to be more willing to offer treatment choices to, and share responsibility and control with, their patients.

At the same time, a number of studies in oncology and other settings report that patients vary substantially in their preference for participation in decision making (e.g., Arora & McHorney, 2000; Beisecker & Beisecker, 1990; Blanchard et al., 1988; Degner & Sloan, 1992; Gattellari et al., 2001; Sutherland, Llewellyn-Thomas, Lockwood, Tritchler, & Till, 1989). Not all patients want to share or assume responsibility for treatment decisions, and a number of them prefer physicians to make decisions on their behalf. Given that patients vary in their preference for involvement in medical decision making, it has been recommended that physicians evaluate each patient's "level of readiness" for participation and tailor their decision-making approach accordingly (Arora, Ayanian, & Guadagnoli, 2003; Guadagnoli & Ward, 1998).

PHYSICIAN COMMUNICATION AND THE CANCER CARE CONTINUUM

Zapka, Taplin, Solberg, and Manos (2003) describe the continuum of cancer care as including the following distinct phases: risk assessment, primary prevention, early detection/cancer screening, diagnosis, treatment, long-term surveillance during survivorship, and end-of-life care. The continuum of cancer care provides a useful framework for examining physician communication within the context of cancer. In this section we discuss findings from the literature that highlight the significance of the role of physicians' communication behavior during each phase of the continuum of cancer care.

Risk Assessment

Primary care physicians are in a unique position to identify patients at high risk for certain cancers. The process of cancer risk assessment begins with the acquisition of detailed information about relevant risk factors, which may include age, family history of cancer, smoking status, dietary intake, and other lifestyle factors that may influence cancer risk (Caro, 1999; Penson et al., 2000; Stefanek, 1990). During this consultation, attention should be paid to both informational and emotional factors (Stefanek, 1990).

The development of genetic tests for predicting cancer susceptibility, such as tests for breast and ovarian cancer syndromes, hereditary retinoblastoma, and colon cancer, brings to the fore the importance of physician counseling regarding cancer risk (Taylor, 2000). Increasing availability and public knowledge of genetic tests challenges primary care physicians to remain abreast of available genetic testing options (Taylor, 2000; Velicer & Taplin, 2001). Physicians can play an important role in identifying potential candidates for genetic testing and offering patients credible advice (Taylor, 2000; Velicer & Taplin, 2001). Physicians should be prepared to discuss the benefits and limitations of genetic testing and make referrals for formal genetic counseling for interested patients.

Investigations examining the impact of physician communication about cancer risk and genetic risks have shown decreases in various measures of psychological distress among patients who receive risk counseling (Lerman et al., 1996; Meiser et al., 2001; Meiser & Halliday, 2002). Improvements in accuracy of perceived risk and increases in knowledge following physician counseling about risk have also been documented (Meiser et al., 2001; Meiser & Halliday, 2002). The impact of risk assessment on screening outcomes has been mixed. Schwartz, Rimer, Daly, Sands, and Lerman (1999) found that among women with lower levels of education, mammography use decreased following risk counseling, whereas there was no evidence of an intervention effect among participants with higher education. Decreases in clinical breast examination among women who received genetic counseling about breast cancer risk have also been documented (Meiser et al., 2001). Further understanding of the influence of physician communication around cancer risk on a variety of patient outcomes, including patients' health behaviors (i.e. diet, exercise, cancer screening) and long-term health outcomes, is needed to inform clinical practice.

Primary Prevention

The physician-patient interaction is vital to assessing cancer risk, educating patients, and motivating preventive measures (Carney, Dietrich, Keller, Landgraf, & O'Conner, 1992; Dube, O'Donnell & Novack, 2000; Hoppe, Farquhar, Henry & Stoffelmayr, 1990). Through promotion of smoking cessation, increased physical activity, and healthy diets, physicians can influence the initiation, maintenance, or alteration of behaviors that are likely to result in improved health outcomes (Brown et al., 1996; Dube et al., 2000; Eaton, Goodwin, & Stange, 2002; Ellerbeck, Ahluwalia, Jolicoeur, Gladden & Mosier, 2001; Fox & Stein, 1991; Fox, Sui, & Stein, 1994; Glanz, Tzirake, Albright, & Fernandes, 1995; Hoppe et al., 1990; Mickey, Vezina, Worden, & Warner, 1997; Ockene et al., 1988; Phillips & Kelly, 1999; Podl, Goodwin, Kikano, & Stange, 1999; Simon et al., 1998; Whitlock, Orleans, Pender & Allan, 2002). There is considerable evidence for the effectiveness of behavioral counseling interventions for smoking cessation, physical activity, dietary change, and cancer screening in health care settings (Eden, Orleans, Mulrow, Pender & Teutsch, 2002; Kottke, Battista, DeFriese, & Brekke, 1988; Ockene et al., 1994; Ockene & Zapka, 1997; Pignone et al., 2003; Silagy & Stead, 2001).

Smoking Cessation

Physician-delivered behavioral counseling regarding smoking cessation may involve discussion around risk according to symptoms and family history, and the delivery of cessation materials with appropriate follow-up (Kottke et al., 1988; Ockene et al., 1994; Ockene et al., 1988; Ockene & Zapka, 1997). A number of strategies have been identified to improve the efficacy of physician-directed smoking cessation efforts (USPSTF, 1996). Published clinical guidelines suggest that smoking cessation messages should be brief, clear, and informative, with emphasis on the short- and long-term benefits of quitting. Physician messages should be tailored to patient's concerns and address patient barriers. Smoking cessation messages should be consistent with the patient's readiness to change. For those patients who are not contemplating cessation, the physician should attempt to motivate the patient to consider quitting. For patients who are contemplating stopping, physicians should encourage them to set a specific "quit date" and discuss withdrawal symptoms. For those patients who have relapsed after a previous quit attempt, physicians should offer the reassurance that most smokers experience several unsuccessful attempts before achieving long-term cessation. During the first two weeks of cessation, relapse is common, thus physicians should encourage their patients to schedule follow-up visits or telephone calls (Kenford, Fiore, & Jorenby, 1994).

The effectiveness of physician-delivered smoking cessation interventions has been demonstrated in several investigations (Kottke et al., 1988; Ockene et al., 1994; Ockene & Zapka, 1997; Silagy & Stead, 2001). Results from these investigations suggest that the greater amount of time physicians spent discussing smoking cessation, and the greater number of providers intervening, the greater the effect. A recent meta-analytic review of 16 trials comparing brief advice to no advice demonstrated a small but significant increase in smoking cessation among patients who received brief physician counseling compared to those who received usual care (Silagy & Stead, 2001).

Physical Activity

Behavioral counseling to increase physical activity should aim to determine patients' current activity levels and assess individual barriers to physical activity. Physicians should discuss the role of physical activity in disease prevention with their patients and assist their patients in selecting appropriate types of physical activity according to their medical needs, interests, and current activity levels (USPSTF, 1996).

Eden et al. (2002) recently conducted a systematic review of randomized trials of interventions focusing on increasing physical activity. This review focused on controlled trials published since 1996, the year the U.S. Preventive Services Task Force (USPSTF) began recommending counseling to promote physical activity in children and adults. This review included seven randomized controlled trials and one nonrandomized controlled trial wherein some component of the intervention was conducted by a primary care clinician. The review yielded mixed results; among the 6 trials considered to be of good or fair quality, two did not show any effect after 6 months of follow-up.

Available evidence regarding the efficacy of physician-delivered behavioral counseling about physical activity is inconclusive. However, given the strength of evidence regarding the benefits of increased physical activity and the degree of risks associated with sedentary lifestyles, even modest changes in physical activity levels could have a large public health impact. Evidence supporting this potential for improving public health corroborates the 1996 USPSTF recommendations.

Dietary Change

Physician-delivered behavioral counseling to initiate dietary change may involve the provision of nutrition education in combination with counseling to assist patients in developing the skills, motivation, and support necessary for dietary change (USPSTF, 2003). Counseling may include discussion of strategies for overcoming barriers to selecting a healthy diet and assistance in developing goals for dietary change. Specific strategies for physician counseling include guiding patients in their food selection and preparation, teaching self-monitoring of food intake, role-playing healthy dietary choices, and arranging for social support (USPSTF, 2003).

Physician counseling has been found to improve dietary outcomes (Beresford et al., 1997; Pignone et al., 2003). A review of randomized controlled trials of physician-delivered nutritional counseling published between 1996 and 2001 was conducted to examine the effectiveness of counseling in producing dietary change (Pignone et al., 2003). A total of 21 studies addressing changes in consumption of dietary fat, fruit and vegetable intake, and fiber were reviewed. The review provided evidence that low- to medium-intensity dietary counseling conducted in primary care settings can produce decreases in dietary fat intake and increases in fruit and vegetable intake.

Early Detection/Cancer Screening

Physicians also play a pivotal role in educating patients about and recommending cancer screening. Conflicting screening recommendations and uncertainty regarding the benefits of certain cancer screening procedures make shared decision making between physicians and patients essential (Dunn, Shridharani, Lou, & Bernstein, 2001). Physicians should provide patients with information about the costs and benefits of screening and facilitate patient involvement in decision making (Dunn et al., 2001; Pellissier & Venta, 1996; Wolf & Becker, 1996). Communication around the patient's risk of developing cancer, the efficacy of screening exams, the possible implications of the results of screening exams, and the likely benefits and potential burdens of screening exams is essential to lay the foundation for informed decision making (Brown, 1991; Wolf & Becker, 1996). Assessing patients' beliefs about screening—and welcoming patient discussion of their goals, values, and preferences—may improve the shared decision-making process (Farrell, Murphy & Schneider, 2002; Pellissier & Venta, 1996; Royak-Schaler et al., 2002; Royak-Schaler, Parr Lemkau, & Ahmed, 2002).

Physician-delivered behavioral counseling about screening has been found to predict adherence to screening guidelines (Brown et al., 1996; Fox & Stein, 1991; Fox et al., 1994; Mickey et al., 1997; Phillips & Kelly, 1999; Simon et al., 1998). For example, Fox and Stein (1991) examined predictors of mammography screening among White, Black, and Hispanic women. Results of their investigation revealed that among each race group, the odds of having had a recent mammogram and of having ever had a mammogram were 6 to 7 times greater among women who reported that their physician talked with them about mammography. In Brown et al.'s (1996) simultaneous examination of patient, physician, and system factors associated with screening, physician recommendation was associated with a 50% increase in the odds of patients having an annual mammogram.

Cancer Diagnosis and Treatment

Upon diagnosis of cancer and during cancer treatment, cancer patients rely on their physicians for support, information, and guidance. McWilliam, Brown, and Stewart (2000) suggest that the feelings of vulnerability, uncertainty, and loss of self that are often experienced by cancer patients may heighten the intensity with which patients "feel the present moments of patient-doctor communication, and render more powerful their positive or, conversely, negative experiences of the interaction" (p. 201). Similarly, Siminoff, Radvin, Colabianchi, and Saunders-Sturm (2000) observe that although the communication process between physicians and cancer patients shares most of the general features of standard physician-patient interactions, the stigma and fear associated with a cancer diagnosis, the complexity of medical information, and uncertainty regarding the course of the disease and treatment adds a greater emotional dimension to the interaction. Thus, patients whose information and support needs are met are likely to experience less disruption in QOL and more favorable health outcomes (Rose, 1990; Schain, 1990).

The difficult task for physicians of "breaking the bad news" of a cancer diagnosis to patients has been addressed in several articles that advise physicians to guide the process of communicating a cancer diagnosis in a way that facilitates psychological adjustment and effective coping among patients (e.g. Baile & Beale, 2001; Bennett & Alison, 1996; Ellis & Tattersall, 1999; Girgis & Sanson-Fisher, 1998; Lee, Back, Block, & Stewart, 2002). In general, these guidelines encourage physicians to make preparations to deliver cancer diagnoses in a private setting with sufficient time set aside to address patient concerns and reactions. Assessing the patient's understanding of their situation and desire for information is also encouraged. It has been recommended that physicians disclose the diagnosis in honest and simple terms, providing medical details consistent with the patient's interest in such detail. Physicians have been advised to facilitate and respond to patients' emotional reactions. Discussing the implications of the diagnosis and offering additional resources is also recommended. Finally, physicians have been encouraged to summarize the discussion and arrange for a follow-up consultation to address patient and family concerns.

Although numerous articles offering advice to physicians regarding communicating difficult news to patients have been published in medical journals, only a few studies have examined the influence of physician communication during diagnosis on patient outcomes (Butow et al., 1996; Mager & Andrykowski, 2002; Omne-Ponten, Holmberg, & Sjoden, 1994; Roberts, Cox, Reintgen, Baile, & Gibertine, 1994). These investigations have demonstrated better psychological adjustment among patients who had their questions answered by their physician during the diagnostic consultation (Roberts et al., 1994), were satisfied with communication in the diagnostic consultation (Butow et al., 1996), and had positive perceptions of the quality of interaction with their physician during the diagnostic consultation (Omne-Ponten et al., 1994). Mager and Andrykowski (2002) found an association between long-term psychological adjustment and patients' perceptions of their physicians use of psychotherapeutic techniques during the diagnostic consultation among women with breast cancer. However, no association between patient satisfaction with the diagnostic consultation and long-term adjustment was found in this investigation (Mager & Andrykowski, 2002). These findings suggest that physician communication at the time of diagnosis influences patients' coping trajectory and psychological adjustment; research is needed to examine the impact of the diagnostic consultation on other patient outcomes, including adherence to treatment regimens and survival.

Critical and difficult decisions about cancer treatment must be made following a cancer diagnosis. Physician communication about available treatments, clinical trails, and the risks and benefits of treatment options is crucial in cancer care because indications for treatment are not always obvious. One study examining the impact of treatment discussions on patient outcomes showed that patients were overwhelmed by and had difficulty comprehending the information provided to them (Siminoff, Fetting, & Abeloff, 1989). This same study revealed that physicians spent little time explaining the pros and cons of treatment options, and that, in turn, patients did not have a good understanding of the pros and cons of available treatment (Siminoff et al., 1989).

Reductions in anxiety and depression and improved physical functioning among patients whose physicians encouraged their involvement in treatment decisions have been documented (Fallowfield, Hall, Maguire, & Baum, 1990; Fallowfield, Hall, Maguire, Baum, & A'Hern, 1994; Morris & Ingham, 1988; Morris & Royle, 1988). Higher levels of QOL have also been observed among patients who believed they were given decisional control about their cancer treatment (Street & Voigt, 1997), and among patients for whom there was consistency between their preferences for decisional control and actual control (Gattellari et al., 2001). These findings emphasize the primacy of the shared decision-making model and suggest that encouraging patient involvement in treatment decisions has a positive impact on their psychological adjustment and QOL.

Follow-up Cancer Care During Survivorship

Cancer survivors often experience late and/or long-term complications due to their cancer treatments, which may be physiological or psychosocial in nature (Campbell, Marbella, & Layde, 2000; Fernsler & Fanuele, 1998; Gotay & Muraoka, 1998; Hancock & Hoppe, 1996). Although research on cancer survivors is beginning to receive more attention, the extent to which physicians educate their patients about potential health problems they are likely to experience in the future and the extent to which they help their patients in dealing with such problems is not well documented. In general, follow-up care for cancer survivors is understudied and a fertile area for future research (Institute of Medicine, 2003).

Tesauro, Rowland, and Lustig (2002) examined the availability of supportive care and medical follow-up for cancer survivors. Frequently identified physician-led support services included lymphedema management, support groups, and long-term follow-up clinics. Although such services appear to be consistent with the concerns of long-term cancer survivors (Gray et al., 1998; Mullan, 1984), evidence regarding survivors' participation in and the impact of such programs on survivor outcomes is limited. Eiser, Hill, and Blacklay (2000) evaluated a clinic-based intervention for survivors of childhood cancer. The intervention was presented by physicians to patients during routine follow-up care and consisted of an information booklet, treatment summary, and information sheets. Assessment of patients before and after intervention revealed increases in self-efficacy regarding health, greater preparedness for behavioral change, and increased perceptions of susceptibility to future health problems. Other studies show that cancer survivors indeed report a strong preference for receiving follow-up care (Stiggelbout et al., 1997), and survivors who play an active role in follow-up care decisions also report better quality of life (Andersen & Urban, 1999). Clearly, by educating their patients and involving them in the decision-making process, physicians have the potential to positively impact the health outcomes of cancer survivors. Future studies are needed to assess the impact of post-treatment physician-delivered services on cancer survivors' health and well-being.

End-of-Life Care

Several studies have documented a need for improvements in the quality of end-of-life care in the United States. (AMA Council on Scientific Affairs, 1996; Institute of Medicine, 1998; SUPPORT Principal Investigators, 1995). Specifically, the need for improvement in physician communication with the patient at the end of life has been consistently recommended (Hanson, Danis, & Garrett, 1997; Steinhauser et al., 2000). Curtis et al. (2001) developed a conceptual framework based on focus group interviews with seriously ill patients, including cancer patients, to describe domains of physicians' skills in providing quality end-of-life care. Not surprisingly, communication skill was one of the key domains to be consistently identified by the patients.

Despite growing recognition of the importance of physician communication during end-of-life care, the impact of physician communication on patients' QOL and well-being at the end of life has not been extensively studied. Higginson and Costantini (2002) conducted a series of prospective cohort studies to assess physician communication during end-of-life care and to describe factors associated with problematic communication. Results of this investigation revealed problematic communication among 40% of the patients; what is more, communication problems were associated with a shorter time in care, greater spiritual need, need for care planning, poorer patient and family insight, and hospice death. Detmar, Muller, Wever, Schornagel, and Aaronson (2001), in a study of physician communication with cancer patients who had an incurable cancer and were receiving palliative care, report that in 20% to 54% of the consultations in which patients experienced significant problems in several domains of their health-related quality of life, the physicians did not devote any time to discussing those problems with their patients. The high prevalence of communication problems and their resulting negative impact on patient outcomes underscores the importance of physician communication during the end of life.

LIMITATIONS OF EXISTING RESEARCH AND FUTURE DIRECTIONS

This section describes limitations of existing research on physician-patient communication and offers recommendations for future studies emphasizing the following key areas: measurement, conceptual refinement, study design, and study content.

Measurement

Two approaches have commonly been used to measure physician communication. In the observational approach, medical encounters are recorded by way of standardized observation, audiotape, or videotape. Observed behaviors in the actual medical encounter are analyzed and coded using one of several interaction analysis systems (IAS), also called *observational instruments* (e.g., Bertakis et al., 1993; Blanchard et al., 1988; Cegala, 1997; Maguire et al., 1996; Ong et al., 1995; Roter & Larson, 2002; Stewart, 1984). An alternative approach assesses patient perceptions of physician behavior via surveys wherein patients are asked to either rate on a rating scale, or report the occurrence or nonoccurrence of specific physician behaviors (e.g., Buller & Buller, 1987; Cegala, Coleman, & Turner, 1998; DiMatteo & Hays, 1980; Falvo & Smith, 1983; Lerman et al., 1990; Weaver, Ow, Walker, & Degenhardt, 1993; Wolf, Putnam, James, & Stiles, 1978).

Both the behavioral/observational and the perceptual measures of physician behavior have relative strengths and weaknesses. The behavioral/observational approach is more objective in its assessment of actual physician-patient behaviors. In this approach, elements of physician behavior are coded in terms of frequencies, durations, or ratios of their occurrence. However, in the perceptual approach, patient perceptions of physician behavior may reflect both qualitative and quantitative dimensions. For example, although the observational measures may reliably capture the amount of time spent by physicians in information-giving activities, they fail to assess whether the information was easily understood by patients or whether it addressed their main concerns. Observational measures may not adequately reflect patients' perspective or fully capture the subjective impact of physician-patient communication on patient outcomes (Street, 1992, 1993).

On the other hand, perceptual measures are more subjective in nature and may be influenced by other factors such as patients' health status (Hall, Milburn, Roter, & Daltroy, 1998). Therefore, assessment of physician behavior using perceptual measures may skew the "reality" of the consultation. However, arguments in favor of measuring patient perceptions assert that patients' outcomes likely depend on how they perceive and interpret events of their medical visits; therefore, patient perceptions may influence patient outcomes more so than actual physician behavior (Cleary et al., 1991; Street, 1992). This argument is supported by the Institute of Medicine's "Quality Chasm" report, which identifies patient experience as the fundamental source for quality-of-care evaluation (Berwick, 2002).

Although the use of both behavioral/observational and perceptual measures of physician-patient communication would be ideal, such studies are limited (see Blanchard et al., 1990; Street, 1992) and need to be encouraged. Furthermore, the state of the science of measurement in this area of research is in need of advancement and refinement. For example, although a number of interaction analysis systems for coding physicians' communication behavior, as well as a number of different survey-based assessment tools of physician behavior, have been developed, mapping the different observational measures onto their perceptual counterparts would advance these efforts and provide a fuller description of physician-provider interactions. Simultaneous application of observational and perceptual methodological approaches will require greater understanding of the conceptual overlap in the elements of physicians' communication behavior as assessed by these distinct, yet complementary, measurement approaches.

Finally, although the relative strengths and weaknesses of different IAS have been evaluated (Frankel, 2001; Rimal, 2001), a state-of-the-science evaluation of the published literature on survey-based perceptual measures of physician-patient communication has not been conducted. Utilizing existing conceptual frameworks (e.g., the elements of physician behavior identified in the Kalamazoo Consensus Statement, Makoul, 2001), existing gaps in the science could be identified by comparing identified measures on several criteria within a state-of-the-science evaluation of the published literature. Evaluation criteria may include the following: sources of item generation, elements of behavior assessed, conceptually driven versus empirically driven strategies for item reduction and classification, evidence of misclassification, and strength of psychometric properties in terms of reliability, validity, and sensitivity to change.

Validity of measures in their application to cancer studies should also be assessed. Such a review would inform future instrument development and evaluation efforts.

Conceptual Refinement

Several of the investigations examining the impact of physician communication on patient outcomes do not report the use of theory-driven hypotheses (e.g., Kottke et al., 1988; Ockene et al., 1994; Silagy & Stead, 2001). The predominantly exploratory nature of patient-physician communication research is often cited as a limitation (Inui & Carter, 1985; Roter & Hall, 1991). Some attempts at gaining conceptual clarity, such as Roter and Hall's reciprocity theory (Hall, Roter, & Katz, 1988; Roter & Hall, 1991, 1992) have failed to receive empirical support in subsequent studies (see Roberts & Aruguete, 2000). It has been argued that that the lack of a valid conceptual framework and theoretically driven hypotheses makes it difficult to translate research findings into improved clinical practice (Leventhal, 1985).

Research examining the underlying mechanisms by which physicians' communication influences patient outcomes is likely to contribute to improvements in the delivery of care. As discussed in Arora (2003), examination of several mediating and moderating relationships can help achieve conceptual refinement; however, the focus of research exploring the link between physician communication and patient health outcomes has largely been on main effects.

Mediation Effects

According to Mishel's theory of "uncertainty in illness," patients who perceive their physician as a credible information source use that information to reduce uncertainty and construct a meaningful illness experience, thereby improving health outcomes (Mishel, 1999; Mishel & Braden, 1987). Evidence supporting a mediation effect of uncertainty has been found in studies in noncancer settings, which have independently demonstrated empirical relationships between information adequacy in patient-physician interactions and uncertainty reduction (Sheer & Cline, 1995) and reduced uncertainty and improved QOL (Padilla, Mishel, & Grant, 1992), respectively. Mishel and Braden (1987) also found uncertainty to mediate the relationship between social support and adjustment among women diagnosed with gynecological cancer.

Similarly, conceptual frameworks of personal control (Averill, 1973; Reid, 1984) describe informational and decisional control as key mechanisms used by individuals confronting stressful situations (e.g., invasive cancer screening procedures or a cancer diagnosis) to regain a sense of control over their health and life. Qualitative research confirms that patients perceive a greater sense of control when they are satisfied with their physicians' efforts to inform and involve them in decision making (Bakker et al., 2001; McWilliam et al., 2000). A positive relationship between personal control and health outcomes has been established in studies conducted in noncancer settings (e.g. Affleck, Tennen, Pfeiffer, & Fifield, 1987). Although limited available evidence to date suggests that patient perceptions of uncertainty and personal control mediate the relationship between physicians' communication behavior and patient outcomes, empirical tests of such mediational relationships in cancer research have not been conducted and are encouraged.

Moderation Effects

Several existing theoretical frameworks could be used to generate theoretically driven moderation hypotheses. Models focusing on the role of expectations, such as the expectancy-value model (Linder-Pelz, 1982), expectancy theory (Burgoon, Birk, & Hall, 1991), and reinforcement expectancy theory (Klingle & Burgoon, 1995) assert that individuals' expectations function as perceptual filters that influence their evaluation of the communicator's message. According to these theoretical perspectives, the influence of physician's communication behavior on patient outcomes depends not only on the quality of the physician's behavior but also on the patient's expectations concerning that particular behavior. Given the substantial variability in patients' preference for participation in treatment decision making, it seems reasonable to assume that only those patients who *prefer* an active role in decision making would *expect/want* physicians to involve them. A hypothesis following from this theoretical perspective is that physicians' facilitation of patient involvement in decision making would positively influence patient outcomes, but only among those patients who prefer an active role. Thus, patients' preferences for involvement in decision making may moderate the relationship between physicians' decision-making approach and patient outcomes. Although moderation hypotheses of this sort have been recently tested in a noncancer sample (Arora, 2002), their evaluation is lacking from cancer studies and is encouraged.

Evaluation of theoretically driven mediating and moderating relationships will enhance the validity of the hypotheses tested; these efforts can be further enhanced by conducting them within the context of an overarching conceptual framework. The "Transformation Model of Communication and Health Outcomes" developed by Kreps, O'Hair, and Clowers' (1994) is an example of one such framework. This model provides a useful framework for integrating and examining the interplay between antecedent conditions such as physician and patient attitudes and preferences, communication between physician and patient, and patient health outcomes. Existing empirical evaluations have seldom used such conceptual frameworks to guide research efforts. The application of such frameworks would provide a context for generating and testing theoretically driven hypotheses, and is encouraged.

Study Design

The predominant use of cross-sectional designs is a limitation of the body of research assessing physician-patient interactions. A majority of studies provide a "snapshot" view of the physician-patient encounter derived from assessments made during a single clinical encounter. Inferences about the impact of physician behavior drawn from a single clinical encounter assume stability in physician-patient interactions and fail to adequately address the likely variation in structure and content of medical visits over time. Although the physician-patient relationship is usually long-term in chronic illness situations such as cancer, very few longitudinal investigations have examined the physician-patient interaction; thus, it is difficult to assess from existing literature how communication between physicians and patients evolves over time, and, in turn, how this evolution influences patient outcomes. Understanding the evolution of the physician-patient relationship is key to assessing the long-term impact of physician communication on patient health outcomes.

Other limitations in study design include small sample sizes reported by several studies (e.g., Morris and Royle, 1988, $n = 30$). Results from these studies may not be representative of the wider population and must be interpreted with caution. Intervention adherence rates were often low (below 50%), threatening the validity of the results; in some cases intervention adherence rates were not reported, making it difficult to judge the quality of these studies (see Eden et al., 2002). Another methodological limitation that may restrict the generalizability and clinical relevance of reported findings was the use of global health measures, or measures lacking psychometric rigor; such measures may not adequately capture patients' QOL and/or health status (Fogarty, Curbow, Wingard, McDonnell, & Somerfield, 1999). Many investigations also reported bivariate analyses only, without accounting for potentially confounding factors that may be significantly associated with patient outcomes, such as sociodemographic characteristics, severity of illness, possible comorbidities, and treatment regimen (Street & Voigt, 1997). Future research efforts should strive to address the limitations identified in past research by conducting prospective, longitudinal evaluations of the physician-patient interaction utilizing large, representative, and diverse samples and analyzing the data using multivariate statistical techniques.

Study Content

Consideration of physician-patient interaction across the cancer care continuum reveals important gaps in our understanding of the impact of physician communication on patient outcomes. Although considerable research has been conducted to examine the influence of physician communication on patient outcomes for cancer prevention, early detection, and treatment, fewer investigations have explored this association beyond the active phase of care. Thus, the impact of physician communication on the well being of cancer survivors and patients facing the end of life is less well understood. Additional research efforts are needed to explore the impact of physician communication on patient outcomes during cancer survivorship and end of life.

CONCLUSIONS

Examination of the empirical evidence regarding the influence of physician communication behaviors on patient outcomes reveals that physician communication is vital during all stages in the continuum of cancer care from risk assessment, primary prevention, early detection, diagnosis and treatment, and survivorship, to end of life. Each phase in the continuum of cancer care represents an opportunity for physicians to inform, support, and engage patients in their cancer-relevant health care. The methodological and conceptual limitations of existing research identified in this review offer potential guidance for future investigations of physician-patient interactions. Advancing our understanding of the impact of elements of physician communication behavior on patient outcomes through longitudinal examination of objective and perceptual qualities of the physician-patient interaction promises to improve clinical services and promote patient health.

REFERENCES

Affleck, G., Tennen, H., Pfeiffer, C., & Fifield, J. (1987). Appraisals of control and predictability in adapting to a chronic disease. *Journal of Personality and Social Psychology, 53*(2), 273-279.

AMA Council on Scientific Affairs. (1996). Good care of the dying patient. *Journal of the American Medical Association, 275*, 474-478.

Andersen, M. R., & Urban, N. (1999). Involvement in decision-making and breast cancer survivor quality of life. *Annals of Behavioral Medicine, 21*, 201-209.

Arora N. K. (2002). *Physician communication and patient outcome experiences*. Paper presented at the International Conference on Communication in Healthcare, Warwick, UK.

Arora N. K. (2003). Interacting with cancer patients: The significance of physicians' communication behavior. *Social Science & Medicine, 57*, 791-806.

Arora N. K., Ayanian, J. Z., & Guadagnoli, E. (2003). *Examining correlates of patient participation in medical decision-making*. Paper presented at the Second International Shared Decision Making Conference, Swansea, UK.

Arora, N. K., & McHorney, C. A. (2000). Patient preferences for medical decision making: Who really wants to participate? *Medical Care, 38*(3), 335-341.

Averill, J. R. (1973). Personal control over aversive stimuli and its relationship to stress. *Psychological Bulletin, 80*, 286-303.

Baile, W. F., & Beale, E. A. (2001). Giving bad news to cancer patients: Matching process and content. *Journal of Clinical Oncology, 19*, 2575-2577.

Bakker, D. A., Fitch, M. I., Gray, R., Reed, E., & Bennett, J. (2001). Patient-health care provider communication during chemotherapy treatment: The perspectives of women with breast cancer. *Patient Education and Counseling, 43*, 61-71.

Balint, J., & Shelton, W. (1996). Regaining the initiative: Forging a new model of the patient-physician relationship. *Journal of the American Medical Association, 275*, 887-891.

Ballard-Reisch, D. S. (1990). A model of participative decision making for physician-patient interaction. *Health Communication, 2*, 91-104.

Beisecker, A. E. (1996). Older persons' medical encounters and their outcomes. *Research on Aging, 18*(1), 9-31.

Beisecker, A. E., & Beisecker, T. D. (1990). Patient information-seeking behaviors when communicating with doctors. *Medical Care, 28*(1), 19-28.

Bennett, M., & Alison, D. (1996). Discussing the diagnosis and prognosis with cancer patients. *Postgraduate Medical Journal, 72*(843), 25-9.

Bensing, J. M., & Dronkers, J. (1992). Instrumental and affective aspects of physician behavior. *Medical Care, 30*, 283-290.

Beresford, S. A. A., Curry, S. J., Kristal, A.R., Lazovich, D., Feng, Z., & Wagner, E. H. (1997). A dietary intervention in primary care practice: The eating patterns study. *American Journal of Public Health, 87*, 610-616.

Bertakis, K. D., Callahan, E. J., Helms, L. J., Azari, R., & Robbins, J. A. (1993). The effect of patient health status on physician practice style. *Family Medicine, 25*, 530-535.

Berwick, D. M. (2002). A user's manual for the IOM's "Quality Chasm" report: Patients' experiences should be the fundamental source of the definition of "quality." *Health Affairs, 21*(3), 80-90.

Blanchard, C. G., Labrecque, M. S., Ruckdeschel, J. C., & Blanchard, E. B. (1988). Information and decision-making preferences of hospitalized adult cancer patients. *Social Science and Medicine, 27*, 1139-1145.

Braddock, C. H., Edwards, K. A., Hasenberg, N. M., Laidley, T. L., & Levinson, W. (1999). Informed decision making in outpatient practice: Time to get back to basics. *Journal of the American Medical Association, 282*, 2313-2320.

Brown, H. G. (1991). The messages primary care physicians should convey to their patients about mammography. *Women's Health Issues, 1,* 74-77.

Brown, R. L., Baumann, L. J., Helberg, C. P., Han, Y., Fontana, S. A., & Love, R. R. (1996). The simultaneous analysis of patient, physician and group practice influences on annual performance. *Social Science and Medicine, 43,* 315-324.

Buller, M. K., & Buller, D. B. (1987). Physicians' communication style and patient satisfaction. *Journal of Health and Social Behavior, 28,* 375-388.

Burgoon, M., Birk, T. S., & Hall, J. R. (1991). Compliance and satisfaction with physician-patient communication: An expectancy theory interpretation of gender differences. *Human Communication Research, 18,* 177-208.

Butler, N. M., Campion, P. D., & Cox, A. D. (1992). Exploration of doctor and patient agendas in general practice consultations. *Social Science & Medicine, 35,* 1145-1155.

Butow, P. N., Kazemi, J. N., Beeney, L. J., Griffin, A. M., Dunn, S. M., & Tattersall, M. H. (1996). When the diagnosis is cancer: Patient communication experiences and preferences. *Cancer, 15, 77(12),* 2630-22637.

Campbell, B. H., Marbella, A., & Layde, P. M. (2000). Quality of life and recurrence concern in survivors of head and neck cancer. *Laryngoscope, 110,* 895-906.

Carney, P. A., Dietrich, A. J., Keller, A., Landgraf, J., & O'Conner, G. T. (1992). Tools, teamwork, and tenacity: An office system for cancer prevention. *Journal of Family Practice, 35,* 388-394.

Caro, S.W. (1999). Breast and ovarian cancer: Issues in risk assessment. *Advances for Nurse Practitioners, 7,* 26-32.

Cassileth, B. R., Zupkis, R. V., Sutton-Smith, K., & March, V. (1980). Information and participation preferences among cancer patients. *Annals of Internal Medicine, 92,* 832-836.

Cegala, D. J. (1997). A study of doctors' and patients' communication during a primary care consultation: Implications for communication training. *Journal of Health Communication, 2,* 169-194.

Cegala, D. J., Coleman, M. T., & Turner, J. W. (1998). The development and partial assessment of the medical communication competence scale. *Health Communication, 10,* 261-288.

Chaitchik, S., Kreitler, S., Shaked, S., Schwartz, I., & Rosin, R. (1992). Doctor-patient communication in a cancer ward. *Journal of Cancer Education, 7,* 41-54.

Charles, C., Gafni, A., & Whelan, T. (1997). Shared decision-making in the medical encounter: What does it mean? (or it takes at least two to tango). *Social Science & Medicine, 44,* 681-692.

Charles, C., Gafni, A., & Whelan, T. (1999). Decision-making in the physician-patient encounter: Revisiting the shared treatment decision-making model. *Social Science & Medicine, 49,* 651-661.

Chewning, B., & Sleath, B. (1996). Medication decision-making and management: A client-centered approach. *Social Science & Medicine, 42,* 389-398.

Cleary, P. D., Edgman-Levitan, S., Roberts, M., Moloney, T. W., McMullen, W., Walker, J. D., & Delbanco, T. L. (1991). Patients evaluate their hospital care: A national survey. *Health Affairs, 10,* 254-267.

Curtis, J. R., Wenrich, M. D., Carline, J. D., Shannon, S. E., Ambrozy, D. M., & Ramsey, P. G. (2001). Understanding physicians' skills at providing end-of-life care perspectives of patients, families, and health care workers. *Journal of General Internal Medicine, 16*(1), 41-49.

Degner, L. F., Kristjanson, L. J., Bowman, D., Sloan, J. A., Carriere, K. C., O'Neil, J., Bilodeau, B., Watson, P., & Mueller, B. (1997). Information needs and decisional preferences in women with breast cancer. *Journal of the American Medical Association, 277,* 1485-1492.

Degner, L. F., & Sloan, J. A. (1992). Decision making during serious illness: What role do patients really want to play? *Journal of Clinical Epidemiology, 45,* 941-950.

Detmar S. B., Muller, M. J., Wever, L. D. V., Schornagel, J. H., & Aaronson, N. K. (2001). Patient-physician communication during outpatient palliative treatment visits: An observational study. *Journal of the American Medical Association, 285,* 1351-1357.

DiMatteo, M. R. (1994). The physician-patient relationship: Effects on the quality of health care. *Clinical Obstetrics and Gynecology, 37,* 149-161.

DiMatteo, M. R., & Hays, R. (1980). The significance of patient' perceptions of physician conduct: A study of patient satisfaction in a family practice center. *Journal of Community Health, 6,* 18-34.

DiMatteo, M. R., & Lepper, H. S. (1998). Promoting adherence to courses of treatment: Mutual collaboration in the physician-patient relationship. In L. D. Jackson & B. K. Duffy (Eds.), *Health communication research: A guide to developments and directions* (pp. 75-86). Westport, CT: Greenwood Press.

Dube, C. E., O'Donnell, J. F., & Novack, D. H. (2000). Communication skills for preventive interventions. *Academic Medicine, 75,* S45-S54.

Dunn, A. S., Shridharani, K. V., Lou, W., & Bernstein, J. (2001). Physician-patient discussions of controversial cancer screening tests. *American Journal of Preventive Medicine, 20,* 130-134.

Eaton, C. B., Goodwin, M. A., & Stange, K. C. (2002). Direct observation of nutrition counseling in community family practice. *American Journal of Preventive Medicine, 23,* 174-179.

Eden, K. B., Orleans, C. T., Mulrow, C. D., Pender, N. J., & Teutsch S. M. (2002). Does counseling by clinicians improve physical activity? A summary of the evidence for the U.S. Preventive Services Task Force. *Annals Internal Medicine, 137,* 208-15.

Eiser, C., Hill, J. J., & Blacklay, A. (2000). Surviving cancer; what does it mean for you? An evaluation of a clinic based intervention for survivors of childhood cancer. *Psychooncology, 9*(3), 214-220.

Ellerbeck, E. F., Ahluwalia, J. S., Jolicoeur, D. G., Gladden, J., & Mosier, M. C. (2001). Direct observation of smoking cessation activities in primary care practice. *Journal of Family Practice, 50,* 688-693.

Ellis, P. M., & Tattersall, M. H. N. (1999). How should doctors communicate the diagnosis of cancer to patients? *Annals of Medicine, 31,* 336-341.

Emanuel E. J., & Emanuel, L. L. (1992). Four models of the physician-patient relationship. *Journal of the American Medical Association, 267,* 2221-2226.

Fallowfield, L. J., Hall, A., Maguire, G. P., & Baum, M. (1990). Psychological outcomes of different treatment policies in women with early breast cancer outside a clinical trial. *British Medical Journal, 301,* 575-580.

Fallowfield, L. J., Hall, A., Maguire, P., Baum, M., & A'Hern, R. P. (1994). Psychological effects of being offered choice of surgery for breast cancer. *British Medical Journal, 309,* 448.

Falvo, D. R., & Smith, J. K. (1983). Assessing residents' behavioral science skills: Patients' views of physician-patient interaction. *The Journal of Family Practice, 17,* 479-483.

Farrell, M. H., Murphy, M. A., & Schneider, C. E. (2002). How underlying patient beliefs can affect physician-patient communication about prostrate-specific antigen testing. *Effective Clinical Practice.* Available: http://.acponline.org/journals/ecp/mayjun02/farrell.htm. Accessed February 2003.

Fernsler, J., & Fanuele, J. S. (1998). Lymphomas: Long-term sequelae and survivorship issues. *Seminars in Oncology Nursing, 14,* 321-328.

Finney Rutten L. J., Arora, N. K., Bakos, A. D., Rowland J., & Aziz N. (2004). Cancer patients' information needs and information sources: A systematic review of the literature. *Patient Education and Counseling* (under review).

Finset, A., Smedstad, L. M., & Ogar, B. (1997). Physician-patient interaction and coping with cancer: The doctor as informer or supporter? *Journal of Cancer Education, 12,* 174-178.

Fogarty, L. A., Curbow, B. A., Wingard, J. R., McDonnell, K., & Somerfield, M. R. (1999). Can 40 seconds of compassion reduce patient anxiety? *Journal of Clinical Oncology, 17,* 371-379.

Fox, S., & Stein, J. A. (1991). The effect of physician-patient communication on mammography utilization by different ethnic groups. *Medical Care, 29,* 1065-1082.

Fox, S., Siu, A.L., & Stein, J. A. (1994). The importance of physician communication on breast cancer screening of older women. *Archives of Internal Medicine, 154,* 2058-2068.

Frankel, R. M. (2001). Cracking the code: Theory and method in clinical communication analysis. *Health Communication, 13*(1),101-10.

Gattellari, M., Butow, P. N., & Tattersall, M. H. N. (2001). Sharing decisions in cancer care. *Social Science & Medicine, 52,* 1865-1878.

Gattellari, M., Butow, P. N., Tattersall, M. H. N., Dunn, S. M., & MacLeod, C. A. (1999). Misunderstanding in cancer patients: Why shoot the messenger? *Annals of Oncology, 10,* 39-46.

Gattellari, M., Voigt, K. J., Butow, P. N., & Tattersall, M. H. N. (2002). When the treatment goal is not cure: Are cancer patients equipped to make informed decisions? *Journal of Clinical Oncology, 20,* 503-513.

Girgis, A., & Sanson-Fisher, R. W. (1998). Breaking bad news 2: Current best advice for clinicians. *Behavioral Medicine, 24,* 53-59.

Glanz, K., Tziraki, C., Albright, C. L., & Fernandes, J. (1995). Nutrition assessment and counseling practices: Attitudes and interests of primary care physicians. *Journal of General Internal Medicine, 10,* 89-92.

Golin, C. E., DiMatteo, M. R., & Gelberg, L. (1996). The role of patient participation in the doctor visit. *Diabetes Care, 19,* 1153-1164.

Gotay, C. C., & Muraoka, M. Y. (1998). Quality of life in long-term survivors of adult-onset cancers. *Journal of the National Cancer Institute, 90,* 656-667.

Gray, R. E., Fitch, M., Greenberg, M., Hampson, A., Doherty, M., & Labrecque, M. (1998). The information needs of well, longer-term survivors of breast cancer. *Patient Education and Counseling, 33*(3), 245-55.

Guadagnoli, E., & Ward, P. (1998). Patient participation in decision-making. *Social Science & Medicine, 47,* 329-339.

Hall, J. A., Roter, D. L., & Katz, N. R. (1988). Meta-analysis of correlates of provider behavior in medical encounters. *Medical Care, 26,* 657-675.

Hall, J. A., Milburn, M. A., Roter, D. L., & Daltroy, L. H. (1998). Why are sicker patients less satisfied with their medical care? Tests of two explanatory models. *Health Psychology, 17,* 70-75.

Hancock, S. L., & Hoppe, R. T. (1996). Long-term complications of treatment and causes of mortality after Hodgkin's disease. *Seminars in Radiation Oncology, 6,* 225-242.

Hanson, L. C., Danis, M., & Garrett, J. (1997). What is wrong with end-of-life care? Opinions of bereaved family members. *Journal of the American Geriatric Society, 45*(11), 1339-1344.

Higginson, I. J., & Costantini, M. (2002). Communication in end-of-life cancer care: A comparison of team assessments in three European countries. *Journal of Clinical Oncology, 20*(17), 3674-82.

Hoppe, R. B., Farquhar, L. J., Henry, R., & Stoffelmayr, B. (1990). Residents' attitudes towards and skill in counseling. *Journal of General Internal Medicine, 5,* 415-420.

Institute of Medicine (1998). Approaching death: Improving care at the end of life. *Health Services Research, 33*(1), 1-3.

Institute of Medicine. (2003). *Childhood cancer survivorship: Improving care and quality of life.* Washington, DC: National Academy Press.

Inui, T. S., & Carter, W. B. (1985). Problems and prospects for health services research on provider-patient communication. *Medical Care, 23,* 521-538.

Jenkins, V., Fallowfield, L., & Saul, J. (2001). Information needs of patients with cancer: Results from a large study in UK cancer centers. *British Journal of Cancer, 84,* 48-51.

Kaplan, S. H., Greenfield, S., Gandek, B., Rogers, W. H., & Ware, J. E. (1996). Characteristics of physicians with participatory decision-making styles. *Annals of Internal Medicine, 124,* 497-504.

Keller, V. F., & Carroll, J. G. (1994). A new model for physician-patient communication. *Patient Education and Counseling, 23,* 131-140.

Kenford, S. L., Fiore, M. C., & Jorenby, D. E. (1994). Predicting smoking cessation: Who will quit with and without the nicotine patch. *Journal of the American Medical Association, 271,* 589-594.

Klingle, R. S., & Burgoon, M. (1995). Patient compliance and satisfaction with physician influence attempts: A reinforcement expectancy approach to compliance-gaining over time. *Communication Research, 22,* 148-187.

Kottke, T. E., Battista, R. N., DeFriese, G. H., & Brekke, M. L. (1988). Attributes of successful smoking cessation interventions in medical practice: A meta-analysis of 39 controlled trials. *Journal of the American Medical Association, 259,* 2882-2889.

Kottke, T. E., Edwards, B. S., & Hagen, P. T. (1999). Counseling: Implementing our knowledge in a hurried and complex world. *American Journal of Preventive Medicine, 17,* 295-298.

Kreps, G. L. (2003). The impact of communication on cancer risk, incidence, morbidity, mortality, and quality of life. *Health Communication, 152,* 161-169.

Kreps, G. L., O'Hair, D., & Clowers, M. (1994). The influences of human communication on health outcomes. *American Behavioral Scientist, 38,* 248-256.

Lazare, A., Eisenthal, S., & Wasserman, L. (1975). The customer approach to patienthood: Attending to patient requests in a walk-in clinic. *Archives of General Psychiatry, 32,* 553-558.

Lee, S.J., Back, A.L., Block, S.D., & Stewart, S.K. (2002). Enhancing physician-patient communication. *Hematology,* 464-483.

Lerman, C. E., Brody, D. S., Caputo, G. C., Smith, D. G., Lazaro, C. G., & Wolfson, H. G. (1990). Patients' perceived involvement in care scale: Relationship to attitudes about illness and medical care. *Journal of General Internal Medicine, 5,* 29-33.

Lerman, C., Daly, M., Walsh, W. P., Resch, N., Seay, J., Barsevick, A., Birenbaum, L., Heggan, T., & Martin, G. (1993). Communication between patients with breast cancer and health care providers: Determinants and implications. *Cancer, 72,* 2612-2620.

Lerman, C., Schwartz, M.D., Miller, S.M., Daly, M., Sands, C., & Rimer, B.K. (1996). A randomized trial of breast cancer risk counseling: Interacting effects of counseling, educational level, and coping style. *Health Psychology, 15*(2), 75-83.

Leventhal, H. (1985). The role of theory in the study of adherence to treatment and doctor-patient interactions. *Medical Care, 23,* 556-563.

Levine, D.M. (1987). The physician's role in health-promotion and disease prevention. *Bulletin of the New York Academy of Medicine, 63,* 950-956.

Linder-Pelz, S. (1982). Toward a theory of patient satisfaction. *Social Science & Medicine, 16,* 577-582.

Lobb, E. A., Butow, P. N., Kenny, D. T., & Tattersall, M. H. (1999). Communicating prognosis in early breast cancer: Do women understand the language used? *Medical Journal of Australia, 171,* 290-294.

Mager, W. M., & Andrykowski, M. A. (2002). Communication in the cancer 'bad news' consultation: Patient perceptions and psychological adjustment. *Psychooncology, 11*(1), 35-46.

Maguire, P., Booth, K., Elliott, C., & Jones, B. (1996). Helping health professionals involved in cancer care acquire key interviewing skills—the impact of workshops. *European Journal of Cancer, 32S,* 1486-1489.

Makoul, G. (2001). Essential elements of communication in medical encounters: The Kalamazoo consensus statement. *Academic Medicine, 76,* 390-393.

McWilliam, C. L., Brown, J. B., & Stewart, M. (2000). Breast cancer patients' experiences of patient-doctor communication: A working relationship. *Patient Education and Counseling, 39,* 191-204.

Meiser, B., Butow, P. N., Barratt, A. L., Schnieden, V., Gattas, M., Kirk, J., Gaff, C., Suthers, G., & Tucker, K. (2001). Long-term outcomes of genetic counseling in women at increased risk of developing hereditary breast cancer. *Patient Education and Counseling, 44*(3), 215-25.

Meiser, B., & Halliday, J. L. (2002). What is the impact of genetic counseling in women at increased risk of developing hereditary breast cancer? A meta-analytic review. *Social Science and Medicine, 54*(10), 1463-70.

Mickey, R. M., Vezina, J. L., Worden, J. K., & Warner, S. L. (1997). Breast screening behavior and interactions with health care providers among lower income women. *Medical Care, 35,* 1204-1211.

Mishel, M. H. (1999). Uncertainty in chronic illness. *Annual Review of Nursing, 17,* 269-294.

Mishel, M. H., & Braden, C. J. (1987). Uncertainty: A mediator between support and adjustment. *Western Journal of Nursing Research, 9,* 43-57.

Morris, J., & Ingham, R. (1988). Choice of surgery for early breast cancer: Psychosocial considerations. *Social Science & Medicine, 27,* 1257-1262.

Morris, J., & Royle, G. T. (1988). Offering patients a choice of surgery for early breast cancer: A reduction in anxiety and depression in patients and their husbands. *Social Science & Medicine, 26,* 583-585.

Mullan, F. (1984). Re-entry: The educational needs of the cancer survivor. *Health Education Quarterly, (10* Suppl), 88-94.

Ockene, J. K., Kristeller, J., Goldberg, R., Amick, T. L., Pekow, P. S., Hosmer, D., Quirk M., & Kalan, K. (1994). Increasing the efficacy of physician-delivered smoking interventions: A randomized clinical trial. *Journal of General Internal Medicine, 6,* 1-8.

Ockene, J., Quirk, M. E., Goldberg, R. J., Kristeller, J. L., Donnelly, G., Kalan, K. L., Gould, B., Greene, H. L., Harrison-Atlas, R., Pease, J., Pickens, S., & Williams, J. W. (1988). A residents' training program for the development of smoking intervention skills. *Archives of Internal Medicine, 148,* 1039-1045.

Ockene, J. K., & Zapka, J. G. (1997). Physician-based smoking intervention: A rededication to a five-step strategy to smoking research. *Addictive Behavior, 22,* 835-848.

Omne-Ponten, M., Holmberg, L., & Sjoden, P.O. (1994). Psychosocial adjustment among women with breast cancer stages I and II: Six-year follow-up of consecutive patients. *Journal of Clinical Oncology, 12*(9), 1778-1782.

Ong, L. M. L., de Haes, J. C. J. M., Hoos, A. M., & Lammes, F. B. (1995). Doctor-patient communication: A review of the literature. *Social Science & Medicine, 40,* 903-918.

Padilla, G. V., Mishel, M. H., & Grant, M. M. (1992). Uncertainty, appraisal, and quality of life. *Quality of Life Research, 1,* 155-165.

Parsons, T. (1951). *The social system.* Glencoe, IL: The Free Press.

Pellissier, J. M., & Venta, E. R. (1996). Introducing patient values into the decision making process for breast cancer. *Women and Health, 24,* 47-67.

Penson, R. T., Seiden, M. V., Shannon, K. M., Lubratovich, M. L., Roche, M., Chabner, B. A., & Lynch, T. J. (2000). Communicating genetic risk: Pros, cons, and counsel. *The Oncologist, 5,* 152-161.

Phillips, R., & Kelly, K. T. (1999). Practice-based or community-based smoking cessation counseling? *Journal of Family Practice, 48*(12), 941-2.

Pignone, M.P., Ammerman, A., Fernandez, L., Orleans, C.T., Pender, N., Woolf, S., Lohr, K.N., & Sutton, S. (2003). Counseling to promote a healthy diet in adults: A summary of the evidence for the U.S. Preventive Services Task Force. *American Journal of Preventive Medicine, 24*(1), 75-92.

Podl, T. R., Goodwin, M. A., Kikano, G. E., & Stange, K. C. (1999) Direct observation of exercise counseling in community family practice. *American Journal of Preventive Medicine, 17,* 207-210.

Quill, T. E., & Brody, H. (1996). Physician recommendations and patient autonomy: Finding a balance between physician power and patient choice. *Annals of Internal Medicine, 125,* 763-769.

Reid, D. (1984). Participatory control and the chronic-illness adjustment process. In H. M. Lefcourt (Ed.), *Research with the locus of control construct: Extensions and limitations* (Vol. 3, pp. 361-389). Orlando: Academic Press.

Richards, M. A., Ramirez, A. J., Degner, L. F., Fallowfield, L. J., Maher, E. J., & Neuberger, J. (1995). Offering choice of treatment to patients with cancers: A review based on a symposium held at the 10th annual conference of The British Psychosocial Oncology Group, December 1993. *European Journal of Cancer, 31A,* 112-116.

Rimal, R. N. (2001). Analyzing the physician-patient interaction: An overview of six methods and future research directions. *Health Communication, 13*(1), 89-99.

Roberts, C. A., & Aruguete, M. S. (2000). Task and socioemotional behaviors of physicians: A test of reciprocity and social interaction theories in analogue physician-patient encounters. *Social Science & Medicine, 50,* 309-315.

Roberts, C. S., Cox, C. E., Reintgen, D. S., Baile, W. F., & Gibertini, M. (1994). Influence of physician communication on newly diagnosed breast patients' psychologic adjustment and decision-making. *Cancer, 74*(1 Suppl), 336-341.

Rose, J. H. (1990). Social support and cancer: Adult patients' desire for support from family, friends, and health professionals. *American Journal of Community Psychology, 18,* 439-464.

Rosenblum, D. (1994). Listening to people with cancer. *Seminars in Oncology, 21,* 701-704.

Roter, D. (2000). The enduring and evolving nature of the patient-physician relationship. *Patient Education and Counseling, 39,* 5-15.

Roter, D., & Larson, S. (2002). The Roter interaction analysis system (RIAS): Utility and flexibility for analysis of medical interactions. *Patient Education and Counseling, 46*, 243-251.

Roter, D. L., & Hall, J. A. (1991). Health education theory: An application to the process of patient-provider communication. *Health Education Research, 6*, 185-193.

Roter, D. L., & Hall, J. A. (1992). *Doctors talking with patients; Patients talking with doctors: Improving communication in medical visits.* Westport, CT: Auburn House.

Royak-Schaler, R., Klabunde, C.N., Greene, W.F., Lannin, D.R., DeVellis, B., Wilson, K.R., & Cheuvront, B. (2002a). Communicating breast cancer risk: Patient perceptions of provider discussions. *Medscape Women's Health eJournal, 7*, 1-10.

Royak-Schaler, R., Parr Lemkau, J., & Ahmed, S.M. (2002b). Discussing breast cancer risk in primary care. *Journal of the American Medical Women's Association, 57*, 115-116.

Schain, W. S. (1990). Physician-patient communication about breast cancer: A challenge for the 1990s. *Surgical Clinics of North America, 70*, 917-935.

Schwartz, M.D., Rimer, B.K., Daly, M., Sands, C., & Lerman, C. (1999). A randomized trial of breast cancer risk counseling: The impact on self-reported mammography use. *American Journal of Public Health, 89*(6), 924-926.

Sheer, V. C., & Cline, R. J. (1995). Testing a model of perceived information adequacy and uncertainty reduction in physician-patient interactions. *Journal of Applied Communication Research, 23*, 44-59.

Silagy, C., & Stead, L.F. (2001). Physician advice for smoking cessation. *Cochrane Database System Review, 2*, CD000165.

Silliman, R. A., Dukes, K. A., Sullivan, L. M., & Kaplan, S. H. (1998). Breast cancer care in older women: Sources of information, social support, and emotional health outcomes. *Cancer, 83*, 706-711.

Siminoff, L.A., Fetting, J.H., & Abeloff, M.D. (1989). Doctor-patient communication about breast cancer adjuvant therapy. *Journal of Clinical Oncology, 7*(9), 1192-200.

Siminoff, L. A., Ravdin, P., Colabianchi, N., & Sauders-Sturm, C. M. (2000). Doctor-patient communication patterns in breast cancer adjuvant therapy discussions. *Health Expectations, 3*, 26-36.

Simon, M.S., Gimotty, P.A., Coombs, J., McBride, S., Monsrease, A., & Burack, R.C. (1998). Factors affecting participation in a mammography screening program among members of an urban Detroit Health Maintenance Organization. *Cancer Detection and Prevention, 22*, 30-38.

Simpson, M., Buckman, R., Stewart, M., Maguire, P., Lipkin, M., Novack, D., & Till, J. (1991). Doctor-patient communication: The Toronto consensus statement. *British Medical Journal, 303*, 1385-1387.

Stefanek, M. E. (1990). Counseling women at high risk for breast cancer. *Oncology, 4*, 27-33.

Steinhauser, K. E., Clipp, E. C., McNeilly, M., Christakis, N. A., McIntyre, L. M., & Tulsky, J. A. (2000). In search of a good death: Observations of patients, families, and providers. *Annals of Internal Medicine, 132*(10), 825-832.

Stewart, M. A. (1984). What is a successful doctor-patient interview? A study of interactions and outcomes. *Social Science & Medicine, 19*, 167-175.

Stiggelbout, A. M., de Haes, J. C. J. M., Vree, R., van de Velde, C. J. H., Bruijninckx, C. M. A., van Groningen, K., & Kievit, J. (1997). Follow-up of colorectal cancer patients: Quality of life and attitudes towards follow-up. *British Journal of Cancer, 75*, 914-920.

Street, R. L. (1992). Analyzing communication in medical consultations: Do behavioral measures correspond to patients' perceptions? *Medical Care, 30*, 976-988.

Street, R. L. (1993). Analyzing messages and their outcomes: Questionable assumptions, possible solutions. *The Southern Communication Journal, 58*, 85-90.

Street, R. L., & Voigt, B. (1997). Patient participation in deciding breast cancer treatment and subsequent quality of life. *Medical Decision Making, 17*, 298-306.

Strull, W. M., Lo, B., & Charles, G. (1984). Do patients want to participate in medical decision making? *Journal of the American Medical Association, 252*, 2990-2994.

SUPPORT Principal Investigators (1996). A controlled trial to improve care for seriously ill hospitalized patients. The study to understand prognoses and preferences for outcomes and risks of treatments (SUPPORT). *Journal of the American Medical Association, 274*(20), 1591-1598. (Erratum in: *Journal of the American Medical Association, 275*(16), 1232.)

Sutherland, H. J., Llewellyn-Thomas, H. A., Lockwood, G. A., Tritchler, D. L., & Till, J. E. (1989). Cancer patients: Their desire for information and participation in treatment decisions. *Journal of the Royal Society of Medicine, 82,* 260-263.

Szasz, T. S., & Hollender, M. H. (1956). A contribution to the philosophy of medicine: The basic models of the doctor-patient relationship. *Archives of Internal Medicine, 97,* 585-592.

Taylor, M.R.G. (2001). Genetic testing for inherited breast and ovarian cancer syndromes: Important concepts for the primary care physician. *Postgraduate Medicine, 77,* 11-15.

Tesauro, G. M., Rowland, J. H., & Lustig, C. (2002). Survivorship resources for post-treatment cancer survivors. *Cancer Practice, 10*(6), 277-83.

U.S. Preventive Services Task Force (1996). Guide to clinical preventive services (2nd ed.). Washington, DC: U.S. Department of Health and Human Services.

U.S. Preventive Services Task Force (2003). Behavioral counseling in primary care to promote a healthy diet. *American Journal of Preventive Medicine, 24,* 93-100.

Valente, C. M., Sobal, J., Muncie, H. L., Jr., Levine, D. M., & Antlitz, A. M. (1986). Health promotion: Physicians' beliefs, attitudes, and practices. *American Journal of Preventive Medicine, 2,* 82-88.

Velicer, C. M., & Taplin, S. (2001). Genetic testing for breast cancer: Where are health care providers in the decision process? *Genetics in Medicine, 3,* 112-119.

Weaver, M. J., Ow, C. L., Walker, D. J., & Degenhardt, E. F. (1993). A questionnaire for patients' evaluations of their physicians' humanistic behaviors. *Journal of General Internal Medicine, 8,* 135-139.

Whitlock, E. P., Orleans, T., Pender, N., & Allan, J. (2002). Evaluating primary care behavioral counseling interventions: An evidence-based approach. *American Journal of Preventive Medicine, 22,* 267-284.

Wolf, A. M. D., & Becker, D. (1996). Cancer screening and informed patient discussions: Truth and consequences. *Archives of Internal Medicine, 156,* 1069-1072.

Wolf, M. H., Putnam, S. M., James, S. A., & Stiles, W. B. (1978). The Medical Interview Satisfaction Scale: Development of a scale to measure patient perceptions of physician behavior. *Journal of Behavioral Medicine, 1,* 391-401.

Zapka, J. G., Taplin, S. H., Solberg, L. I., & Manos, M. M. (2003). A framework for improving the quality of cancer care: The case of breast and cervical cancer screening. *Cancer Epidemiology, Biomarkers and Prevention, 12*(1), 4-13.

3 | Health Care Partnership Model of Doctor–Patient Communication In Cancer Prevention and Care Among the Aged

Eva Kahana
Case Western Reserve University

Boaz Kahana
Cleveland State University

In the attempt to improve communication between doctors and patients related to cancer prevention and care, there has been relatively little patient-driven data, particularly based on elderly patients, to help in developing better communication guidelines (Dowsett et al. 1999, Thorne, 1988). Present recommendations are largely based on expert (physician) opinions about desirable approaches to communication (Ellis & Tattersall, 1999; Fallowfield, 1993). We present a model that aims to address this gap in knowledge. Our discussion goes beyond the typical focus of the health communication literature on only dyadic interactions, to consideration of interactions among members of a health care triad of physician, patient, and health significant other (HSO).

Research has documented that older adults are an underserved population in terms of communication regarding cancer prevention and control (Fox, Roetcheim, & Kington, 1997; Goldberg & Chavin, 1997). In terms of prevention, doctors are less likely to discuss preventive practices and recommend cancer screening tests to elderly patients than to middle aged individuals (Breen & Kessler, 1996; Giles, Williams & Couplard, 1990). In terms of cancer care, physician communication has been found to be largely inadequate in meeting older patients' needs (Butow, Kazemi, Griffin, Dunn & Tattersall, 1996), Maguire, 1999a), based on both insufficient information given to patients (Ellis & Tattersall, 1999; Rothenbacher, Lutz, & Porzsolt, 1997) and information presented in a manner too difficult to understand (Lobb, Butow, Kenny, & Tattersall). To better understand factors influencing cancer prevention and care in elderly populations, we propose a comprehensive and testable model of health communication (Fig. 3.1).

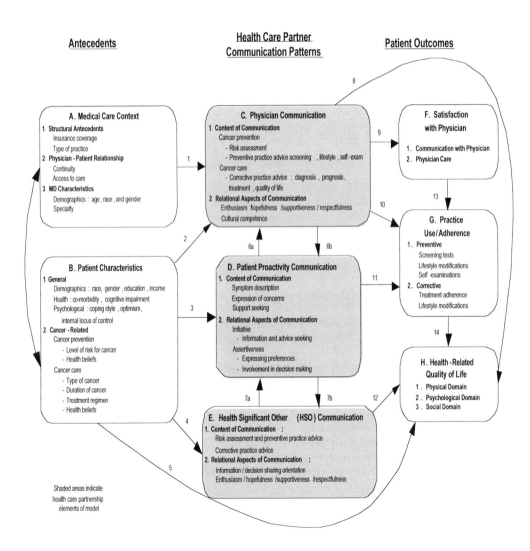

FIGURE 3.1   Health Care Partnership Model of Communication in Cancer Prevention and Care

AN OVERVIEW OF THE HCP MODEL

The integrated *Health Care Partnership* (HCP) model we have developed is predicated on understanding the influence of communication among health care partners on patient outcomes in both cancer prevention and cancer care. This model considers not only content and relational aspects of doctor-patient communication (Kreps, O'Hair, & Clowers. 1994), but also the proactive roles played by patients in information gathering and communication (Kahana & Kahana, 2003).

The role of *health significant others* (HSOs) in providing advocacy and support is also explored. Communication has been identified as the primary process that can close the gap in power between health care providers and consumers (Kreps, 1996). In our prior work, we have urged a paradigm shift from patients and families "patiently" awaiting good care to their taking greater responsibility for getting optimal health care (Kahana & Kahana, 2003). Thus, we are particularly interested in ways that proactive communication by patients and involvement of HSOs in communication can improve patient outcomes. The HCP model proposed here is an effort toward development of comprehensive models of health communication in the context of both cancer prevention and care.

The proposed model stops short of including communication between nonphysician health care providers (e.g., nurses or social workers) and physicians or patients. Nevertheless, it strives for greater comprehensiveness than typical in empirical research on doctor-patient communication. It is our hope that this model can thus pave the way to the development of other testable, comprehensive models in the field of cancer communication. We recognize that there are both divergences and overlap in the types of variables and causal linkages relevant to communication in cancer prevention and in cancer care. Our model affords flexibility in considering relationships salient to each of these two areas of communication. At the same time it maps how communication may span these two distinct areas. Employing longitudinal designs, researchers can test causal sequences proposed in the HCP Model of doctor-patient communication (including reciprocal causal relationships).

The Health Care Partnership model builds on prior conceptual models. Thus, we incorporate elements from Andersen and Newman's (1973) Health Care Utilization Model, as we consider the "enabling factors" of continuity and access to medical care and the "need factors" represented by cancer risk or comorbidity. We draw on the Health Belief Model (Becker, 1974; Janz & Becker, 1984; Rosenstock, 1966), as we consider the role of patient beliefs in susceptibility to illness. This model also sheds light on patients' views about the benefits of interventions and their resulting adherence to physician's recommendations regarding cancer prevention or cancer care. We also apply Query and Kreps' (1996) "Relational Health Communication Competence Model" to older patient-provider communication. In our consideration of physician-patient and HSO-patient communication, we focus on two key dimensions proposed in Query and Kreps' communication model: content and relationship. Query and Kreps' model, which posits that the consumer is at the center of the "communication wheel," is further developed in our depiction of the mutual influences among health care partners. An innovative focus of the HCP model is the inclusion of proactive health care consumerism, considered under the conceptual rubric of proactive adaptations, which has been articulated in our conceptualizations of successful aging (Kahana & Kahana, 1996, 2003). Because we visualize older people as crafting strategies to optimize their health that synthesize lay and professional resources (Pescosolido & Kronenfeld, 1995), we move from a passive model of health care to a participatory or collaborative view that recognizes opportunities for active participation and proactive adaptations by patients.

THE RATIONALE FOR MODEL COMPONENTS

Figure 3.1 outlines the key causal relationships posited in our model, including reciprocal causal relationships occurring in communication among health care partners. Shaded boxes (Boxes C, D, & E) designate central model components representing communication among the three health care partners. The model depicts antecedents as well as sequelae of health care provider communication. However, for ease of presentation, our model does not depict all hypothesized causal linkages between antecedents and dimensions of health care provider communication. Additionally, we do not depict those causal relationships between antecedents and health outcomes, which are not mediated by communication (e.g., relationships between patient characteristics and health-related quality of life). Moderating relationships and expectations of congruence reflecting interaction terms are also not shown in the model.

The focus of our model is on communication among health care partners (Boxes C, D, & E) and the sequelae of their communication in terms of patient outcomes (Boxes F, G, & H). A secondary focus of the model is on antecedents of health care partner communication (particularly of physician-patient communication) (Boxes A & B). Discussion of our rationale for model components begins by describing how communication of each health care partner relates to patient outcomes in terms of cancer prevention and cancer care. Subsequently, we turn to discussing the antecedents of health care partner communication. Our consideration of patient health outcomes is multidimensional, encompassing patient satisfaction, practice use (also referred to as adherence) (DiMatteo, Hays, & Sherbourne, 1992), and health-related quality of life.

RELATIONSHIP OF HEALTH CARE PARTNERSHIP COMPONENTS TO PATIENT OUTCOMES

Physician Communication (Component C): Prevention

Efforts at cancer prevention subsume early detection, which may be accomplished by screening practices, recommendations for patient self-examination, and early symptom reporting, as well as maintenance of protective lifestyles involving risk avoidance (Champion, 1994; Rimer, Jones, Wilson, Bennett, & Engstrom, 1983). There is consensus about appropriate cancer prevention recommendations for many common cancers, particularly breast, colorectal, and skin cancer (NCI, 2001a-d). Yet, there is insufficient "evidence-based" information for making recommendations to persons in old-age groups to permit clear prevention guidelines for physicians (U.S. Preventive Services Task Force, 1996). Nevertheless, studies indicate (e.g., Herman, Hoffman, & Altobelli, 1999) that even when the scientific basis for using screening tests for older patients is uncertain, the standard of care in U.S. communities includes the administration of tests generally recommended by the American Cancer Society (2000).

Physicians play a critical role in counseling patients about cancer prevention and in ordering screening tests for their patients. In making preventive recommendations physicians must consider potential costs and benefits of cancer screening, as well as values and preferences of the patient (Walter & Covinsky, 2001). Thus, communication between older patients and physicians assumes particular importance. Risk assessment, patients' health beliefs, as well as patient initiatives in discussing preferences regarding preventive practices, can influence specific preventive recommendations made by the physician, and patient adherence to recommendations (Hawley, Earp, O'Malley, & Ricketts, 2000; Rakowski, Assaf, Lefebvre, & Lasater, 1990).

Physician communication is defined by two elements proposed in Query and Kreps' (1996) communication model: content and relational aspects of communication. We recognize that both aspects of communication exert their influence on patient outcomes. For influencing practice use, the content of communication (i.e., the specific practices recommended by the physicians) is most important (Fox et al. 1991), with relational aspects of communication, such as enthusiasm in recommending a screening test, also playing a role (Fox et al. 1994). Advice regarding preventive lifestyles and screening practices may range from lack of communication about prevention to advice for or against given preventive practices. The type of advice given is likely to differ depending on perceived familial or lifestyle-related risk of a given patient for the type of cancer being considered (Tominaga, 1999), and based on costs and benefits of screening practices recommended (McCaul & Tulloch, 1999). Growing attention in the literature to health care dispositions reflected in physician communication with lower SES patients and with patients who are members of racial and ethnic minorities, has also called attention to the important physician characteristic of cultural competence in communication (Smedley, Stith, & Nelson, 2003; Kahana, Kahana, King, Meehan, Lovegreen, & Brown, 2005).

Physicians' communications to their patients during medical visits is an important determinant of satisfaction with care (Path 9 in Figure 3.1) (Coe, 1987). Physicians who elicit patients' opinions about diagnostic or treatment options receive higher ratings of patient satisfaction with care (Stewart, Brown, Boon, Galajda, Meredith, & Sangster, 1999). Physician communication also impacts on preventive practice use (Path 10). Patients are more likely to adhere to instructions and advice from physicians who give clear and enthusiastic communication, and who show emotional support and concern (Bartlett et al. 1984; Heszen-Klemens & Kapinska, 1984; Stewart et al. 1999). Adherence to professionally prescribed prevention regimens is also enhanced when older people and their physicians share understandings of appropriate health care strategies and goals (Leventhal et al. 1992). The supportiveness and respectfulness of physicians' communication are also expected to contribute to improved health-related quality of life among patients (Braddock, Fihn, Levinson, Jonsen, & Pearlman, 1997) (Path 8).

Care

In the cancer care component of our model, we primarily focus on the patient's experience with three key areas of physician communication: disclosure of cancer diagnosis, decision making about treatment, and discussions about maintenance of quality of life. Both content and relational aspects of communication are expected to influence patient outcomes in cancer care (Path 8, 9, & 10). We consider content of communication in terms of the amount of information disclosed by the physician and the involvement of the patient in decision making. Additionally, relational components of communication are considered in terms of support, respectfulness, and hopefulness expressed by the physician during communication about disclosure of diagnosis and decision making about treatments.

Diagnosis of cancer is one of the most traumatic events a patient may ever encounter, as it influences life expectancy as well as quality of life (Mills & Sullivan, 1999). Most patients want to be told about the diagnosis of cancer and the nature of their disease (Maguire, 1999b; Meredith, Symonds, Webster, Lamont, Pyper, Gillis, & Fallowfield, 1996). Most physicians in the United States disclose the cancer diagnosis to patients, but there are inconsistencies in the amount and type of information provided to patients about prognosis, treatment options, and quality of life (Butow et al., 1996). Because patients diagnosed with cancer are typically in a crisis situation, the content of physicians' communication is anticipated to be more complex than in encounters dealing with prevention (Bloch, 1994; Krant, 1981). Relational components of communication, such as support and reassurance, are expected to assume particular importance (Butow et al., 1996). Sensitivity to cultural traditions of the patient, which we refer to as respect and cultural competence (in Figure 3.1), also plays an important role in insuring good relational communication (Smedley, Stith, & Nelson, 2003; Kahana, Kahana, King, Meehan, Lovegreen, & Brown, 2005). Greater cultural competence of physician communication leads to empowerment of patients and fosters patient proactivity (Path 6b).

Physician communication affects patients' satisfaction with cancer care (Path 9). For example, physicians who communicate personal interest, empathy, mutual respect, honesty, and are not overly pessimistic are more likely to have satisfied patients (Ellis & Tattersall, 1999; Loge, Kaasa & Hytten, 1997). Similarly, physician communication to cancer patients, particularly in terms of level of support and amount of information provided, have been found to be significant predictors of patient adherence to treatment regimens and lifestyle modifications (Butler, Rollnick, & Stott, 1996; Mills & Sullivan, 1999) (Path 10).

Physicians' communications regarding cancer diagnosis and treatment options also have a major influence on cancer patients' health-related quality of life (Harrison, Galloway, Graydon, Palmer-Wickham & Rich-van der Bij, 1999) (Path 8). Communication of information to patients about their disease and treatment options is important in allowing patients to gain a sense of control (Mills & Sullivan, 1999) and maintain psychological well-being (Maguire, 1998; Bloch, 1994). Because all cancer patients are likely to benefit from affective support, positive relational communication is expected to have a "main effect" on outcomes. In contrast, patients differ in their preferences for communication of information, and hence, the latter construct is viewed in "interaction" terms. Positive relational communication reflecting support, respect and hope is expected to flow from physician to patient. Multiple physicians, including surgeons, procedural specialists, and oncologists, are likely to be involved in cancer diagnosis and care. We anticipate that the support patients perceive from formal health care partners (e.g., primary care physician and oncologist) should be cumulative in its positive effects on outcomes. In testing the proposed model, studies should ideally incorporate data on health care partner communications, including at least key treating physicians. In terms of cancer prevention, focus may be on primary care physicians and key treating specialists. In terms of cancer care focus could most profitably be placed on oncologists and other key treating physicians. Although increasing the number of physicians considered will add to comprehensiveness, it also complicates analyses of data for empirical studies.

Patient Proactivity in Communication (Component D): Prevention

Our HCP model of communication is predicated on the understanding that the more actively patients are involved in health communication with their physicians, the better their health outcomes will be (Kreps & O'Hair, 1995). Specifically, we focus on two key, relational elements of patient's health communication: initiative and assertiveness. Initiative is reflected in patients seeking out medical information from multiple sources, including HSOs and the media (Kreps, 1996). Additionally, patient proactivity in communication involves assertiveness in expressing preferences to the physician and to the HSO and in seeking to take an active role in medical decision making. Collectively, we refer to these behaviors as patient proactivity reflecting health care consumerism (Kahana & Kahana, 2002). Whereas older patients may be less proactive than their younger counterparts, increasingly, educated cohorts of older adults have been assuming more active orientations in their interactions with their doctors (Beisecker, 1988). In addition to the innovative focus of our model on patient proactivity we also recognize that content of communication of patients may range widely, reflecting support seeking, expression of fear, or even helplessness.

We anticipate that patients' proactivity in communicating with their physicians and HSOs will affect the communication they receive as well as their satisfaction, practice use, and quality of life. Patients who elicit the active involvement of their physicians are likely to receive encouragement for expressing their screening preferences (Path 6a). We recognize that the medical sociological and health services literature typically places responsibility on the physician for assessing patients' preferences (Stewart et al., 1999). When physicians encourage patients to voice their views and preferences, patient proactivity is likely to be reinforced (Path 6b). Nevertheless, studies suggest that physicians take limited initiatives to solicit patient input (Delbanco, 1993; Rosenfeld, 2002). Consequently, we present a consumer-focused model of patient-physician communication suggesting patient empowerment, proactivity, and initiative as critical facilitators of satisfactory doctor-patient communication and important avenues for enhancing patient-responsive care (Kahana & Kahana, 2002). Similarly patients who actively solicit opinions from their HSOs will be more likely to receive advice on asking physicians the appropriate questions (Path 7a). HSO communication that reflects an information and decision-sharing orientation will also enhance patient proactivity (Path 7b). Furthermore, patients who are more assertive and involved in communication with their physicians are expected to be more adherent to cancer screening recommendations (Rimer, Davis, Engstrom, Myers, Rosan, Fox, & McLaughlin, 1988) (Path 11). A patient's proactivity in communication with his or her HSO is likely to play a secondary, but still important, facilitative role in contributing to patient satisfaction with care, adherence to preventive practice recommendations, and a higher quality of life.

Seeking information from the media is another strategy utilized by proactive patients. The Internet provides immediate access to desired information about cancer prevention. In fact, searching for health information or health-related support are among the most frequent reasons for older adults' use of the Internet, with over one half of users spending some time seeking health-related information (Turk-Charles, Meyerowitz, & Gatz, 1997). By using media sources to enhance their understanding of their health risks and improve their knowledge of the availability of health care services older adults can play more active roles in preventive efforts (Gustafson, Hawkins, Boberg, Pingree, Serlin, Graziano, & Chan, 1999). Even as we acknowledge the value of information available through the media, it should also be noted that accurate and user-friendly information is not available for many important decisions involved in cancer prevention (Hibbard & Jewett, 1997).

Care

Proactive information-seeking behavior is also a useful coping strategy for those living with cancer (Van Der Molen, 1999) and is generally expected to elicit responsiveness in communication from both physicians and HSOs (Paths 6a and 7a). The nature of cancer at times makes it difficult for patients to play proactive roles, so the extent of patient proactivity may change with phases of the illness and of treatments. Major areas of investigation concerning physician-patient communication in cancer care involve information sharing and the treatment decision-making process. Most people want to be given full information about their condition, people vary in how much they wish to participate in making decisions about their treatment (Roberts, Cox, Reintgen, Baile, A Gilbertini, 1994; Rothenbacher, et al., 1997; Turner & Maher, 1994). In cancer related communication we also anticipate that physicians and HSOs who communicate in an information and decision-sharing manner will help enhance patient proactivity (6b and 7b).

Even though doctors are preferred as a source of information about cancer treatment, information from the media is also widely used (Bilodeau & Degner, 1996). Older adults who have been socialized not to challenge medical authority may be more comfortable in seeking answers to their care-related questions from informal sources, such as self-help groups and the Internet (Gray, Fitch, Greenberg, Hampson, Doherty, & Labrecque, 1998). At the doctor's office older patients may present information obtained from informal sources incorporate it into their discussions with their physician (Seckin & Kahana, 2005). Accordingly, the older cancer patient, who is an informed health care partner and who shares the decision-making role with their physician, is becoming a more common reality (Benjamin, 2001). We predict that patients who are more informed about cancer care (i.e., seek more advice and information from their physicians) will also demonstrate greater levels of adherence to medication and other treatment regimens (Spiegel, 1997) (Path 11).

HSO Communication (Component E): *Prevention*

Family members and friends serve as powerful influences on the health behaviors of older adults. They provide informational, affective, and instrumental support, which facilitate the pursuit of healthy lifestyles, and adherence to the preventive practice recommendations of physicians (Kahana, Biegel, & Wykle, 1994). HSOs may also facilitate proactive consumer roles of patients by helping them obtain health information from the media (Path 7b). HSOs accompanying an older adult on a medical visit often serve as advocates and make consumerist statements in triadic interactions (Beisecker, 1988). Alternatively, the patient may arrive at the physician's office armed with questions relevant to screening or other preventive services based on suggestions by their HSO.

It has long been recognized that health behaviors occur in a social context. HSOs play potentially important and helpful roles in supporting lifestyle changes that can contribute to prevention of cancer (e.g. using protection in the sun), as well as in secondary prevention activities, such as self-examination and screening (Path 12) (Phillips, 1989). HSOs can also enhance preventive practice use by fostering health beliefs about susceptibility to illness and by encouraging risk assessments (Walter & Covinsky, 2001). HSOs can also influence beliefs in the efficacy of preventive practices, by recommending for or against such services.

Care

When older patients are dealing with cancer diagnosis or treatment, the role of the HSO gains further importance as part of a triadic health care communication structure (Adelman, Greene, & Charon, 1987). The HSO (who may also act as caregiver) is often an integral part of visits to the physician during discussions of treatment plans (Greene, Adelman, & Majerovitz, 1996), and may facilitate patient adherence to physician recommendations about treatment and lifestyle modifications (Spiegel, 1997) (Path 12). HSOs often play an important role in influencing patient decision making by encouraging or discouraging adjuvant chemotherapy or radiation therapy (Haug, 1994).

During medical visits, HSOs may act as allies or advocates for the patient, and may encourage patient proactivity (Path 7b). HSOs also typically accompany patients for radiation and chemotherapy treatments and communicate support, enhancing patients' quality of life. The involvement of an HSO is generally viewed by patients as facilitative. However, at times it could also have a negative impact, as it may reinforce patients' feelings of dependency and loss of personal control, and may be perceived as interfering with communication with physicians (Greene, Hoffman, Charon, & Adelman, 1987).

ANTECEDENTS TO PHYSICIAN COMMUNICATION

Medical Care Context (Component A): *Prevention*

Structural aspects of the medical care context play an important role in the content of preventive recommendations of physicians (Path 1). For example, out-of-pocket costs and lack of supplemental insurance coverage constitute major barriers to obtaining preventive cancer screening, such as mammograms (Blustein, 1995). There are conflicting data, based largely on younger patients, about the influence of health maintenance organization (HMO) versus fee-for-service health care delivery on physicians' preventive practice recommendations. Patients in HMOs have been found to have a higher rate of utilization of cancer screening tests than patients with fee-for-service insurance (Bernstein, Thompson, & Harlan, 1991). Other research (Potosky, Breen, Graubard, & Parsons, 1998) reports that fee-for-service insurance coverage is positively associated with the use of cancer screening tests.

Group practices have been found to have higher compliance scores than solo practices in meeting preventive cancer recommendation guidelines of National Cancer Institute for colorectal screening and breast exams for women over age 50 (Hillman, Ripley, Goldfarb, Nuamah, Weiner, & Lusk, 1998). Access to care and continuity in care have been identified as the strongest predictors of screening for both breast and cervical cancer among older women (Mandelblatt, Yabroff, & Kerner, 1999). Personal characteristics of physicians have also been associated with the content of communication to patients regarding cancer prevention. Thus, women with female physicians were almost twice as likely to receive mammograms during a two-year period than those with male physicians (Andersen & Urban, 1997). Cooper, Fortinsky, Hapke, and Landefeld (1997) found that physician age and board certification affects colorectal cancer screening recommendations, whereas gender and specialty (internal medicine or family practice) had no effect.

Care

Structural constraints on physicians' time may limit attention directed to both content and relational aspects of communication in dealing with patients diagnosed with cancer (Loge et al., 1997). Communication differences have been observed based on both the setting and the specialty of the physician disclosing the diagnosis (Lind et al., 1989; Loge et al., 1997) (Path 1). Having the diagnosis shared by a physician with whom the patient has a long history and continuity of care also appears to enhance satisfaction (Butow et al., 1996). It is noteworthy that patients are often given their cancer diagnosis and initiate treatment with a newly introduced specialist, rather than their regular physician (Lind, DelVecchio-Good, Seidel, Csordas, & Good, 1989). This discontinuity in care may impact the quality of communication between health care partners, as well as adherence to physician recommendations.

Patient Characteristics (Component B): Prevention

In addition to the medical care context, patient characteristics and particularly the personal resources patients bring into the medical encounter, also influence physician communication about care (Path 2). Minority status, low income, and limited education reflect limitations in resources, which, in turn, are related to obtaining less extensive communication from physicians about preventive care. Older men with less education and lower socioeconomic status are less likely to be screened for prostate cancer (Steele, Miller, Maylahn, Uhler, & Baker, 2000). Lower education levels and minority status reduce the likelihood of breast cancer screening of older women (Mor, Pacala, & Rakowski, 1992; Rimer, Ross, Cristinzio, & King, 1992). Chronic illness and cognitive impairment also represent personal limitations, which can serve as barriers to physician communication about preventive service use (Messecar, 2000; Rost & Frankel, 1993). Anxiety or pessimism about cancer diagnosis attributed to older patients by physicians may also influence likelihood of cancer screening (Beisecker, 1988; Fox et al., 1997). Health beliefs of patients can influence providers' recommendations about cancer screening. Thus, physicians are less likely to screen older women who are embarrassed about cancer screening tests and who fear the pain of screening tests (Gulitz, Bustillo, & Kent, 1998).

Care

Personal characteristics of patients are likely to influence physician communication related to cancer care (Path 2). For example, the patient's level of comorbid conditions has been shown to limit the content of communication (Kutner, Zhang, & McClellan, 2000). Similarly, a patient's comorbid conditions tend to decrease physician's recommendation for adjuvant chemotherapy (Kutner et al., 2000). Patients with severe medical conditions and those with illness requiring highly complex decisions tend to receive more participatory decision-making communications from their physicians than their counterparts who are less ill (Gotler, Flocke, Goodwin, Zyzansky, Murray, & Stange, 2000; Hall, Roter, Milburn, & Daltroy, 1996).

Patients' characteristics also influence their orientation to information seeking and medical decision making (Path 3). Many factors may contribute to patients' preferences for involvement in treatment decisions, including the nature and severity of the illness and the type and complexity of the decision being made (Georgiou & Robinson, 1999). Men, individuals with lower SES, and those with limited education tend to prefer to let the doctor decide on the best treatment options (Lobb et al., 1998; Stiggelbout & Kiebert, 1997). Furthermore, psychological characteristics of the patient may also influence their corrective practice use. Being female, having low SES, less education, and psychological coping orientations of blunting have also been found to limit corrective practice use (Benbassat, Pilpel, & Tidhar, 1998; Coulter, 1997).

ANTECEDENTS TO PATIENT PROACTIVITY AND PRACTICE USE

Patient Characteristics (Component B): Prevention

Personal resources represent an important background to patient proactivity (Path 3) with more educated, healthier older adults and those with better coping skills being more likely to engage in proactive adaptations (Kahana & Kahana, 1996, 2003). Both initiative and assertiveness, which are the key components of patient proactivity in our model, are likely to be facilitated by better cognitive functioning, health, and coping resources, including internal locus of control (Norris & Murrell, 1987; Kahana, Kahana, & Zhang, in press). Furthermore, health beliefs reflecting greater appreciation of cancer risk and greater benefits attributed to cancer prevention are likely to contribute to older adults communicating more actively with their physicians and discussing cancer screening services and practice use (Worthern, 1999).

The personal characteristics of older adults are also likely to affect their preventive practice use. Specific psychological characteristics are associated with a lack of adherence to physicians' preventive practice recommendations (Path 5). For example, health anxious individuals tend to not engage in health promotion behaviors (Hadjistavropoulos, Craig, & Hadjistavropoulos, 1998). Persons who exhibit a high degree of monitoring (i.e., vigilant coping styles) are more likely to adhere to protective health behaviors (Miller, Brody & Summerton, 1988). The health beliefs of patients about susceptibility to illness and efficacy of screening also serve as powerful influences to deter or facilitate patient adherence to preventive recommendations (Janz & Becker, 1984).

Care

Demographic, health, and psychological characteristics of patients living with cancer are also related to their proactivity in communication (Path 3). For example, patients' psychological characteristics are likely to impact their orientation to information-seeking and decision making. Specifically, older adults, men, individuals with less education, and those of lower SES (Lobb, Butow, Kenny, & Tattersall, 1999; Maguire, 1998; Meredith, Symonds, Webster, Lamont, Pyper, Gills, & Fallowfield, 1996) prefer to receive less information about their conditions or about chance of cure from their physicians. Similarly, older adults, men, individuals with less education, people with multiple comorbidities, and high blunters/low monitors tend to prefer to let the doctor decide on the best cancer treatment options (Lobb et al., 1999; Maguire, 1998; Stiggelbout & Kiebert, 1997) (Path 5).

ANTECEDENTS TO HSO COMMUNICATION

Patient Characteristics (Component B): *Prevention*

There has been very little research focusing on the way patient characteristics may impact on HSO communication regarding preventive practices or service use (Path 4). More educated older adults and those with higher incomes tend to be provided with more extensive information by their HSOs and are invited to play more proactive and assertive roles in communicating with their physicians (Prohaska & Glasser, 1996). Additionally, research has documented that women tend to have larger social support networks and receive more supportive communication from their HSOs than do men (Pearlin, Aneshensel, Mullan, & Whitlatch, 1996).

Care

Prior research suggests that patient characteristics affect communication from and level of instrumental and affective support provided by HSOs (Path 4). For instance, among cancer patients, women, less educated persons (Prohaska & Glasser, 1996), older adults who have higher levels of dependency, cancer patients who are in treatment longer (Oberst, Thomas, Gass, & Ward, 1989), and patients with mental health problems (McCorkle & Wilkerson, 1991) have been shown to be given more support by HSOs. Consequently, we would expect that HSOs may be more supportive and directive to a physically frail and/or cognitively impaired patient or to a patient who is in the later stages of cancer, or undergoing more aggressive treatments.

CONCLUSIONS

The framework proposed here aims to provide a testable model for describing antecedents, components, and sequelae of communications related to cancer prevention and care among aged patients and their formal and informal health care partners. It is our hope that the availability of such models will facilitate empirical research to enhance scientific understandings of cancer-relevant communication in health services research.

Although the model is focused on elderly patients and their health care partners, we believe that model components are applicable to cancer patients of all ages. We are particularly interested in seeing further model developments in this area. Such models would address life course development relevant to the nature of health care partnerships and to issues of health communication. Our ultimate hope is that model development, research, and dialogue among professionals interested in communication about cancer prevention and cancer care will lead to the development of guidelines for policy and clinical practice that will improve health and quality of life for patients with cancer.

The focus of this chapter has been on previously little emphasized opportunities that patients have in influencing communication with their health care providers,and. particularly, with their physicians. Our interest in highlighting the proactive role of the consumer is not based on a disregard for the critical roles of the physician, other health care providers, and family and friends in fostering good communication. It is clearly seen as desirable for physicians to elicit their patients concerns and respond to them. However, we are also cognizant of research findings about limited communication by physicians and reports of patient dissatisfaction with deficiencies in physician-patient communication.

We believe that patients can directly impact the system without having to wait for structural and educational changes aimed at enhancing health care communication. We urge improvements in health care delivery and physician education, but believe that patients can and must go beyond lamenting the state of affairs in health communication by soliciting, demanding, and reinforcing patient responsive care (Kahana & Kahana, 2002).

REFERENCES

Adelman, R.D., Greene, M.G., & Charon, R. (1987). The physician-elderly patient-companion triad in the medical encounter: The development of a conceptual framework and research agenda. *The Gerontologist, 27*(6), 729-734.

American Cancer Society. (2000). *Cancer medicine* (5th ed.) (R.C. Bast, T. S. Gansler, J.F. Holland, & E. Frei, Eds.) Washington DC: Author.

Andersen, R., & Newman, J. (1973). Societal and individual determinants of medical care utilization in the United States. *Milbank Memorial Fund Quarterly, 51*, 95-124.

Andersen, R.M., & Urban, N. (1997). Physician gender and screening: Do patient differences account for differences in mammography use? *Women and Health, 26*(1), 29-39.

Bartlett, E.E., Grayson, M., Barker, R., Levine, D.M., Golden, A. & Libber, S. (1984). The effects of physician communication skills on patient satisfaction, recall, and adherence. *Journal of Chronic Disease, 37*(9-10), 755-764.

Becker, M.H. (1974). The health belief model and personal health behavior. *Health Education Monographs, 2(4)*, 326-473.

Beisecker, A. (1988). Aging and the desire for information and input in medical decisions: Patient consumerism in medical encounters. *The Gerontologist, 28(3)*, 330-335.

Benbassat, J., Pilpel, D., & Tidhar, M. (1998). Patients' preferences for participation in clinical decision-making: A review of published surveys. *Behavioral Medicine 24*, 81-88.

Benjamin, G. C. (2001). Health care and new technology. *Maryland Medicine, 2*(1), 20-22.

Bernstein, A.B., Thompson, G.B., & Harlan, L.C. (1991). Differences in rates of cancer screening by usual source of medical care. *Medical Care, 29*, 196-209.

Bilodeau, B.A., & Degner, L.F. (1996). Information needs, sources of information and decisional roles in women with breast cancer. *Oncology Nursing Forum, 23*, 691-696.

Bloch, R. (1994). Disclosing cancer diagnosis to a patient. *Journal of the National Cancer Institute*, *86*(11), 868.

Blustein, J. (1995). Medicare coverage, supplemental insurance, and the use of mammography by older women. *New England Journal of Medicine, 332*(17), 1138-1143.

Braddock, C.H., Fihn, S.D., Levinson, W., Jonsen, A.R., & Pearlman, R.A. (1997). How doctors and patients discuss routine clinical decisions. Informed decision making in the outpatient setting. *Journal of General Internal Medicine, 12*(6), 339-345.

Breen, N., & Kessler, L. (1996). Trends in cancer screening–United States, 1987 and 1992. *Mortality Weekly Report, 45*, 57-61.

Butler, C., Rollnick, S., & Stott, N. (1996). The practitioner, the patient and resistance to change: Recent ideas on compliance. *Canadian Medical Association Journal, 154*(9), 1357-1362.

Butow, P.N., Kazemi, J.N., Griffin, A.M., Dunn, S.M., & Tattersall, M.H. (1996). When the diagnosis is cancer: Patient communication experiences and preferences. *Cancer, 77*(12), 2630-2637.

Champion, V. (1994). Strategies to increase mammography utilization. *Medical Care, 32*, 118-129.

Coe, R. (1987). Communication and medical care outcomes: Analysis of conversations between doctors and elderly patients. In R. Ward & S. Tobin (Eds.), *Health in aging* (pp. 180-193). New York: Springer.

Cooper, G.S., Fortinsky, R.H., Hapke, R., & Landefeld, C.S. (1997). Primary care physician recommendations for colorectal cancer screening. *Archives of Internal Medicine, 157*, 1946-1950.

Coulter, A. (1997). Partnerships with patients: The pros and cons of shared clinical decision-making. *Journal of Health Service Research and Policy, 2*, 112-121.

Delbanco, T.L. (1993). Promoting the doctor's involvement in care. In M. Gerteis, S. Edgman-Levitan, J. Daley, & T. L. Delbanco (Eds.), *Through the patient's eyes: Understanding and promoting patient-centered care* (pp. 260-279). San Francisco: Jossey-Bass.

DiMatteo, M.R., Hays, R.D., & Sherbourne, C.D. (1992). Adherence to cancer regimens: Implications for treating the older patient. *Oncology, 6*(2), 50-57.

Dowsett, S., Saul, J., Butow, P., Dunn, S., Boyer, M., Findlow, R., & Dunsmore, J. (1999). Communication styles in the cancer consultation: Preferences for a patient-centered approach. *Psycho-Oncology, 8*, 155-166.

Ellis, P.M., & Tattersall, M.H. (1999). How should doctors communicate the diagnosis of cancer to patients? *Annals of Medicine, 31*(5), 336-341.

Fallowfield, L. (1993) Giving sad and bad news. *Lancet, 341*(8843), 476-478.

Fox, S., Murata, P., & Stein, J. (1991). The impact of physician compliance on screening mammography for older women. *Archives of Internal Medicine, 151*, 50-56.

Fox, S., Murata, P., & Stein, J. (1991). The impact of physician compliance on screening mammography for older women. *Archives of Internal Medicine, 151*, 50-56.

Fox, S., Roetzheim, R., & Kington, R. (1997). Barriers to cancer prevention in the older person. *Clinics in Geriatric Medicine, 13*(1), 79-95.

Fox, S., Siu, A., & Stein, J. (1994). The importance of physician communication on breast cancer screening of older women. *Archives of Internal Medicine, 154*, 2058-2068.

Georgiou, A., & Robinson, M. (1999). *What is the scope for improving health outcomes by promoting patient involvement in decision-making?* Leeds, England: University of Leeds.

Giles, H., Williams, A., & Coupland, N. (1990). Communication, health and the elderly: Frameworks, agenda and a model. In H. Giles, N. Coupland, & J.M. Wiemann (Eds.), *Communication, health, and the elderly* (pp 1-28). New York: St. Martin's Press.

Goldberg, T.H., & Chavin, S.I. (1997). Preventive medicine and screening in older adults. *Journal of the American Geriatric Society, 45*, 344-354.

Gotler, R., Flocke, S., Goodwin, M., Zyzansky, S., Murray, T., & Stange, K. (2000). Facilitating participatory decision-making. What happens in real-world community practice? *Medical Care, 38*(12), 1200-1209.

Gray, R. E., Fitch, M., Greenberg, M., Hampson A., Doherty, M., & Labrecque, M. (1998). The information needs of well, longer-term survivors of breast cancer. *Patient Education and Counseling, 33,* 245-255.

Greene, M.G., Adelman, R.D., & Majerovitz, S.D. (1996). Physician and older patient support in the medical encounter. *Health Communication, 8*(3), 263-279.

Greene, M.G., Hoffman, S., Charon, R., & Adelman, R. (1987). Psychosocial concerns in the medical encounter: A comparison of the interactions of doctors with their old and young patients. *The Gerontologist, 27*(2), 164-168.

Gulitz, E., Bustillo, H.M., & Kent, E.B. (1998). Missed cancer screening opportunities among older women: A provider survey. *Cancer Practice, 6,* 325-332.

Gustafson, D.H., Hawkins, R., Boberg, E., Pingree, S., Serlin, R.E., Graziano, F., & Chan, C.L. (1999). Impact of a patient-centered, computer-based health information/support system. *American Journal of Preventive Medicine, 16*(1), 1-9.

Hadjistavropoulos, H.D., Craig, K.D., & Hadjistavropoulos, T. (1998). Cognitive and behavioral responses to illness information: The role of health anxiety. *Behaviour Research and Therapy, 36*(2) 149-164.

Hall, J.A., Roter, D.L., Milburn, M.A., & Daltroy, L.H. (1996). Patients' health as a predictor of physician and patient behavior in medical visits: A synthesis of four studies. *Medical Care, 34*(12), 1205-1218.

Harrison, D.E., Galloway, S., Graydon, J.E., Palmer-Wickham, S., & Rich-van der Bij, L. (1999). Information needs and preference for information of women with breast cancer over a first course of radiation therapy. *Patient Education and Counseling, 38,* 217-225.

Haug, M.R. (1994). Elderly patients, caregivers, and physicians: Theory and research on health care triads. *Journal of Health and Social Behavior, 35*(3), 1-12.

Hawley, S., Earp, J., O'Malley, M., & Ricketts, T.C. (2000). The role of physician recommendation in women's mammography use. *Medical Care, 38*(4), 392-403.

Herman, C.J., Hoffman, R.M., & Altobelli, K.K. (1999). Variation in recommendations for cancer screening among primary care physicians in New Mexico. *Journal of Community Health, 24*(4), 253-267.

Heszen-Klemens, J. & Kapinska, E. (1984). Doctor-patient interaction, patients' health behavior and effects of treatment. *Social Science and Medicine, 19,* 9-18.

Hibbard, J.H., & Jewett, J.J. (1997). Will quality report cards help consumers? *Health Affairs, 16*(3), 218-228.

Hillman, A.L., Ripley, K., Goldfarb, N., Nuamah, I., Weiner, J., & Lusk, E. (1998). Physician financial incentives and feedback: Failure to increase cancer screening in Medicaid managed care. *American Journal of Public Health, 88*(11), 1699-1701.

Janz, N.K., & Becker, M.H. (1984). The health belief model: A decade later. *Health Education Quarterly, 11,* 1-47.

Kahana, E., Biegel, D.E., & Wykle, M.L. (Eds.). (1994). *Family caregiving across the lifespan.* Thousand Oaks, CA: Sage.

Kahana, E., & Kahana, B. (1996). Conceptual and empirical advances in understanding aging well through proactive adaptation. In V. Bengtson (Ed.), *Adulthood and aging: Research on continuities and discontinuities* (pp. 18-41). New York: Springer.

Kahana, E., & Kahana, B. (2001). On being a proactive health care consumer: Making an "unresponsive" system work for you. *Research in Sociology of Health Care: Changing Consumers and Changing Technology in Health Care and Health Care Delivery, 19,* 21-44.

Kahana, E., & Kahana, B. (2003). Contextualizing successful aging: New directions in age-old search. In R. Settersten, Jr. (Ed.), *Invitation to the life course: A new look at old age* (pp. 225-255). Amityville, NY: Baywood.

Kahana, E., Kahana, B., King, C., Meehan, R., Lovegreen, L., & Brown, J. (2005). The role of health communication in contributing to health disparities in cancer prevention and screening. In S.

RubinellI & J. Haes (Eds.), *Proceedings of Tailoring Health Messages Conference* (pp. 135-142). Lugano, Switzerland: Health Care Communication Laboratory.

Kahana, E., Kahana, B., & Zhang, J. (in press). Motivational antecedents of preventive proactivity in late life: Linking future orientation and exercise. *Journal of Motivation & Emotion.*

Krant, M.J. (1981). Psychosocial impact of gynecologic cancer. *Cancer, 48*(2), 608-612.

Kreps, G.L. (1996). Promoting a consumer orientation to health care and health promotion. *Journal of Health Psychology, 1*(1), 41-48.

Kreps, G.L., & O'Hair, D. (Eds.). (1995). *Communication and health outcomes.* Cresskill, NJ: Hampton Press.

Kreps, G.L., O'Hair, D., & Clowers, M. (1994). The influences of human communication on health outcomes. *American Behavioral Scientist, 38*(2), 248-256.

Kutner, N.G., Zhang, R., & McClellan, W.M. (2000). Patient-reported quality of life early in dialysis treatment: Effects associated with usual exercise activity. *Nephrol Nursing, 27*(4), 357-367.

Leventhal, H., Leventhal, E.A., & Schaefer, P.M. (1992). Vigilant coping and health behavior. In M.G. Ory, R.P. Ables, & P.D. Lipman (Eds.), *Aging, health, and behavior* (pp. 109-140). Newbury Park, CA: Sage.

Lind, S.E., DelVecchio-Good, M., Seidel, S., Csordas, T., & Good, B.J. (1989). Telling the diagnosis of cancer. *Journal of Clinical Oncology, 7*(5), 583-589.

Lobb, E.A., Butow, P.N., Kenny, D.T., & Tattersall, M.H. (1999). Communicating prognosis in early breast cancer: Do women understand the language used? *Medical Journal of Australia, 171*(6), 290-294.

Loge, J.H., Kaasa, S., & Hytten, K. (1997). Disclosing the cancer diagnosis: The patients' experiences. *European Journal of Cancer, 33,* 878-882.

Maguire, G.P. (1999a). Improving communication with cancer patients. *European Journal of Cancer, 35*(10), 1415-1422.

Maguire, G.P. (1999b). Breaking bad news: Explaining cancer diagnosis and prognosis. *Medical Journal of Australia, 171*(6), 288-289.

Maguire, P. (1998). Breaking bad news. *European Journal of Surgical Oncology, 24*(3), 188-191.

Mandelblatt, J.S., Yabroff, K.R., & Kerner, J.F. (1999) Equitable access to cancer services: A review of barriers to quality care, *Cancer, 86*(11), 2378-90.

McCaul, K.D., & Tulloch, H.E. (1999). Cancer screening decisions. *Journal of the National Cancer Institute Monographs, 25,* 52-58.

McCorkle, R., & Wilkerson, K. (1991). *Home care needs of cancer patients and their caregivers* (Final Rep. No. NR01914). Bethesda, MD: National Center for Nursing Research/University of Pennsylvania.

Meredith, C., Symonds, P., Webster, L., Lamont, D., Pyper, E., Gillis, C.R., & Fallowfield, L. (1996). Information needs of cancer patients in west Scotland: Cross sectional survey of patients' views. *British Medical Journal, 313,* 724-726.

Messecar, D.C. (2000). Mammography screening for older women with and without cognitive impairment. *Journal of Gerontological Nursing, 26*(4), 14-24.

Miller, S.M., Brody, D.S., & Summerton, J. (1988). Styles of coping with threat: Implications for health. *Journal of Personality and Social Psychology, 54*(1), 142-148.

Mills, M.E., & Sullivan, K. (1999). The importance of information giving for patients newly diagnosed with cancer: A review of the literature. *Journal of Clinical Nursing, 8*(6), 631-642.

Mor, V., Pacala, J.T., & Rakowski, W. (1992). Mammography for older women: Who uses, who benefits? *Journal of Gerontology, 47,* 43-49.

National Cancer Institute (NCI). (2001a-d). *Prevention of colorectal cancer; Prevention of prostate cancer; Prevention of breast cancer; Prevention of skin cancer.* Bethesda, MD: Author.

Norris, F.H., & Murrell, S.A. (1987). Transitory impact of life-stress on psychological symptoms in older adults. *Journal of Health and Social Behavior, 28,* 197-211.

Oberst, M., Thomas, S., Gass, K., & Ward, S. (1989). Caregiving demands and appraisal of stress among family caregivers. *Cancer Nursing, 12*(4), 209-215.

Pearlin, L.I., Aneshensel, C.S., Mullan, J.T., & Whitlatch, C.J. (1996). Caregiving and its social support. In R.H. Binstock & L. George (Eds.), *Handbook of aging and the social sciences* (4th ed.). San Diego, CA: Academic Press.

Pescosolido, B.A., & Kronenfeld, J.J. (1995) Health, illness, and healing in an uncertain era: challenges from and for medical sociology. *Journal of Health and Social Behavior* [Special Issue], 5-33.

Phillips, B.U. (1989). The forgotten family: An untapped resource in cancer prevention. *Family Community Health, 11*(4), 17-31.

Potosky, A.L., Breen, N., Graubard, B.I., & Parsons, P.E. (1998). The association between health care coverage and the use of cancer screening tests. Results from the 1992 National Health Interview Survey. *Medical Care, 36*, 257-270.

Prohaska, T.R., & Glasser, M. (1996). Patients' views of family involvement in medical care decisions and encounters. *Research on Aging, 18*(1), 52-69.

Query, J.L., & Kreps, G.L. (1996). Testing a relational model for health communication competence among caregivers for individuals with Alzheimer's Disease. *Journal of Health Psychology, 1*(13), 335-351.

Rakowski, W., Assaf, A.F., Lefebvre, R.C., & Lasater, T.M. (1990). Information-seeking about health in a community sample of adults: Correlates and associations with other health related practices. *Health Education Quarterly, 17*, 379-393.

Rimer, B., Davis, S., Engstrom, P.F., Myers, R., Rosan, J., Fox, L., & McLaughlin, R. (1988). An examination of compliance and noncompliance in an HMO cancer screening program. *Progress in Clinical and Biological Research, 278*, 21-30.

Rimer, B., Jones, W., Wilson, C., Bennett, D., & Engstrom, P. (1983). Planning a cancer control program for older citizens. *The Gerontologist, 23*(4), 384-389.

Rimer, B.K., Ross, E., Cristinzio, C.S., & King. E. (1992). Older women's participation in breast screening. *Journal of Gerontology, 47*, 85-91.

Roberts, C.S., Cox, C.E., Reintgen, D.S, Baile, W.F., & Gibertini, M. (1994). Influence of physician communication on newly diagnosed breast patients' psychologic adjustment and decision-making. *Cancer, 74*(1), 336-341.

Rosenfeld, I. (2002). *Power to the patient.* New York: Warner Books.

Rosenstock, I.M. (1966). Why people use health services. *Milbank Memorial Fund Quarterly, 44*, 94-127.

Rost, K., & Frankel, R. (1993). The introduction of the older patient's problems in the medical visit. *Journal of Aging & Health, 5*(3), 387-401.

Rothenbacher, D., Lutz, M.P., & Porzsolt, F. (1997). Treatment decisions in palliative cancer care: Patient's preferences for involvement and doctors' knowledge about it. *European Journal of Cancer, 33*(8), 1184-1189.

Seckin, G., & Kahana, E. (2005, October). *Patient participation and decision making in the age of communication technology.* Paper presented at the International Conference on Communication in Health Care, Northwestern University, Chicago.

Smedley, B.D., Stith, A.Y., & Nelson, A.R. (Eds.). (2003). *Unequal treatment: Confronting racial and ethnic disparities in healthcare.* Washington, DC: National Academies Press.

Spiegel, D. (1997). Psychosocial aspects of breast cancer treatment. *Seminars in Oncology, 24*(1), S1-36-S1-47.

Steele, C.B., Miller, D.S., Maylahn, C., Uhler, R.J., & Baker, C.T. (2000). Knowledge, attitudes, and screening practices among older men regarding prostate cancer. *American Journal of Public Health, 90*(10), 1595-1600.

Stewart, M., Brown, J.B., Boon, H., Galajda, J., Meredith, L., & Sangster, M. (1999). Evidence on patient-doctor communication. *Cancer Prevention and Control, 3*(1), 25-30.

Stiggelbout, A.M., & Kiebert, G.M. (1997). A role for the sick role: Patient preferences regarding information and participation in clinical decision-making. *Canadian Medical Association Journal, 157*, 383-389.

Thorne, S.E. (1988). Helpful and unhelpful communications in cancer care: The patient perspective. *Oncology Nursing Forum, 15*(2), 167-172.

Tominaga, S. (1999). Major avoidable risk factors of cancer. *Cancer Letters, 143*, S19-S23.

Turk-Charles, S., Meyerowitz, B.E., & Gatz, M. (1997). Age differences in information-seeking among cancer patients. *International Journal of Aging and Human Development, 45*(2), 85-98.

Turner, S.L., & Maher, E.J. (1994). Information and choice in decisions about cancer treatment. *British Medical Journal, 309*(6959), 955.

U.S. Preventive Services Task Force. (1996). *Guide to clinical preventive service* (2nd ed.). Baltimore: Williams & Wilkins.

Van Der Molen, B. (1999). Relating information needs to the cancer experience: Information as a key coping strategy. *European Journal of Cancer Care, 8*, 238-244.

Walter, J.C., & Covinsky, K. (2001). Cancer screening in elderly patients. *Journal of American Medical Association, 285*(21), 2750-2778.

Worthen, H.G. (1999). Inherited cancer and the primary care physician: Barriers and strategies. *Cancer, 86*(11), 2583-2588.

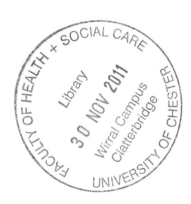

4 | Health Communication Technology and Quality Cancer Care

Linda M. Harris
National Cancer Institute

Gary L. Kreps
George Mason University

Connie Dresser
National Cancer Institute

Effective methods of communication, both among caregivers and between caregivers and patients, are critical to providing high-quality care. . . . IT must play a central role in the redesign of the health care system if a substantial improvement in health care quality is to be achieved during the coming decade. (Institute of Medicine [IOM], 2001)

OVERVIEW

The cancer care process is complex and challenging for all involved, especially for patients, informal caregivers/supporters, and health care providers. A diagnosis of malignant cancer certainly challenges health care consumers who receive the frightening news to come to grips with the diagnosis and its impact on their lives, as well as to make sense of available treatment options for effectively confronting the disease. Family members and friends of the diagnosed individual are also challenged to make sense of cancer and its many influences on their lives and their personal relationships, so they can provide needed support and help as health care advocates. Health care providers are challenged to gather relevant information to make accurate diagnoses, share information about relevant treatment options, facilitate treatment decision making, and help coordinate cancer care. Communication is the critically important social process that helps these individuals confronting cancer to make sense of the disease and its impact on their lives, make relevant cancer care decisions, and respond effectively across the continuum of cancer care, from cancer prevention, through detection and diagnosis, through cancer treatment and survivorship, even to the end-of-life (Kreps, 2003a, 2003b).

The communication demands in cancer care are very high, involving gathering, interpreting, and sharing complex and often emotionally charged information among a network of interdependent caregivers, health care professionals, and patients. Communication technologies (such as interactive computer systems, advanced telecommunications programs, and multimedia educational programs) have been developed, adopted, and adapted to help individuals confronting cancer to meet the unique communication demands of cancer care, access the most relevant and accurate health information, coordinate complex interdependent caregiving activities, gather and provide needed social support, and to facilitate informed decision making. The purpose of this chapter is to examine the uses of health communication technologies, often referred to as e-health, to support cancer care.

SYSTEMIC E-HEALTH RESEARCH AND CANCER CARE TECHNOLOGIES

Scientists working with the Health Communication and Informatics Research Branch at the National Cancer Institute (NCI) have found that systemic e-health research can help guide the use of communication technologies and improve the quality of cancer care. E-health research is conceptualized here as the ongoing interaction of complex adaptive systems in which researcher and subject continually adapt to the other's reciprocal inquiries and feedback. These interactions, when supported with information and communication technologies, can monitor and change the quality of cancer care immediately, automatically, and continuously. Following the lead of the Institute of Medicine's systemic model of health care and recommendations for quality improvement, examples are offered from work supported by the NCI in which e-health research is being conducted to improve the quality of cancer care. One of these research programs, which is highlighted in this chapter and conducted in partnership with the Veterans Health Administration, is designing and implementing an e-health research system to monitor and improve the quality of care for cancer patients receiving chemotherapy. Finally, the implication of this systems approach to health communication technologies for cancer care research and practices in the 21st century is discussed.

DESIGNING FOR QUALITY

In 1998 the Committee on the Quality of Health Care in America was constituted to identify strategies for achieving a substantial improvement in quality health care in the United States. Its dynamic approach invited health communication scientists to apply systemic theoretical and methodological tools to the study of health care in ways that other models of health care have not. First, the Committee viewed health care as a function of the interactions (including electronic) among its participants, rather than as a static institution. This process model of "health care as communication" is complementary with a systems view of health communication and suggests exciting new research directions for communication scientists. Second, it based its claims on the contemporary science of complex, adaptive systems rather than on traditional economic or medical models. This science presumes that changes in quality are continuous events that, although not predictable in detail or direction, are highly predictable in their occurrence. Third, the Committee, in perhaps its most radical claim, asserted that improvements in quality will flow from a patient-centered rather than a medical institution-centered system. Finally, it postulated that systems can be designed to improve quality. Its recommendations are made in terms of design changes, specifically, designs driven by patient needs, not the typically suggested changes in provider incentives or payment methods.

In 2001, the Institute of Medicine published the committee's report on the state of the quality of care in the United States. This report, *Crossing the Quality Chasm: A New Health System for the 21st Century* (2001), offers a challenge and a heuristic model for redesigning the health care system to dramatically improve the quality of care. Meanwhile, at the National Cancer Institute, health communication scientists in the Health Communication and Informatics Branch were developing an e-health research methodology that was in many ways complementary to the IOM's approach and recommendations. This chapter describes how these two approaches, from the IOM and from NCI, are aligned and can be used to enhance the use of health communication technologies in cancer care. One area of alignment is the science of complex, adaptive systems, which informs both approaches to communication, context, and change.

THE SCIENCE OF COMPLEX ADAPTIVE SYSTEMS

Over the past 40 years the science of complex, adaptive systems (CAS) has evolved from von Bertalanffy's original systems theory (1968). This contemporary, interdisciplinary science has a rich history of inquiry, from the human body's immune system (Varela & Coutinho, 1991), the mind (Morowitz & Singer, 1995), the stock market (Mandelbrot, 1999); human organizations (Brown & Eisenhardt, 1998) and human communication patterns (Cronen & Pearce, 1981). The science of complex, adaptive systems has focused on the interactions inherent in multiple systems, including the Internet's rapid world-wide evolution, to VISA card's remarkable self-evolving efficiencies, to the Veterans Health Administration's radical transformation into a sophisticated health care system. A set of defining features of complex adaptive systems has arisen from this research paradigm:

Adaptability. Learning, creativity, and self-change are inherent capabilities of complex adaptive systems;
Interdependence. Systems are interdependent and serve as context for each other;
Synergism. The whole of a system is greater than the sum of its parts. (Plsek, 2001)

According to this model, change and adaptation happen naturally within the context of the relationships among interdependent system agents. Plsek's (2001) model further specifies that one can observe change occurring within the *interactions* of complex, adaptive systems:

> When complex, adaptable systems *interact*, their actions are interconnected such that one system's actions changes the context for the other system. In complex adaptive systems, change (either creativity or error) is an emergent product of the interaction of two components of the system and is the essence of what helps the system organize itself and adapt. (Plsek, Appendix B)

In summary, the unit of analysis is the interaction between systems rather than their structure. Creativity and adaptivity can be observed in action.

People as Complex, Adaptive Systems

The study of human communication, as an interdisciplinary science, has multiple theoretical roots. Communication theory, like CAS, has one set of roots in systems theory. Norbert Wiener, the "father" of cybernetics, observed the continuous flow of information: "I approached information theory from the point of departure of the electrical circuit carrying a continuous current" (1956, p. 23). The continuous feedback loop—the essence of human communication, was first fundamental to cybernetics, the science of maintaining order in a system (Campbell, 1960). From within a systemic model of human communication individuals are conceptualized as complex and adaptive and interdependent systems in which each individual's action is feedback for the other's actions and interpretations.

Human communication is also rooted in phenomenological approaches. Rogers (1994), in his history of communication science, traces this influence back to Dewey, Cooley, Park and Mead, who argued that:

> the individual subjectivity of how a message is perceived is an essentially human quality . . . thus, to these first four American scholars of communication, how an individual makes sense out of information, and thus how meaning is given to a message, was a fundamental aspect of the communication process. (p. 74)

A number of communication theorists have joined systems theory and phenomenology into communication models that conceptualize humans as complex, adaptive systems, and unique among those systems in their ability to make sense of their actions. "The ability to coordinate, give, and read nonverbal and verbal cues makes humans excellent feedback users," according to Cragan and Shields (1994, p. 84). Other communication theorists hold similar views of humans as particular complex systems, in large part due to their ability to create and change meaning (Ray & Donohew, 1990; Kreps, 1990). Cronen, Pearce, and Harris (1979, 1982) extend this model to propose a systemic view of communication in which the source of meaning (or knowledge) is within the interaction of two complex adaptive systems (people). This coordinated creative process is constrained primarily by logical forces (what "makes sense"). Humans, through their interactions, are adapting, creating context for each other and synergistic—all the characteristics of complex, adaptive systems capable of changing the quality of their interactions if they are not satisfied with them.

In summary, humans have inherent capabilities to monitor and correct the quality of their interactions—of what happens between them. The science of human communication offers an organic theoretical and methodological basis from which to observe quality in action. When the context is health care, quality control is, then, a naturally occurring event. It is happening right under our scientific noses.

HEALTH CARE AS HEALTH COMMUNICATION

Another common ground between the IOM Committee on Quality and NCI communication scientists is a shared view of health care as process. The IOM Committee on Quality defines health care as a function of its interdependence and interactions. It conceptualizes health care, not as a static institution, but as "a set of connected or interdependent parts or agents—including caregivers and patients—bound by a common purpose and acting on their knowledge." This acknowledgment does not necessarily make it easier to reshape into a higher quality system. Health care is complex, the IOM Committee continues, because of the great number of interconnections within and among small care systems. And, they argue, health care systems are adaptive because unlike mechanical systems, they are composed of individuals—patients and clinicians who have the capacity to learn and change as a result of experience. Their actions in delivering health care are not always predictable and tend to change both their local and larger environments. In other words, health care systems are complex because human interactions—those inherently creative and unpredictable processes that occur each day, every day—are what drives and shapes them.

This dynamic view of health care is akin to the view of health communication researchers who claim that "health—like politics—is not an institution, but a set of collective behaviors that are formed and influenced through communication processes" (Finnegan & Viswanath, 1990, p. 14). Communication systems, like transportation systems, play a fundamental organizing function. A transportation system is a network of interconnected roads and highways, river ways and other links that determine and reflect the quality of travel, how we use these modes of travel and how efficiently and effectively we travel. Similarly, the kind of communication systems we design can determine the quality of health information and other health care services.

From a systems view in which each person's action is another person's feedback, humans are adapting to each other constantly; during each communication exchange, with each assignment of meaning; each responsive act. In the health care context adaptation is happening when a doctor searches for a patient's reaction on telling her that she has breast cancer. It happens when a patient tries to read a doctor's intention on being told she needs another CAT scan. It happens when a health care organization places patient educational material on their Web site, based on focus group feedback. And, on and on in our daily interactions, emails, phone calls, visits between and among health professionals, patients, families, friends, and yes, even researchers. Even though we may take it for granted much of the time, we humans are rather busy complex systems, adapting to each other all the time in sometimes predictable but sometimes surprising and creative ways.

In summary, the health care system is the sum of the human interactions within it. The quality of interactions serve as measures of its quality. It is daunting to imagine trying to redesign an entire health care system to achieve better quality. It is much more manageable, however, to design patterns of human interactions toward that end.

Health Communication and Designing for Quality

Plsek (2001) has argued that efforts to reduce the health care system to its components have failed at improving the system. From a systems view, whole systems can be designed in a way to harness the ongoing change through a simple set of rules, then observe how it changes rather than isolating its separate components or holding its dynamic characteristics constant. The IOM Committee on Quality concurs and has set forth a few sets of design rules and observing the emergent qualities.

The committee offers six challenges to building quality systems of care:

1. Redesign care processes to serve more effectively the needs of the chronically ill for coordinated, seamless care across settings and clinicians and over time.
2. Make effective use of information technologies to automate clinical information and make it accessible to patients and all members of the care team.
3. Manage the growing knowledge base.
4. Coordinate care across patient conditions, services and settings over time.
5. Continually advance the effectiveness of teams.
6. Incorporate care process and outcome measures into their daily work. (p. 12)

We approach these challenges from a systemic model of human communication in which we see an isomorphism between improving the quality of health interactions and improving the quality of health care. *This model offers a research method for designing human interactions that make up the health care process and observing changes in quality over the course of the interactions.* In other words, the unit of observation is the interaction between health care participants. The research method this invites is the design of human interactions that reflect the characteristics of complex, adaptive systems and allow their inherent capacity for self-improvement.

This interaction, from a systems view, is an organic approach to research. It already has within it two critical components of quality improvement: the capability for creative change and a built in feedback loop for observing and adapting to that change. We believe this is an effective alternative way to conduct outcomes research and test interventions.

The Role of E-Health

E-health is the use of information and communication technologies within the context of health care. The essential ingredient of these technologies is their interactivity; they extend the human ability to create and mange interactions in highly structured ways that are not bound by the constraints of time and place. The potential for e-health to radically change the

IOM RECOMMENDATIONS TO DESIGN TO:	HEALTH COMMUNICATION RESEARCH DESIGN TO:
Make patient centered, coordinated, and seamless	Support ongoing interactions, including frequent feedback opportunities, between caregivers and their patients and family members
Make effective use of IT	Embed outcomes queries into ongoing interactions
Manage the knowledge base	Embed standards based or best-of-breed interventions into ongoing interactions and adapt interventions according to feedback
Coordinate across conditions, services, settings, and time	Integrate human and e-health communication for continual personalization and localization
Continually improve teamwork	Create a web of interactions for all members of each team
Incorporate care process and outcome measures into daily work	Link all team interaction results to computerized patient record.

way health interactions are conducted has yet to be tapped, much less reached (Neuhauser & Kreps, 2003a, 2003b). We illustrate this point later in two research examples. But first, we describe how a systemic health communication research approach, enhanced with e-health tools, can operationalize the IOM's design for quality challenge.

VA PROJECT AND CARE COORDINATION

Organizational problems are cited as key culprits in our efforts to manage chronic care.

> The fact that more than 40% of people with chronic conditions have more than one such condition argues strongly for sophisticated mechanisms to coordinate care. Yet health care organizations, hospitals, and physician groups typically operate as separate "silos," acting without the benefit of complete information about the patient's condition, medical history, services provided in other settings, or medications provided by other clinicians. (Institute of Medicine, 2001, p. 2)

In 2002, the National Cancer Institute and the Veterans Health Administration (VHA) initiated a joint research project for the purpose of developing a model of telehome care for cancer patients and their families. One of the primary goals of this effort is to test the viability of integrating outcomes research into the delivery of care process. The evolving model of cancer care reflects a systemic view of health communication. We describe the contours of this research project here to lend pragmatic support to our earlier theoretical view of health communication as the dynamics involved in organizing health care systems.

The VA—an Exemplary Communication System

The Veterans Health Administration has one of the world's most comprehensive and sophisticated computerized patient record systems. This record is the backbone for organizing interdisciplinary teams of caregivers around a single, real-time view of a patient's health status. In the case of a cancer patient, the radiologist, oncologist, nurse, primary care provider, and so on, have online access to each other's reports, test results, notes, prognosis, and the like. This shared knowledge enables members of the team to engage in efficient and effective communication regarding the patient's status. By extending the computerized patient record to the Web, patients and their families and informal caregivers become part of the communication system that is made up of all the stakeholders in a given patient's well being.

Home Care at the VA

It is within this elaborate e-health communication system that the VA has engaged in a bold effort to extend health care into the homes of thousands of veterans with chronic conditions. Beginning in April 2000, the Veterans Health Administration began testing a model of home-based coordinated chronic care. Designed as an "aging in place" model of care by the Sunshine Network of the VHA (VISN 8 Veterans Integrated Service Network), the aim of this program is to "improve health status, increase program efficiency, and decrease resource utilization" (Meyer, Kobb, & Ryan, 2002, p. 87). After the first two years of operation evaluation results have shown:

- 40% reduction in emergency room visits
- 63% reduction in VHA nursing home admissions
- 88% reduction in nursing home bed days of care

The VHA, like all healthcare systems, is trying to manage the costs of chronic care. They face an increasingly older population and tightening budgets. In a break from traditional hospital-based VHA care, the Community Care Coordination Service (CCCS) in VISN 8 designed a working model of care that places communication and e-health at the heart of their community-based system of care.

Over 1.5 million veterans live in the VISN 8 service area, 45% of whom are 65 years of age or older. Four percent of these veterans were found to be consuming over 40% of the network's resources (Veterans Integrated Service Network [VISN8]. Strategic plan. Department of Veterans Affairs, Bay Pines, FL, 2001). This group was identified as "high risk, high use, high cost" (Meyer, 2002, p. 88), and the new coordinated care model was deployed to improve quality while managing costs.

Coordinated Home Care

The CCCS strategic model includes business and clinical components. It links care coordinators and communication technologies to the 7 hospitals, 10 multispeciality outpatient clinics, and 28 community-based primary care clinics in the Florida and Puerto Rico VISN. In the coordinated care model at the VHA, each high-cost, high-risk, high-use veteran is "assigned a care coordinator for the entire continuum of care. Care coordinators monitor patient problems and help resolve them whenever and wherever they arise" (Meyer, 2002, p. 88)

"The role of the care coordinator is a key factor in ensuring appropriate, timely patient data—which constitutes the most vital part of clinical decision-making—are communicated to the healthcare provider" (Meyer, 2002, p. 88). Care coordinators have been trained as social workers, nurse practitioners, and/or registered nurses. Each is empowered to assess and make decisions across departments to enhance access to care and eliminate bureaucratic barriers that sometimes prevent timely symptom management. The communication technologies are used to maintain frequent and timely communication between the care coordinator and the patient at home.

Feedback: The Essence of Care Coordination

Ongoing communication between patient and care coordinator and between care coordinator and providers of care from across the VHA is the central dynamic of this innovative model. The infrastructure is in place to support communication involving three continually repeated activities: assessment, matching, and monitoring.

- First, care coordinator and patient talk about the patient's clinical needs, functional status, and the social and environmental context in which care occurs.
- Second, the care coordinator, in communication with various care providers, matches the services to the needs of the patient.
- Third, an ongoing feedback loop is installed in each patient's home to monitor patient's health status, quality of life, patient satisfaction, and need for new or modified services. Various information and communication technologies are deployed, depending on the fit with each patient's situation.

This model has improved patient/provider relationships and patient satisfaction. Self-management is another key component of this model. Technologies were chosen that supported patient compliance and provided educational opportunities to enhance self-management.

In a preliminary study, the CCCS program was compared with usual VHA care, which does not involve coordinated care or communication technologies. Data analysis for the intervened group from the first year to the second year showed a reduction in ER visits by 40%, hospital admissions by 63%, and hospital BDOC by 60%. Nursing home admissions declined by 64%, and nursing home DCOC were reduced by 88%. In the comparison group, nursing home admissions increased by 106%. Patients enrolled in the CCCS program were 77.7% less likely to be admitted to a nursing home care unit than those not enrolled in the program. Quality of life and functional liability as measured by the SF 36V indicated significant improvements in the physical, pain, social functional, emotional, and mental composite scores. On performance dimensions, such as compliance with medication (93%) and appropriate, timely communication between primary care provider and the care coordinator (85%), scores are also impressive.

Overall, when comparing the intervened group findings to the comparison group, it was found that the intervened group showed considerably greater improvements on all measures.

This communication system is proving to be effective in designing a proactive healthcare model that facilitates patient-oriented and cost-effective delivery of services. VHA is so impressed it is planning to roll out to the care coordination system nationwide.

Coordinated Cancer Care

The National Cancer Institute has joined with the VHA in further elaborating on this coordinated care model to develop a model of home-based coordinated cancer care. Together, these two agencies will help meet two of the VHA's high-priority goals as they design quality home-based systems of care that meet their growing need for deinstitutionalized health care:

1. A strategy for developing home-tele-health that is explicit and evidence based.
2. A set of uniform standards for home-tele-health in the VA.

This collaborative research project will also help meet two of the eNCI's high priority goals of focusing on the chronic nature of cancer and those who must manage this condition over time:

1. Develop quality standards for information and communication technologies that can be used to support providers, patients, and caregivers.
2. Develop models of coordinated and secure systems of cancer care that are patient-centered and patient-friendly.

The proposed VISN 8 Home & Community Care Model is central to veterans and caregivers. The entry point of the veteran into home care can be anywhere along the continuum of care, for example, acute care, nursing home, or primary care settings. This continuum of care framework is supported and strengthened by focusing on clinical outcomes and quality, use of state-of-the-art technology, and ongoing education and research with special emphasis on customer satisfaction and good communication. Services available will be standardized across the network through new program developments including telemedicine clinics, a network Telephone Care Program, in-home respite services, consolidated contracting for services, and new partnerships. The care coordinator will have both a clinical and administrative background and experience and will be responsible for following patients to assure timely and appropriate movement through all levels of the care continuum. The care coordinator will be knowledgeable about all services accessible to patients and caregivers in the home, including those available through newly emerging technology. The coordinator, directly responsible to the VISN Home Care leadership, will be located at the local pilot site and serve as a link between the hospitals, discharge planning team, primary care provider, home care staff, and other professionals involved in the patients' care. The care coordinator, assisted by the Network Telephone Care Program, will assure the patient is provided support 24 hours a day, 7 days a week.

Long-range program goals include:

*   Expanding the use of patients' homes as alternate clinic sites through the use of technology; this will allow full development of the primary care concept with the team involved in all facets of patients' care outside an in-patient stay.

- Developing a process for managing all VA and VA-sponsored visits to patients' residences.
- Exploring and developing new resources to enable patients to remain in their homes.
- Exploring and developing the care coordinator role to impact on high-risk, high-cost patients' care through the continuum of cancer care.

Research as Dialogue

One of the defining characteristics of the care coordination model is the ongoing dialogue between the care coordinator and patients. Every qualifying veteran in VISN 8 is assigned a care coordinator for the duration of his chronic condition. Although the care coordinator is an infrequent visitor in the veteran's home, they communicate on a daily basis via a variety of technologies, including telephone, picture phone, and/or "dialogue boxes." The dialogue box makes it viable to integrate outcomes research into this ongoing flow of communication.

The dialogue box is a small in-home messaging device. It is a web-based, store-and-forward application that connects to the care coordinator through the Internet from the patient's home via a toll-free number, requiring no technology know-how. The dialogues are highly structured questions and answers regarding symptom management, self-management, and disease knowledge for a variety of chronic conditions. This dialogue is highly structured (standards driven) and partly automated, using a communication technology placed in the patient's home, along with personal communication when needed. This system accomplishes a number of things at once:

1. It monitors compliance, health status, and quality of life on a daily basis.
2. It collects and stores baseline patient data against which daily adjustments can be made.
3. Behavioral interventions, health promotion, and patient education are incorporated into the dialogue when appropriate.
4. Data collection occurs in the context of an ongoing relationship between the patient-trusted care coordinator.
5. Patients who normally would have to have extensive nursing home or hospital care can stay at home.

Each veteran is expected to engage in a brief dialogue each day. Care coordinators are able to access the answers over a secured Web site in near real time. Using this communication process care coordinators receive ongoing feedback concerning the health status and knowledge-based resources available to each patient. Answers become data that, collected in an outcomes database over time, reveals a highly accurate profile of the patient's progress. If a particular answer is outside the latitude of an acceptable health condition, according to the standard of care, an alert automatically becomes part of the patient's response. The care coordinator, on receiving the alert, can inquire further and/or contact a health care provider immediately.

The dialogue box holds, in microcosm, the essence of systemic communication in which ongoing reciprocated feedback facilitates adjustments and adaptations in an ongoing basis. In it communication and outcomes research become a fully integrated process on which interventions can be tested, altered, and tried again as part of the daily exchange between patient and care coordinator.

E-HEALTH TECHNOLOGY AND CANCER CARE

E-health technologies provide a unique opportunity for establishing meaningful interactions between health care providers and consumers, as well as with health researchers who seek to learn more about the role of communication in providing high-quality care. The electronic interactions among the participants in the modern health care system allow development of evolving cooperative relationships, sharing of relevant information, identification of emergent health problems and issues, and the ability to intervene early to ameliorate these problems before they spiral out of control. This opportunity for meaningful health care dialogue provides consumers with greater access to their different health care providers, allows them to ask questions to guide health maintenance activities, and empowers them to take care of themselves. E-health dialogues provide health care providers with the opportunity to educate consumers, learn about their responses to treatment, track their clients' changing conditions, and answer any questions that arise, both from consumers and local caregivers. Thus, electronic communication has the potential to help increase reach, influence, and coordination for all members of the health care system.

The crucial issue is that communication technologies have the potential to revolutionize cancer care by promoting greater cooperation among consumers, providers, and caregivers in the delivery of cancer care. Information technologies, such as those used in the care coordination programs at the VHA, provide timely and relevant feedback to consumers and providers. Health care providers use the technologies (both telecommunications equipment and computerized analyses of patient data) to effectively monitor their clients' physical and emotional responses to cancer care. When problems arise, the use of e-health technologies facilitates rapid provider (or guided patient/caregiver) interventions to arrest health problems, improve quality of care, and ultimately enhance the quality of life for individuals confronting cancer. The future is bright for the development of new communication technologies to support provision of relevant health information and the delivery of high-quality cancer care.

REFERENCES

Brown, S. L., & Eisenhardt, K. M. (1998). *Competing on the edge: Strategy as structured chaos.* Cambridge, MA: Harvard Business School Press.

Campbell, D. T. (1960). Blind variation and selective retention in creative thought as in other knowledge processes. *Psychological Review, 67,* 380-400.

Cragan, J. F., & Shields, D. C. (1998). *Understanding communication theory: The communicative forces for human action.* Boston: Allyn & Bacon.

Cronen, V. E. & Pearce, W. B. (1981). Logical force in interpersonal communication: A new concept of the "necessity" of social behaviour. *Communication, 6,* 5-67.

Cronen, V. E., Pearce, W. B., & Harris, L. M. (1979). The logic of the coordinated management of meaning: A rules-based approach to the first course in interpersonal communication. *Communication Education, 28,* 22-38.

Cronen, V. E., Pearce, W. B., & Harris, L. M. (1982). The coordinated management of meaning: A theory of communication. In E. X. Dance (Ed.), *Human communication theory; comparative essays* (pp. 61-89). New York: Holt, Rinehart & Winston.

Finnegan, J. R., & Viswanath, K. (1990). Health and communication: Medical and public health influences on the research agenda. In E. B. Ray & L. Donohew (Eds.), *Communication and health: Systems and applications* (pp. 9-24). Hillsdale, NJ: Erlbaum.

Institute of Medicine. (2001). *Crossing the quality chasm: A new health system for the 21st century.* Washington, DC: National Academy of Sciences.

Kreps, G. L. (1990). *Organizational communication: Theory and practice* (2nd ed.). New York: Longman.

Kreps, G. L. (2003a). Guest editor's foreword. E-Health: Technology-mediated health communication. *Journal of Health Psychology, 8*(1), 5-6.

Kreps, G. L. (2003b). The impact of communication on cancer risk, incidence, morbidity, mortality, and quality of life. *Health Communication, 15*(2), 163-171.

Mandelbrot, B. B. (1999, February). A multifractal walk down Wall Street. *Scientific American,* pp. 50-53.

Meyer, M., Kobb, R., & Ryan, P. (2002). Virtually healthy: Chronic disease management in the home. *Disease Management, 5*(2), 87-94.

Morowitz, H. J., & Singer, J. L. (Eds.). (1995). *The mind, the brain, and complex adaptive systems.* Boston: Addison-Wesley.

Neuhauser, L., & Kreps, G. L. (2003a). The advent of e-health: How interactive media are transforming health communication. *Medien & Kommunikations-wissenschaft, 51*(3-4), 541-556.

Neuhauser, L., & Kreps, G. L. (2003b). Rethinking communication in the e-health era. *Journal of Health Psychology, 8*(1), 7-22.

Plsek, P. (2001). Redesigning health care with insights from the science of complex adaptive systems. In Institute of Medicine (Ed.), *Crossing the quality chasm: A new health system for the 21st century* (Appendix B, pp. 322-335). Washington, DC: National Academy of Sciences.

Ray, E. B., & Donohew, L. (1990). *Communication and health: Systems and applications.* Hillsdale, NJ: Erlbaum.

Rogers, E. M. (1994). *A history of communication study: A biographical approach.* New York: Free Press.

Varela, F. J., & Coutinho, A. (1991). Second generation immune networks. *Immunology Today, 12,* 159-166.

von Bertalanffy, L. (1968). *General system theory.* New York:Brazillier.

Wiener, N. (1956). *I am a mathematician.* Garden City, NY: Doubleday.

5 | Communication, Adherence, And Outcomes of Cancer Prevention and Treatment

Recommendations for Future Research

M. Robin DiMatteo
University of California, Riverside

Cancer care, from prevention and early detection to the successful management of survivorship, requires effective provider-patient communication. Much evidence exists, in this volume and elsewhere, that enhanced communication leads to better health care outcomes. One important mediating factor that may account for the communication-outcome connection is patient adherence to providers' recommendations. A health professional's clear and sensitive counsel for a mammogram, for example, can lead to early detection of breast cancer and improved odds for survival only if the patient adheres to the recommendation. Relatedly, patient adherence is essential to connect a complex medication regimen to tumor shrinkage and increased functional status. In general, patient adherence is a critical mediating factor between health recommendations and their outcomes.

Although studies show that better adherence is not perfectly correlated with better treatment outcomes (DiMatteo, Giordani, Lepper, & Croghan, 2002), the delivery of medical care is generally based on the assumption that adhering to a providers' advice is better for the patient than ignoring it, and that medical care recommendations, although not perfect, have an appreciable efficacy. It is often argued that noncompliance causes patients to become sicker, and among patients with potentially life-threatening diseases such as cancer, nonadherence can be fatal. At the very least, patient nonadherence can be a source of frustration for all. Although the precise connection between cancer care/ prevention recommendations and their outcomes requires regular examination and update, the goal of this chapter is to assess the relationship between health professional-patient communication and patient adherence in the context of prevention and treatment of cancer and the management of long-term cancer survival.

DEFINING ADHERENCE

Nonadherence can take many forms depending on the regimen to be followed and the disease to be dealt with (DiMatteo & DiNicola, 1982; DiMatteo, Reiter, & Gambone, 1994; Epstein & Cluss, 1982). Patients may fail to take medication or to correctly follow dietary restrictions or other behavioral recommendations. They may fail to keep follow-up medical appointments or persist in lifestyles that endanger their health. They may forego medical treatment entirely (Meichenbaum & Turk, 1987). In a meta-analysis of the adherence literature from 1948-1998, on average only about 80% of cancer patients were found to be at least moderately adherent to recommendations (DiMatteo, 2004a). Adherence to cancer treatment appeared to be higher than adherence to treatment for diabetes, pulmonary disease, end-stage renal disease, and sleep disorders; however, adherence to behavioral treatments for cancer (as opposed to medication) was particularly low (roughly 73%). There were no differences between various types of cancers in terms of adherence, but various methodological factors (such as measurement choices) did affect documented adherence rates.

ADHERENCE AND PROVIDER-CONSUMER COMMUNICATION

A great deal of evidence points to the value of effective health provider-patient (consumer) communication as to the latter's willingness and ability to follow health care recommendations. Communication involves the unimpeded flow of information and meaning between individuals and requires understanding (DiMatteo & DiNicola, 1982). In the realm of primary prevention, for example, patients must understand the costs and benefits of behavioral protocols to reduce their cancer risks. This understanding requires clear explanation as well as encouragement and facilitation, especially when radical lifestyle changes are required. Screening may require the health professional to help overcome patient skepticism and inertia, and even to provide reminders, such as for yearly mammograms. Cancer diagnosis and treatment necessitate even more complex communication involving exploration of patients' preferences for the process of care and various possible outcomes. Diagnosis and treatment planning require trust in the provider-patient relationship, empathic support of the patient and family, and encouragement to adhere to sometimes difficult, challenging, and uncomfortable therapies. Adjusting to the aftermath of cancer treatments and coping with the loneliness and alienation of cancer survival require communication with and emotional support from the provider (Little et al., 1998).

Nearly every theoretical model of patient adherence relies on at least one component of effective provider-patient communication. Communication can sway the patient's belief in the value and importance of the regimen and in his or her own ability to carry it out; communication can affect the degree to which the provider exerts social influence and affects the patient's perception that adherence will reduce any threat to his or her health. The Health Belief Model, for example, emphasizes the role of thoughts about the risks and benefits of a recommended course of health action (Janz & Becker 1984). The Theory of Reasoned Action adds social influences and intentions to this equation, and the Theory of Planned Behavior adds behavioral control and perceived barriers to action (Ajzen & Fishbein, 1980; Schifter & Ajzen, 1985). Attribution theories include concepts such as locus of control (internal versus external), stability, and universality (Wallston, Stein, & Smith, 1994). The Transtheoretical Model proposes stages of behavior modification and maintenance (Prochaska & DiClemente 1983), and self-regulatory models view the patient as an active problem solver (Leventhal & Cameron, 1987). What these various theoretical models have in common is that each depends on some combination of information delivery, trust, encouragement, reframing of information, identification of health threat, outcome appraisal, development and implementation of an action plan, and problem- and/or emotion-focused coping. Health professionals can have an immense influence on these factors that affect patient adherence and directly shape patients' beliefs and ways of thinking (about the regimen, the disease, and the self), as well as their habits, social and cultural norms, family and social support, cognitive functioning, optimism, constructive problem solving, and mood. Although these theoretical models propose that thoughts and actions are initiated and maintained by the individual, the health professional's role is clear. Effective provider-patient communication is essential to the establishment of the thoughts and actions necessary to achieve patient adherence.

Theoretical models of adherence are, of course, useful in guiding our thinking about communication, and they provide the theoretical underpinning for research. Their weakness in practice, however, has been their lack of integration with empirical findings. The corpus of literature on adherence is enormous; however, it consists primarily of theory, opinion, and selective review. Approximately one tenth of Medline and PsycLit citations on patient adherence (or patient compliance) involve empirical research (DiMatteo, Giordani et al., 2002). Analysis of this empirical literature over the past 50 years is what is most valuable, and it too shows that patient adherence is affected by many factors related to provider-patient communication (DiMatteo, 2004a, 2004b). For example, empirical support is strong that nonadherence to cancer treatment may result from the patients' disbelief in its efficacy and the presence of barriers such as side effects and financial constraints (Dolgin, Katz, Doctors, & Siegel, 1986). Nonadherence may also result from a lack of help and support from family members (DiMatteo, 2004b). One of the strongest and most consistent correlates of patient nonadherence is mood disorder, particularly depression, which can impair cognitive focus, energy, and motivation, and limit social support (DiMatteo, Lepper, & Croghan, 2000). This is particularly true of cancer. Three empirical studies have shown that depression is strongly associated with both discontinuation of therapy (Blotcky, Cohen, Conaster, & Klopovich, 1985; Gilbar & DeNour, 1989) and missed doses of medication (Lebovits et al., 1990). Demographic factors, such as low income and limited education, have low but consistent correlations with nonadherence and, like depression, are barriers that can be overcome. If acknowledged and dealt with sensitively through good health professional-patient communication, these barriers can be treated before they seriously reduce adherence. Depression, once recognized by the clinician in the patient's words and behavior, can be treated with support, psychotherapy, and medication. Likewise, although a patient's income and educational level cannot be changed, additional resources such as generic medications or samples, and free or low cost mammograms, can be provided; clear explanations and education specifically about health maintenance and disease management can be given.

Contextual and organizational factors are not irrelevant in this equation, of course. The time necessary for communication and problem solving needs to be available, and support must be provided for health professionals to be willing to offer such care to their patients. In cancer care, the advanced, and sometimes frightening, technological interventions of cancer treatment can make effective communication particularly difficult to achieve. There are now so many occasions to do things to patients that often there is little time to talk with patients and their families about the effects and after effects of cancer care (Little et al., 1998). Health professionals, particularly physicians, are often quite separated from patients by their different perspectives on the illness (Kleinman, 1988). Effective communication is essential for health professionals to learn about the beliefs, commitment, supports, difficulties, and outcome preferences of patients and the dynamics of family members' relationships to each other and to the cancer treatment regimen and its outcomes. All these issues must be addressed in order to enhance patient adherence to recommended cancer treatments and provide effective care for patients as whole individuals.

THE NEED FOR RESEARCH ON ADHERENCE AND COMMUNICATION

Most empirical research on patient adherence demonstrates that doing something to help patients adhere is better than doing nothing, and that adherence can usually be found to correlate with a characteristic of the patient (e.g., motivation), the regimen (e.g., its complexity), or the interaction between patient and health professional (e.g., their communication). Despite the existence of a fairly substantial collection of studies on adherence, this work has not been particularly systematic and there are surprisingly few clear empirical answers not only about how adherence is achieved but also about how communication affects patient adherence (in the care of all diseases, as well as cancer). There are several constructs worth further study, several variables that show promise, and several questions worth posing. These are examined in the remainder of this chapter.

One important question involves trust in the therapeutic relationship—what role it plays in adherence and how therapeutic trust is achieved. It is often argued that trust is important, particularly in the care of diseases such as cancer, because patients' lives and well-being are threatened and treatment regimens are challenging (Roter & Hall, 1992). It is argued that patients' adherence is dependent on their satisfaction with the physician-patient relationship, including the health professionals' positive expectations for healing (Brody, 2000). Provider sensitivity to the adherence barriers that patients struggle with, as well as expressions of respect, rapport, empathy, and acceptance of patients' emotional experience, are likely to build trust and enhance patients' satisfaction (DiMatteo et al., 1993; DiMatteo, Hays, & Prince, 1986; DiMatteo, Linn, Chang, & Cope, 1985; Squier, 1990), but the precise effect that these would have on patient adherence to various kinds of recommendations, and under what circumstances these effects would occur, remain to be determined. It is also likely that trust would foster the active analysis necessary for patient commitment to the regimen (Katz, 1984), and commitment is a prerequisite to behavior change according to several models

(Ajzen & Fishbein, 1980; Prochaska & DiClemente, 1983). Future research should document precisely how effective provider communication can help to build patient trust and commitment to lifestyle change for cancer prevention, adherence to screening recommendations and treatment, and vigilance in survivorship. Research should also address the role of new technologies in fostering versus jeopardizing trust and commitment. For example, how is health professional-patient communication affected by patients' use of the Internet for information about cancer? What happens when patients challenge their providers' recommendations based on what they have learned? Does a health professional's availability by e-mail enhance the therapeutic relationship? Do Internet "chat rooms" and interactive Web sites reduce patient loneliness and improve adherence by helping patients to overcome their fear, passivity, forgetfulness, or denial? Do they enhance their commitment to health action?

A second important element of communication that needs further study in many areas of care, and in cancer care in particular, involves the instrumental communication that is necessary for patients to understand what they are being asked to do by their health professionals. Research in many realms shows that the quantity and quality of information actually provided to medical patients is often surprisingly inadequate, and that communication of the therapeutic regimen is often unclear, inexplicit, and vague (Faden et al., 1981; Ley, 1979; Waitzkin & Stoeckle, 1976). In some settings, insufficient time is available for patients to ask the questions necessary to support their beliefs in and positive expectations for the course of treatment (Glasgow, Wilson, & McCaul, 1985; Leedham, Meyerowitz, Muirhead, & Frist, 1995; Stanton, 1987). How can these problems be remedied? How much and what sorts of information can patients deal with at various stages of their diagnosis and treatment? How might that information best be communicated to them? Addressing these questions is critical for future research on communication in cancer care.

A third factor has figured prominently in the adherence literature, although its precise role is still controversial. Theory proposes, and empirical data generally support, the role of patients' beliefs in regimen adherence and the probability that health professionals can affect these beliefs. The belief that a regimen is effective and that the patient is susceptible to serious consequences of not adhering appears to promote adherence, and if perceived costs (in terms of time, attention, difficulty, distress, and finances) outweigh perceived benefits, adherence is unlikely (Hampson, Glasgow, & Toobert, 1990; Leedham et al., 1995; Stanton, 1987). Empirical support for these effects is not unequivocal, however. For example, many health professionals accept, and models based on "rational thinking" have argued, that patients who believe they have more serious diseases will be most compliant with treatment recommendations. Some studies of adults with very serious illnesses, for example, vision loss due to glaucoma (Kugelmann & Bensinger, 1983; Patel & Spaeth, 1995), potentially fatal complications of end-stage renal disease (Bame, Petersen, & Wray, 1993; Wolcott, Maida, Diamond, & Nissenson, 1986), and HIV/AIDS (Singh et al., 1996; Slavkin, 1996) suggest, however, that nonadherence is common and may be fostered by denial, survivor guilt, and other complex, irrational, or illogical factors (Sensky, Leger, & Gilmour, 1996). Would this be the case for cancer as well? Do poorer prognoses bring poorer adherence? Do patients' idiosyncratic beliefs about the seriousness of cancer, whether or not they are correct, affect adherence? Furthermore, how do social and cultural norms regarding the meaning of illness, medication, and self-care activities guide patients' beliefs and their subsequent responses to medical recommendations (Hampson et al., 1990)? What role might patients general skepticism about medical care and their embarrassment about care-seeking affect their acceptance or avoidance of preventive strategies such as mammography or Pap screening? And, how can the health professional influence these concerns through instrumental communication as well as the building of therapeutic trust? How do patients' choices of alternative and complimentary therapies fit into this equation, particularly when their health professionals do not share their beliefs?

In the treatment of cancer, a fourth issue that deserves further study is the role of effective communication in helping patients fit the regimen into their family life and habits. Past adherence behavior (i.e., habit) is a strong predictor of future adherence (Brownell, Marlatt, Lichtenstein, & Wilson, 1986; DiMatteo et al., 1993). Effective therapeutic communication requires recognition of and work with patients' and families' habitual response patterns and the reinforcements that have maintained them. Chronic daily stress in patients' lives can be a major barrier to adherence and, in some cases, can affect health outcomes dramatically (Cox & Gonder-Frederick, 1992; Everett et al., 1995). Effective health professional-patient communication can be essential in assisting patients to deal with the emotional strains and physical challenges of their treatment, including exhaustion, frustration, and interference with treasured activities (Kleinman, 1988), but what form that communication should take in the management of barriers to cancer prevention and treatment adherence is yet to be determined.

In a fifth arena of research concern, there is growing evidence that provider-patient partnerships matter, and that patients usually desire to be involved in decision making and to be given information and choices. In research on diabetes, indigent patients were most satisfied when they received as much information and as many opportunities for participation and involvement as they desired. Their satisfaction was also high when they received more information and participation than they initially stated they wanted (Golin et al., 2002). Participation may be important for several reasons. The patient, not the health professional, must live each day with the results of medical choices and may implicitly (if not explicitly) view nonadherence as a rational choice after weighing the costs and benefits of adhering to recommendations (Donovan & Blake, 1992; Lynn & DeGrazia, 1991). Research suggests that health professionals and patients often have different preferences for treatments and their outcomes, and that in cancer care patients tend to select more conservative, less invasive, and less expensive treatment strategies than do their physicians (McNeil, Weischelbaum, & Pauker, 1978; Wennberg, 1990). Research on consumers' treatment and outcome preferences in cancer care is in its early stages. The extent to which mutual decision making by providers and patients can lead to higher levels of patient adherence and health status has yet to be explored fully (Greenfield, Kaplan, & Ware, 1985). Because many cancer therapies are complex, demanding, and invasive, it is particularly important to examine the consumer's perspective and the role of informed collaborative choices (DiMatteo, Reiter, & Gambone, 1994).

A sixth area of research endeavor involves the role of emotional distress in cancer care and its management through effective communication. Meta-analytic work has recently shown that patient depression is strongly related to lower levels of adherence to treatment, probably because emotional distress can impair cognitive focus, energy, motivation, and social support (DiMatteo et al., 2000). This work needs to be extended further, particularly to the role that provider-patient communication can play in recognizing and helping to treat depression. Furthermore, research has suggested the importance of social support to adherence in both cancer prevention and rehabilitation (DiMatteo et al., 1993), as well as the role of family cohesion in preventing dropout from cancer therapy (Gilbar & DeNour, 1989). More research on this topic is encouraged. Relatedly, in three decades of adherence literature (1968-1998), there were only five studies of the relationship between adherence and treatment outcomes in cancer (DiMatteo, Giordani et al., 2002), and all five involved medication adherence. Additional research on various regimens using a variety of measurement strategies is needed to explore the effects of adherence on outcomes in cancer care. It is recommended that future research on cancer prevention and treatment include effective assessments of patient adherence to understand the possible attenuating role of nonadherence and provide abundant data for future quantitative reviews. The independent effects of adherence on achieving health outcomes, functional status, psychological and social well-being, and all aspects of health-related quality of life need to be examined. In addition, data are limited on variations in adherence among different cancers and levels of cancer care. Although preliminary evidence from meta-analysis suggests a trend for prevention adherence to be slightly lower than treatment adherence, the reasons for this difference, including the role of provider-patient communication, need to be explored (DiMatteo, 2004a).

A continuing research challenge in the study of adherence in general, and specifically in the realm of cancer care, involves adherence measurement. Assessment of adherence in research and in clinical practice has typically relied on the technique of patient self-report despite the potential biases of patients' self-presentation and fears of reprimand by the health professional. Reports by spouses or by health professionals tend to be used, although they vary in accuracy. More "objective" approaches like pill counts, patient behavioral diaries, and electronic recording devices may be subject to patient manipulation if the patient is of a mind to conceal nonadherence. Tests, such as urine or blood assay, may be useful for medication, but reflect only recent consumption, and chart entries are often inconsistent and based on unclear criteria (DiMatteo et al., 2003). Despite a great deal of research, the most accurate method for measuring adherence is still unknown, and the ways in which various measurement options relate to each other are yet to be explored. Furthermore, the precise implications of measurement choices are as yet unidentified, although research has found that the role of adherence in health care outcomes depends strongly on the sensitivity of the adherence measurement (DiMatteo, Giordani et al., 2002). It is important to note that in research or in clinical settings, reliable and valid assessments of adherence depend on effective communication. Trust is essential for patients to be forthcoming in their self-reports of adherence and honest about their difficulties in following treatment suggestions (DiMatteo, 2001; Hays & DiMatteo 1987).

Finally, despite several decades of research on patient adherence to treatment, there remain serious gaps in the literature, particularly in the area of cancer care. Research findings on adherence and communication are in need of systematic compilation and quantitative review, such as with meta-analysis. Selective qualitative reviews, currently plentiful, are of limited value. The models guiding research on adherence and communication, in cancer and in other areas, are almost solely theoretical (DiMatteo, 2001). There has been little empirical research that is multifaceted enough to reflect the complexity of the adherence construct. The many factors that influence adherence need to be studied simultaneously because they interact with each other and with variations in population and measurement. Unless the phenomenon of adherence to cancer treatment is fully understood in all its complexity, it will be impossible to know when, where, and how it might be best to intervene to help patients adhere. Broader methodological approaches, such as narrative and observational techniques, are also needed in order to examine the entire picture of adherence and communication in the context of the lives of patients and providers, who are themselves functioning in the context of more complex health care organizations. Finally, the organization of research in this area according to a purely biomedical focus has made it difficult to identify psychosocial trends across medical conditions, although a purely psychosocial focus, without regard to disease and regimen, would ignore important disease variations. A combined "biopsychosocial" approach would allow the analysis of psychosocial factors in the context of specific diseases and treatment conditions, such as the levels of cancer care, in order to understand the complex and sometimes evasive process by which patients adhere to medical care.

REFERENCES

Ajzen, I., & Fishbein, M. (1980). *Understanding attitudes and predicting social behavior*. Englewood Cliffs, NJ: Prentice-Hall.

Bame, S. I., Petersen, N., & Wray, N. P. (1993). Variation in hemodialysis patient compliance according to demographic characteristics. *Social Science and Medicine, 37,* 1035-1043.

Blotcky, A. D., Cohen, D. G., Conaster, C., & Klopovich, P. (1985). Psychosocial characteristics of adolescents who refuse cancer treatment. *Journal of Consulting and Clinical Psychology, 53,* 729-731.

Brody, H. (2000). *The placebo response.* New York: Harper Collins.

Brownell, K. D., Marlatt, G. A., Lichtenstein, E., & Wilson, G. T. (1986). Understanding and preventing relapse. *American Psychologist, 41,* 765-782.

Cox, D. J., & Gonder-Frederick, L. (1992). Major developments in behavioral diabetes research. *Journal of Consulting and Clinical Psychology, 60,* 628-638.

DiMatteo, M. R. (2001). Patient adherence to health care regimens. In N.J. Smelser & P.B. Baltes (Eds.), *International encyclopedia of the social and behavioral sciences.* Oxford, UK: Pergamon/Elsevier.

DiMatteo, M. R. (2004a). Variations in patients' adherence to medical recommendations: A quantitative review of 50 years of research. *Medical Care, 42*(3), 200-209.

DiMatteo, M.R. (2004b). Social support and patient adherence to medical treatment: A meta-analysis. *Health Psychology, 23*(2), 207-218.

DiMatteo, M.R., Giordani, P. J, Lepper, H. S., & Croghan, T. W. (2002). Patient adherence and medical treatment outcomes: A meta-analysis. *Medical Care, 40,* 794-811.

DiMatteo, M. R., Hays, R. D., Gritz, E. R., Bastani, R., Crane, L., Elashoff, R. et al. (1993). Patient adherence to cancer control regimens: Scale development and initial validation. *Psychological Assessment, 5,* 102-112.

DiMatteo, M. R., Hays, R. D., & Prince, L. M. (1986). Relationships of physicians nonverbal communication skill to patient satisfaction, appointment noncompliance, and physician workload. *Health Psychology, 5,* 581-594.

DiMatteo, M. R., Lepper, H. S., & Croghan T. W. (2000). Depression is a risk factor for noncompliance with medical treatment: A meta-analysis of the effects of anxiety and depression on patient adherence. *Archives of Internal Medicine, 160,* 2101-2107.

DiMatteo, M. R., Linn, L. S., Chang, B. L., & Cope, D. W. (1985). Affect and neutrality in physician behavior. *Journal of Behavioral Medicine, 8,* 397-409.

DiMatteo M. R., & DiNicola, D.D. (1982) *Achieving patient compliance.* Elmsford, NY: Pergamon.

DiMatteo, M. R., Reiter, R. C., & Gambone, J. C. (1994). Enhancing medication adherence through communication and informed collaborative choice. *Health Communication, 6,* 253-265.

DiMatteo, M.R., Robinson, J.D., Heritage, J., Tabbarah, M., & Fox, S.A. (2003). Correspondence among patients' self reports, chart records, and audio/videotapes of medical visits. *Health Communication, 15,* 393-413.

Dolgin, M. J., Katz, E. R., Doctors, S. R., & Siegel, S. E. (1986). Caregivers' perceptions of medical compliance in adolescents with cancer. *Journal of Adolescent Health Care, 7,* 22-27.

Donovan, J. L., & Blake, D. R. (1992). Patient non-compliance: Deviance or reasoned decision-making? *Social Science & Medicine, 34,* 507-513.

Epstein, L. H., & Cluss, P. A. (1982). A behavioral medicine perspective on adherence to long-term medical regimens. *Journal of Consulting and Clinical Psychology, 50* , 950-971.

Everett, K. D., Brantley, P. J., Sletten, C., Jones, G. N., & McKnight, G. T. (1995). The relation of stress and depression to interdialytic weight gain in hemodialysis patients. *Behavioral Medicine. 21,* 25-30.

Faden, R., Becker, C., Lewis, C., Freeman, J., & Faden, A. (1981). Disclosure of information to patients in medical care. *Medical Care, 19,* 718-733.

Gilbar, O., & DeNour, A. K. (1989). Adjustment to illness and dropout of chemotherapy. *Journal of Psychosomatic Research, 33,* 1-5.

Glasgow, R.E., Wilson, W., & McCaul, K. D. (1985). Regimen adherence: A problematic construct in diabetes research. *Diabetes Care, 8,* 300-301.

Golin, C., DiMatteo, M.R., Duan, N., Leake, B., & Gelberg, L. (2002). Impoverished diabetic patients whose doctors facilitate their participation in medical decision-making are more satisfied with their care. *Journal of General Internal Medicine, 17,* 1-10.

Greenfield, S., Kaplan, S., & Ware, J. E., Jr. (1985). Expanding patient involvement in care: Effects on patient outcomes. *Annals of Internal Medicine, 102,* 520-528.

Hampson, S. E., Glasgow, R. E., & Toobert, D. J. (1990). Personal models of diabetes and their relations to self-care activities. *Health Psychology, 9,* 632-646.

Hays, R. D., & DiMatteo, M.R. (1987). Key issues and suggestions, sources of information, focus of measures, and nature of response options. *Journal of Compliance in Health Care, 2,* 37-53.

Janz, N.K, & Becker, M H. (1984). The Health Belief Model: A decade later. *Health Education Quarterly, 11,* 1-47.

Katz, J. (1984). *The silent world of doctor and patient.* New York: The Free Press.

Kleinman, A. (1988*). The illness narratives: Suffering, healing, and the human condition.* New York: Basic Books.

Kugelmann, R., & Bensinger, R. E. (1983). Metaphors of glaucoma. *Culture, Medicine, and Psychiatry, 7,* 313-328.

Lebovits, A.H., Strain, J.J., Schleifer, S.J., Tanaka, J.S., Bhardwaj, S., & Messe, M.R. (1990). Patient non-compliance with self-administered chemotherapy. *Cancer, 65,* 17-22.

Leedham, B., Meyerowitz, B. E., Muirhead, H., & Frist, W. H. (1995). Positive expectations predict health after heart transplantation. *Health Psychology, 14,* 74-79.

Leventhal, H., & Cameron, L. (1987). Behavioral theories and the problem of compliance. *Patient Education and Counseling, 10,* 117-138

Ley, P. (1979). Memory for medical information. *British Journal of Social & Clinical Psychology, 18,* 245-255.

Little, M., Jordens, C.F., Paul, K., Montgomery, K., & Philipson, B. (1998). Liminality: A major category of the experience of cancer illness. *Social Science and Medicine, 47,* 1485-1494.

Lynn, J., & DeGrazia, D. (1991). An outcomes model of medical decision making. *Theoretical Medicine, 12,* 325-343.

McNeil, B. J., Weichselbaum, R., & Pauker, S. G. (1978). Fallacy of the five-year survival in lung cancer. *New England Journal of Medicine, 299,* 1397-1401.

Meichenbaum, D., & Turk, D.C. (1987*). Facilitating treatment adherence: A practitioner's guidebook.* New York: Plenum.

Patel, S. C., & Spaeth, G. L. (1995). Compliance in patients prescribed eyedrops for glaucoma. *Ophthalmic Surgery, 26,* 233-236.

Prochaska, J. O., & DiClemente, C. C. (1983). Stages and processes of self-change of smoking: Toward an integrative model of change. *Journal of Consulting and Clinical Psychology, 51,* 390-395.

Roter, D. L., & Hall, J. A. (1992). *Doctors talking with patients/patients talking with doctors.* Westport: Auburn House.

Schifter, D.E., & Ajzen, I. (1985). Intention, perceived control, and weight loss: An application of the theory of planned behavior. *Journal of Personality & Social Psychology, 49,* 843-851.

Sensky, T., Leger, C., & Gilmour, S. (1996). Psychosocial and cognitive factors associated with adherence to dietary and fluid restriction regimens by people on chronic haemodialysis. *Psychotherapy and Psychosomatics, 65*, 36-42.

Singh, N., Squier, C., Sivek, M., Wagener, M., Nguyen, M. H., & Yu, V. L. (1996). Determinants of compliance with antiretroviral therapy in patients with immunodeficiency virus: Prospective assessment with implications for enhancing compliance. *AIDS Care, 8*, 261-269.

Slavkin, H. C. (1996). An update on HIV/AIDS. *Journal of the American Dental Association, 127*, 1401-1404

Squier, R. W. (1990). A model of empathic understanding and adherence to treatment regimens in practitioner-patient relationships. *Social Science & Medicine, 30*, 325-339.

Stanton, A. L. (1987). Determinants of adherence to medical regimens by hypertensive patients. *Journal of Behavioral Medicine, 10*, 377-394.

Waitzkin, H., & Stoeckle, J. D. (1976). Information control and the micropolitics of health care: Summary of an ongoing research project. *Social Science and Medicine, 10*, 263-276.

Wallston, K. A., Stein, M. J., & Smith, C. A. (1994). Form C of the MHLC Scales: Condition specific measures of locus of control. *Journal of Personality Assessment, 63*, 534-553.

Wennberg, J. E. (1990). Outcomes research, cost containment, and the fear of health care rationing. *New England Journal of Medicine, 323*, 1202-1204.

Wolcott, D. L., Maida, C. A., Diamond, R., & Nissenson, A. (1986). Treatment compliance in end-stage renal disease patients on dialysis. *American Journal of Nephrology, 6*, 329-338.

II CONTEXTUAL ISSUES

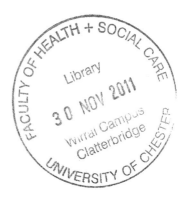

6 Communication in Context

New Directions in Cancer Communication Research

J. M. Bensing
NIVEL, The Netherlands

A. M. van Dulmen
NIVEL, The Netherlands

K. Tates
NIVEL, The Netherlands

Communication research is sometimes described as analyzing the black box of the doctor's healing power (Bensing, 2000; White, 1988), but, every now and then you get a flash which shows communication researchers analyzing this black box as if it was found in the bush after a plane crash: as an object in itself, completely devoid of the broader context of the medical dialogue. Most communication research has been exclusively focused on the dialogue between patient and doctor or nurse in itself, without taking account of its context. However, such a dialogue does not take place in a vacuum. There is a whole world surrounding it. Researchers too often seem to ignore both the context of the patient system and the context of the health care system which have so much to offer for understanding and interpreting the value of the medical dialogue. We strongly believe that this narrow focus blinds communication researchers to many relevant issues and hampers the progress of knowledge as well as the implementation of knowledge in clinical practice. Thus, the central statement in this chapter is: *We have acquired enough knowledge in general of the value of communication skills. Now it is time to focus our attention to the study of specific contextual conditions that may broaden our knowledge and may help, hinder, or complicate the application of this knowledge in everyday practice.*

FOCUS ON CANCER COMMUNICATION

Although we believe that this central statement is valid for all or most communication research, we elaborate on it specifically for the domain of cancer care. After all, apart from general practice, there is no medical setting with a stronger tradition in communication research than the oncological setting. The reasons are obvious. For one thing, cancer care is always laden with emotions. Although in many cases the prognosis is better than it used to be, the diagnosis of cancer still tends to disrupt patients' lives in an extremely painful and powerful way, meaning that patients need emotional support in addition to the best of bio-medical care. Moreover, patients are often confronted with difficult choices that put high demands on informed consent procedures and information-giving. The recent emphasis in communication research on patient-centered care and the relevance of shared decision making also has firm roots in cancer care. Oncologists and oncology nurses, who see so much suffering among their patients, have always shown an interest in communication as an essential part of high-quality care. Probably because of its uncontested relevance in cancer care, communication researchers have always been attracted to this field, and they have provided the field with good empirical descriptions of prevalent and/or adequate communication behaviors. In general, there is much agreement—among teachers as well as researchers—on the basics of good communication in cancer care. Open-ended questions (Maguire, Booth, Elliot, & Jones, 1996), empathy (Razavi et al., 2002), truth-telling (Fallowfield, Jenkins, & Beveridge, 2002), and room for emotional disclosure and psychosocial counselling (Maguire, 1999; Rutter, Iconomou, & Quine, 1996), all are unchallenged elements of good communication. Additionally, much effort has been put into finding empirical evidence for good communication in specific situations, such as bad-news delivery (Fallowfield, Lipkin, & Hall, 1998; Ford, Fallowfield, & Lewis, 1995), palliative care (Detmar et al., 2001), and genetic counselling (Sarangi, 2002). Communication research seems to be firmly rooted within the domain of cancer care.

However, notwithstanding the steady flow of publications, we believe that we should be modest about the real progress that has been made in the development of real evidence-based knowledge about the essentials of high-quality communication in oncology. Much of what is published seems to be a bit more of the same. The problem is this may help "believers" to feel warmly united and committed to a common pursuable aim, but it certainly does not convince "nonbelievers" or more cynical people of the central place communication should have in clinical practice, as well as in medical education and research programs. The community of communication researchers should feel challenged to look for new roads to win the central position in the health care arena that they so often claim.

FUTURE CHALLENGES

A running thread in this chapter is the call for attention to the context of communication. We are convinced that communication has to be studied in its context, the context of aims and targets, the context of persons and organizations, the context of place and time. By doing so we hope to bridge the gap between evidence-based medicine and patient-centered medicine

(Bensing, 2000). Only in this way research can help us find empirical evidence for the mechanisms that foster or hinder patients' well-being, apart from the direct effects of the medical intervention itself. These mechanisms are known to be part of the much-discussed but little-researched placebo- and nocebo-effects in health care (van Dulmen & Bensing, 2001).

There is, however, yet another challenge to meet, the challenge of theory-driven research. Much communication research is still descriptive in nature, more dictated by available methodology than by rigorous application of dedicated theories. Descriptive research is useful in the earlier stages of knowledge-production, when the domain-under-study still has to be charted. Real breakthroughs in knowledge are, however, only possible by systematic testing of theory-guided hypotheses on the presumed mechanisms behind the (positive and negative) effects of communication with cancer patients. We believe that in cancer care the phase of exploratory and descriptive research should and could be over.

Taken together, these two challenges can help to define a research agenda for the next decade. Within the field of communication in context, three four lines of investigation should be distinguished:

1. The context of *goals* or *targets* that are aimed at by both parties in the medical encounter (patient and physician or nurse), referring to the use of communication as a tool.
2. The context of *time* in relation to continuity of care, which necessitates the investigation of not only one single visit but consideration of the role and influence of previous and future consultations, as well as the patient's medical history.
3. The broader *organizational* context in which the dialogue takes place, colored by policies regarding teamwork, time constraints, and implicit and explicit priorities within the medical staff.
4. The context determined by what both *multifaceted parties*—on the one hand, the patient and accompanying spouse or child, and on the other, the physician and/or the nurse—bring to the health care visit: needs, expectations, knowledge and attitudes, and experience and skills, respectively.

Each of these points is elaborated and put in the proper theoretical perspective.

From General to Specific

There is now ample evidence that communication should be considered as perhaps the most powerful tool in medicine, not only in establishing a workable relationship with the patient, but also in both the diagnostic and therapeutic process (Bensing, 1991; Crow et al., 1999; Lipkin, Putnam, & Lazare, 1995; Roter & Hall, 1992; White, 1988). It also works the other way around: Good technical quality care, provided in an unsatisfactory environment and with unsatisfactory interactions, will not produce healthier patients (Koehler, Fottler, & Swan, 1992), and negative expectancies increase the frequency with which patients report all kind of symptoms (Crow et al., 1999). Consciously or unconsciously, communication plays a crucial role in medicine. Sometimes this role is positive and leads to better understanding and coping, to better therapeutic decisions, and more compliance; sometimes, however, the role of communication is negative and leads to misunderstanding, dissatisfaction, wrong decisions, and sometimes even malpractice suits (Levinson, Roter, Mullooly, Dull, & Frankel, 1997; Roter & Hall, 1992). The success or lack of success can often be ascribed to communication processes.

It is important that doctors, nurses, and other health care professionals be aware of the effects of their communication behavior and learn to use it as the powerful tool it can be. At least as important is that communication researchers explore, unravel, and test specific communication behaviors in relation to set medical and nursing goals to provide health care professionals with empirical evidence for the singular items of their tool-box in relation to the problems at hand. Communication is a powerful tool, but only when it is used as a tool, or rather, a set of tools, as consciously planned and targeted interventions.

Aside from its well-known and widely trained generic characteristics (creating a good interpersonal relationship, exchange of information), concrete communication strategies and behaviors can be used to reach specified goals within medical and nursing care. As was shown by many researchers, there is a multitude of different specific goals and subgoals within health care (Lazare, Putnam, & Lipkin, 1995; Lipkin et al., 1995; Ong, de Haes, Hoos, & Lammes, 1995; Roter & Hall, 1992). Depending on phase of treatment and/or patient needs, medical encounters may vary in what both participants aim at: getting or giving reassurance; finding and giving the right diagnostic label; establishing a common agenda; weighing diagnostic and/or risk information; valuing preferred therapeutic options and alternative solutions; making patient preferences more explicit; reaching a medical decision (shared or not); strengthening self-efficacy in maintaining difficult therapeutic regimens; acknowledging, fighting, or relieving anxiety and depression; and giving moral support, comfort, and strength in accepting the unacceptable. Even within one medical visit, different targets can be distinguished. It is essential that researchers be aware of these multiple goals in health care encounters and realize that different goals ask for varied communication strategies that are based on a variety of theoretical frameworks.

Let us give one example: how to create a good interpersonal relationship can best be predicted from psychotherapeutic theories with their heavy accent on affective communication behaviors: friendliness, social courtesies, empathy, showing respect and understanding, and "unconditional positive regard" (Rogers, 1961). However, these theories might be worthless and their accompanying behaviors sometimes even contraproductive when trying to tackle noncompliance, the best hidden taboo in medical encounters. Based on self-regulatory theories (Leventhal, Safer, & Panagis, 1983), it can be predicted that enhancing compliance asks for active problem-solving behaviors, combined with active stress reduction: motivating patients to take responsibility, helping to set realistic and taylor-made personal goals and to list possible barriers, showing understanding for incidental events of noncompliance, and showing partnership in creative problem solving. A good example of what this might mean for communication research is shown by Roter and Hall (1994).

Different problems ask for specific tools and, thus, for specific communication strategies and behaviors. This positions communication researchers for methodological as well as theoretical challenges. Methodological challenges are to be found in subdividing medical encounters in meaningful elements, and in innovative ways of analyzing communication data (sequential analysis, pattern analysis, critical incident analysis, cue responding, etc.). Theoretical challenges are to be found in applying theories that have been developed in clinical psychology, social psychology, and health psychology to the field of communication research and vice versa. As an additional advantage, this could help to explain under which conditions theoretically based behavioral intervention programs are more or less successful when implemented in everyday practice. For, as stated earlier, good technical quality care, provided in an unsatisfactory environment and with unsatisfactory interactions, will not produce healthier patients.

The issue is further complicated by the fact that there are often individual differences in the targets patients may have. Again an example using the recent paradigm on shared decision making might be illustrative. There is ample evidence that patients diagnosed with cancer want to be adequately informed of their diagnosis and prognosis, but that many (but not all) relinquish decisional control (Coulter, 1997; Fallowfield et al., 2002; Stiggelbout & Kiebert, 1997). Patients may feel burdened by the significance and consequences of making treatment decisions and prefer the physician to be accountable for the choices made. Therefore, advocating increased patient involvement for every patient in every situation may well endanger rather than safeguard patient autonomy (Gattellari, Voigt, Butow, & Tattersall, 2002).

Towards a Time Perspective

In most research literature, there is hardly any recognition of past or future. Continuity of care (with the same or other health care providers) is a central issue in health care—especially in complex care settings such as cancer care—but it is hardly an issue in communication research (van Dulmen, Verhaak, & Bilo, 1997). Most dialogues are studied as if previous consultations did not leave the patient with specific uncertainties, hopes, and expectancies, and as if everything has to take place during the consultation under study. From the patient's perspective, receiving bad news may reflect the process of being diseased by cancer, whereas research on breaking bad news primarily focuses on how to provide information in the course of a single diagnostic consultation (Salander, 2002). In addition, previous contacts set the agenda for future contacts and should be taken into consideration when examining the content, process, and effects of a single encounter.

Theories from research into the placebo effect of the provider-patient encounter (Crow et al., 1999; Di Blasi et al., 2001; van Dulmen & Bensing, 2002) could well complement the theoretical and methodological insights gathered so far in studies into communication in oncology. Investigating the role of conditioning and expectancies in ongoing oncological encounters could bring forward a new field of study not yet explored within the field of communication in oncology. The theory of classical conditioning can, for instance, be used to explain why one patient suffers from serious side-effects from chemotherapy and another one does not, or why patients with serious complaints respond positively to a treatment and others with the same complaints do not. Apparently, previous experiences with certain treatments, hospitals, or doctors influence the way patients respond to future experiences. In view of conditioning theory, a current treatment may be associated with an earlier experience that resulted in a reduction in negative symptoms. This earlier experience is said to be positively conditioned as far as recovery and anxiety reduction is concerned. This makes it extremely important to not only look at patients' medical history but also what actually happened in former visits and at the way physicians have attended to patients' experiences with health care. Eliciting patients' past experiences with the health care system, including these subjective experiences, can help the clinician to understand patients' reactions to treatment proposals, personal preferences, and unspoken resistances.

The role of expectancies, the other central placebo theory, has more to do with explaining why experiences in the present influence future treatment outcome (Crow et al., 1999). Response expectations appear to be triggered by the information a person receives (Thomas, 1987). Research shows that physicians—by their communication behavior—are able to influence patients' expectations in a positive as well as a negative direction.

From the neurocognitive sciences it is known that the brain can be blocked from acquiring new information when persons are under stress (Bremner, 1999; Newcomer et al., 1999). This means that in stressful situations information-giving must be carefully dosed, repeated, and spread over more visits. It can be experimentally tested what delay is necessary to allow for new information to be given to the patient. The role of stress-reducing communication techniques in this process is another topic of research. It is worthwhile to look for opportunities to combine this line of research with neuro-imaging techniques, such as PET or MRI scans.

Between Knowing and Doing

Cancer care goes hand in hand with strong emotions and much uncertainty. Doctors and nurses may feel barriers in emotion-laden communication because it produces stress. From stress-coping theories it can be hypothesized that experienced stress in doctors and nurses will lead to blocking behaviors as a coping strategy while facilitating communicative behaviors are needed from the patients' point of view (de Valck, Bruynooghe, Hulsman, Kerssens, & Bensing, 2001; Kruijver, Kerkstra, Bensing, & van de Wiel, 2000). This could explain the discrepancy between doctors attitudes, which tend to be rather patient-centered in general, and patients' assessments of the quality of care, which stresses problems in information-giving and personal care (de Valck, 2002).

Doctors and nurses may not only feel stressed as a result of not being able to relieve the burden of the disease from their patients' shoulders, but also as a result of organizational demands. Time constraints and schedules, treatment protocols, and institutional norms and values may all distract attention from a patient's needs for individualized care. Time constraints, for instance, force many physicians to interrupt their patients' flow of speech at the beginning of the consultation (Marvel, Epstein, Flowers, & Beckman, 1999). Providers, convinced that they know patients' reasons for the encounters, may incorrectly focus on an issue that is not the patient's main concern. This may engender the risk of making incorrect diagnoses and giving inappropriate advice on the part of the physician, and dissatisfaction, noncompliance, and second opinion-seeking on the part of the patient. A recent study showed that cancer patients indeed often seek a second opinion because they are dissatisfied with the way they have been treated by the first physician (Mellink et al., 2003). Although the issue of time has frequently been attended to in communication research, it has, so far, mostly been examined in a retrospective way, that is, by examining the communication process in relation to consultation length (DeVeugele, Derese, van den Brink-Muinen, Bensing, & De Maeseneer, 2002). Less attention has been given to the influence of time pressure experienced by a health care provider at the beginning of the visit on the actual communication process.

In addition, treatment protocols and guidelines developed to improve and standardize the information exchange may also hinder a patient-centered process. Institutionalized norms and values, reflected in a supervisor's attitude toward good health care, is also likely to color the actual communication process. A supervisor may play a fairly prominent role in explaining why communication skills thoroughly acquired in training are not observed in real-life nursing care (Kruijver, 2001). The extent to which a supervisor supports the nurse's communication style appears to have a large impact on the actual communication process. Especially affective communication, highly needed in cancer care, suffers from such contextual constraints.

From the theory of cognitive dissonance it can be hypothesized that doctors and nurses who are highly dependent on organizational norms and values will tend to conform to them at the cost of care tailored to the patient, whereas doctors (and to a lesser degree nurses) who prioritize patient care above institutional demands probably show more patient-centered communication behavior.

Beyond the Dialogue

Traditionally, research on provider-patient communication has focused on the doctor-patient dyad. Yet, in daily medical practice, physicians often find themselves forced to communicate with an elaborate and complicated patient system. Many health care visits, especially those with a strong emotional component such as oncological visits, involve more than two participants—an elderly patient accompanied by a spouse or adult child, couples visiting a doctor, parents consulting a doctor for their child, or, in case of non-native speakers, interpreters supporting a patient.

Due to the myopic dyadic perspective there has been little empirical exploration on the role and influence of a third (or fourth) person's presence on the process, content, and outcome of the medical visit. The scarce research on multiparty medical interactions within the setting of pediatrics (Aronsson, 1991; van Dulmen, 1998; Wissow et al., 1998), geriatrics (Greene, Majerovitz, Adelman, & Rizzo, 1994), dietary counseling (Pyörälä, 2000), and the general practitioner's surgery (Tates, Meeuwesen, Elbers, & Bensing, 2002), showed that merely the presence of a third person changes the dynamics of the medical interaction, no matter how small the third person's conversational contribution to the actual visit. After all, in attending a health care provider, patients have their agenda (needs and expectations) as do the people accompanying the patient. In order to communicate effectively, the health care provider should not only consider the patients' viewpoints but those of their relatives as well.

In the emotionally laden context of communication with cancer patients, caregivers or relatives are likely to make themselves especially felt. Therefore, an appropriate avenue for future communication research in oncology would be to explore the implications regarding participant roles and responsibilities beyond the scope of the medical dialogue. In light of social support theory, the relative's presence should not be ignored but rather encouraged for its positive impact on the patient's quality of life (Kamarck, Peterman, & Raynor, 1998).

Fruitful theoretical frameworks may be derived from social psychology, in particular from social support theories (Cutrona, 1996) and theories on family coping (Coyne & Smith, 1994). Many of these theories lead to explicit assumptions about communication behaviors that are beneficial or detrimental for the patients' well-being.

But patients are only part of a larger system, even within the consultation room. Future research should also pay attention to the multifaceted character of the health care system. Patients diagnosed with cancer are confronted with a broad range of health care providers, such as oncologists, nurses, and radiologists. These providers are likely to differ in attitudes, experience, and skills. Inadequate communication, due to discordance in information or insufficient fine-tuning of information conveyed by the various providers, can lead to confusion for patients about the diagnosis, the prognosis, and future management plans. Indeed, studies in nononcological settings show that patients often feel overwhelmed by contradictory advice or an overload of information supply emanating from multidisciplinary sources (van Weert, van Dulmen, Bär, & Venus, 2002). Not only may this cause unnecessary stress for patients, but also for health care providers themselves. After all, effective communication has been shown to be important for the efficiency, morale, and work satisfaction of the individual providers (Jenkins, Fallowfield, & Poole, 2001). So far, however, few data are available on how the process of information exchange between provider and patient is influenced by factors such as task distribution and delegation and fine-tuning and checking of the information conveyed. Research into the expectations of team members of their own and each other's roles in providing information to women with breast cancer showed that even the members of these multidisciplinary teams were not completely acquainted with the informational roles and responsibilities of their colleagues (Jenkins et al., 2001). These findings may cause concern, as one of the tenets of multidisciplinary oncological care is the provision of comprehensive and consistent information. Further research is required to capture health care providers' views on what they consider to be their individual task and responsibility in the process of exchanging and tailoring the information supply.

Decontextualized dyadic analyses are bound to fail in fully exposing the dynamics of multiparty medical communication. By acknowledging the multiparty character of medical communication, future research will have to take into account the context of medical communication both on the patient's and on the provider's side. Fruitful areas of research might also be communication studies on small group interactions and organizational theory on interdisciplinary collaboration. New advances must be made in order to capture the impact of these contextual factors on the course and outcome of the medical "dialogue."

CONCLUSION

In this chapter we expand the focus of cancer communication research and incorporate the broader context in which a single health care visit takes place. Such a broader perspective is necessary to find out why health care professionals do not always act in conformity with the generally approved standards of high quality communication—although they are known to have mastered the skills in training, how the factor of time span can be used more effectively in the medical encounter, and what the reasons are why patients do not always disclose their concerns assessed prior to the health care visit. Eventually, a broader context view will bridge the existing gap between theory and practice.

REFERENCES

Aronsson, K. (1991). Facework and control in multiparty talk: A pediatric case study. In I. Markovà & K Foppa (Eds.), *Asymmetries in dialogue* (pp. 49-74). New York: Harvester.

Bensing, J.M. (1991). *Doctor-patient communication and the quality of care. An observational study into affective and instrumental behavior.* Utrecht: NIVEL.

Bensing, J.M. (2000). Bridging the gap. The separate worlds of evidence-based medicine and patient-centered medicine. *Patient Education and Counseling, 39,* 17-25.

Bremner, J.D. (1999). Does stress damage the brain? *Biological Psychiatry, 45,* 797-805

Coulter, A. (1997). Partnerships with patients: The pros and cons of shared clinical decision-making. *Journal of Health Service Research Policy, 2*(2), 112-121.

Coyne, J.C., & Smith, D.A. (1994). Couples coping with a myocardial infarction: Contextual perspective on patient self-efficacy. *Journal of Family Psychology, 8,* 43-54.

Crow, R., Gage, H., Hampson, S., Hart, J., Kimber, A., & Thomas, H. (1999). The role of expectancies in the placebo effect and their use in the delivery of health care: A systematic review. *Health Technology Assessment, 3,* 1-96.

Cutrona, C.E. (1996). Social support in couples. In *Marriage as a resource in times of stress.* Thousand Oaks, CA: Sage.

Detmar, S.B., Muller, M.J., Wever, L.D.V., Schornagel, J.H., & Aaronson, N.K. (2001). Patient-physician communication during outpatients palliative treatment visits. An observational study. *JAMA, 285,* 1351-1357.

deValck, C. (2002). *Responding to patient cues in a video simulated bad news consultation.* Leuven.

de Valck, C., Bruynooghe, R., Hulsman, R.L., Kerssens, J.J., & Bensing, J.M. (2001). Cue responding in a simulated bad news situation. *Journal of Health Psychology, 6*(5), 585-596.

DeVeugele, M., Derese, A., van den Brink-Muinen, A., Bensing, J., & De Maeseneer, J. (2002). Consultation length in general practice: Cross sectional study in six European countries. *BMJ, 325*(7362), 472.

Di Blasi, Z., Harkness, E., Ernst, E., Georgiou, A., & Kleijnen, J. (2001). Influence of context effects on health outcomes: A systematic review. *Lancet, 357,* 757-762.

Dulmen, A.M. van. (1998). Children's contribution to pediatric outpatient encounters. *Pediatrics, 102,* 563-568.

Dulmen, A.M. van, & Bensing, J.M. (2001). *The effect of context in healthcare; a programming study.* RGO, The Hague.

Dulmen, A.M. van, & Bensing, J.M. (2002). Health promoting effects of the physician-patient encounter. *Psychology, Health, and Medicine, 7,* 289-300.

Dulmen, A.M. van, Verhaak, P.F.M., & Bilo, H.J.G. (1997). Shifts in doctor-patient communication during a series of outpatient consultations in non-insulin-dependent diabetes mellitus. *Patient Education Counseling, 30,* 227-237.

Fallowfield, L.J., Jenkins, V.A., & Beveridge, H.A. (2002). Truth may hurt, but deceit hurts more: Communication in palliative care. *Palliative Medicine, 16,* 297-303.

Fallowfield, L., Lipkin, M., & Hall, A. (1998). Teaching senior oncologists communication skills: Results from phase 1 of a comprehensive longitudinal program in the United Kingdom. *Journal of Clinical Oncology, 16,* 1961-1968.

Ford, S., Fallowfield, L., & Lewis, S. (1995). Doctor-patient interactions in oncology. *Social Science and Medicine, 42,* 1511-1519.

Gattellari, M., Voigt, K.J., Butow, P.N., & Tattersall, M.H. (2002). When the treatment goal is not cure: Are cancer patients equipped to make informed decisions? *Journal of Clinical Oncology, 20,* 503-513.

Greene, M.G., Majerovitz, S.D., Adelman, R.D., & Rizzo. C. (1994). The effects of the presence of a third person on the physician-older patient medical interview. *Journal of the American Geriatric Society, 42,* 413-419.

Jenkins, V.A., Fallowfield, L.J., & Poole, K. (2001). Are members of multidisciplinary teams in breast cancer aware of each other's informational roles? *Quality in Healthcare, 10,* 70-75.

Kamarck, T.W., Peterman, A.H., & Raynor, D.A. (1998). The effects of the social environment on stress-related cardiovascular activation: Current findings, prospects, and implications. *Annals of Behavioral Medicine, 20,* 247-256.

Koehler, W.F., Fottler, M.D., & Swan, J.E. (1992). Physician-patient satisfaction: Equity in the health services encounter. *Medical Care Review, 49*(4), 455-484.

Kruijver, I.P.M. (2001). *Communication between nurses and admitted cancer patients: The evaluation of a communication training program* (thesis). Utrecht: Nivel.

Kruijver, I.P.M., Kerkstra, A., Bensing, J.M., & van de Wiel, H.B.M. (2000). Nurse-patient communication in cancer care. *Cancer Nursing, 23,* 20-31.

Lazare, A., Putnam, S.M., & Lipkin. M. (1995). Three functions of the medical interview. In M. Lipkin, S.M. Putnam, & A. Lazare (Eds.), *The medical interview. Clinical care, education and research.* New York, Berlin, Heidelberg: Springer Verlag.

Leventhal, H., Safer, M.A, & Panagis, D.M. (1983). The impact of communications on the self-regulation of health beliefs, decisions, and behavior. *Health Education Quarterly, 10*(1), 3-29.

Levinson, W., Roter, D.L., Mullooly, J.P., Dull, V., & Frankel, R.M. (1997). Physician-patient communication. The relationship with malpractice claims among primary care physicians and surgeons. *JAMA, 277,* 553-559.

Lipkin, M., Putnam, S.M., & Lazare, A. (1995). *The medical interview. Clinical care, education and research.* New York, Berlin, Heidelberg: Springer Verlag.

Maguire, P. (1999). Improving communication with cancer patients. *European Journal of Cancer, 35,* 1415-1422.

Maguire, P., Booth, K., Elliot, C., & Jones, B. (1996). Helping health professionals involved in cancer care acquire key interviewing skills—the impact of workshops. *European Journal of Cancer, 32A,* 1486-1489.

Marvel, M.K., Epstein, R.M., Flowers, K., & Beckman, H.B. (1999). Soliciting the patient's agenda: Have we improved? *JAMA, 281,* 283-287.

Mellink, W.A.M., Dulmen, A.M. van, Wiggers, T., Spreeuwenberg, P.M.M., Eggermont, A.M.M., & Bensing, J.M. (2003). Cancer patients seeking a second opinion: Results of a study on motives, needs and expectations. *Journal of Clinical Oncology, 21,* 1992-1997.

Newcomer, J.W., Selke, G., Melson, A.K., Hershey, T., Craft, S., Richards, K., & Alderson, A.L. (1999). Decreased memory performance in healthy humans induced by stress-level cortisol treatment. *Archives of General Psychiatry, 56,* 527-533.

Ong, L.M., de Haes, J.C., Hoos, A.M., & Lammes, F.B. (1995). Doctor-patient communication: A review of the literature. *Social Science and Medicine, 40*(7), 903-918.

Pyörälä, E. (2000). *Interaction in dietary counselling of diabetic children and adolescents* (thesis). Helsinki: Helsinki University Press.

Razavi, D., Delvaux, N., Marchal, S., Durieux, J.F., Farvacques, C., Dubus, L., & Hogenraad, R. (2002). Does training increase the use of more emotionally laden words by nurses when talking with cancer patients? A randomised study. *British Journal of Cancer, 87,* 1-7.

Rogers, C.R. (1961). The characteristics of a helping relationship. In C.R. Rogers (Ed.), *On becoming a person: A therapists' view of psychotherapy.* Boston: Houghton Mifflin.

Roter, D.L., & Hall, J.A. (1992). *Doctors talking with patients; patients talking with doctors. Improving communication in medical visits.* Westport, CT: Auburn House.

Roter, D.L., & Hall, J.A. (1994). Strategies for enhancing patient adherence to medical recommendations. Clinical guidelines. *JAMA, 271*(1), 80.

Rutter, D.R., Iconomou, G., & Quine, L. (1996). Doctor-patient communication and outcome in cancer patients: An intervention. *Psychology and Health, 12,* 57-71.

Salander, P. (2002). Bad news from the patient's perspective: An analysis of the written narratives of newly diagnosed cancer patients. *Social Science and Medicine, 55,* 721-732

Sarangi, S. (2002). The language of likelihood in genetic counseling discourse. *Journal of Language and Social Psychology, 21,* 7-31.

Stiggelbout, A.M., & Kiebert, G.M. (1997). A role for the sick role. Patient preferences regarding information and participation in clinical decision-making. *CMAJ, 157*(4), 383-389.

Tates, H., Meeuwesen, L., Elbers, E., & Bensing J. (2002). "I've come for his throat": Roles and identities in doctor-parent-child communication. *Child: Care, Health Development, 28*, 109-116.

Thomas, K.B. (1987). General practice consultations: Is there any point in being positive? *British Medical Journal, 294*, 1200-1202.

Weert, J.C.M. van, Dulmen, A.M. van, Bär, P., & Venus, E. (2003). Multidisciplinary preoperative patient education in cardiac surgery. *Patient Education Counseling, 49*, 105-114.

White, K. (1988). *The task of medicine.* Menlo Park, CA: The Henry J. Kaiser Family Foundation.

Wissow, L.S., Roter, D., Bauman, L.J., Crain, E., Kercsmar, C., Weiss, K., Mitchell, H., & Mohrs, B. (1998). Patient-provider communication during the emergency department care of children with asthma. *Medical Care, 36*, 1439-1450.

7 | Environmental Influences On Cancer Care and Communication

Gerald Ledlow
*Central Michigan University
and Sisters of Mercy Health System*

Scott D. Moore
California State University, Fresno

H. Dan O'Hair
University of Oklahoma

As many of the chapters in this volume suggest, cancer patients face a myriad of challenges beginning with symptoms and diagnosis, progressing through to treatment and maintenance of care, and eventually to some outcome of the disease state (i.e., cure, cancer-free, palliative, hospice, end-of-life). Some of the more daunting challenges that cancer patients face, beyond the disease itself, are those imposed by the environment, and the systems and organizations that become part of the cancer care delivery mechanism (for related chapters consult Richey & Brown and Villagran, Jones, & O'Hair, this volume). Others have made meaningful contributions by using other terms such as *institutional contexts* (Lammers, Duggan, & Barbour, 2003) and *ecological perspectives* (Street, 2003).

Environmental influences on cancer care emanate from a variety of sources. It would be impossible to review all of these in one chapter; instead we have chosen to discuss those most relevant to issues involving direct patient communication challenges. Employing the term *environment* carries with it a risk of portraying cancer care and communication too broadly. However, our goal is to demonstrate the extent to which forces—whether cognitive, symbolic, informational, structural, or processual—impact cancer patients' communicative abilities to secure a desired level of care. A common viewpoint on environments is that it is often characterized as "a source of resources or as a source of information" (Sutcliffe, 2001, p. 199). Environmental influences also involve social, professional, or institutional pressures that have some impact, either direct or indirect, on the quality or duration of the delivery of cancer care. In the following sections, we briefly describe some of the more prominent environmental influences: (a) the disease context which include types of cancer, pain management, and standards of cancer care, (b) sociocultural with a focus on cultural competence of cancer care delivery systems and poverty's sociolinguistic influence, (c) institutional/regulatory with related discussions on HIPPA, and FMLA, (d) paying for care with directed attention on insurance and managed care, and (e) cancer care delivery systems including provider privileging, cancer care teams, and clinical trials programs.

DISEASE CONTEXT

Cancer patients confront a number of phenomena that loom prominently on the care delivery landscape. Some of these issues involve the disease and resultant treatment whereas others present themselves as outcomes from the predispositions, trends, perceptions, and biases that develop as part of the cancer care delivery system. Three phenomena are discussed in this section: (a) the type of cancer inflicting the patient; (b) issues involving pain management; and (c) national standards of care for cancer.

Type of Cancer

It is commonly known that cancers differ in terms of their familiarity, prevalence, prognosis, treatment protocols, and even their reputation. Breast, lung, and prostate cancer are well known, although they do vary in terms of their prognosis for recovery or even cure. On the other hand, pancreatic, sarcoma, brain, and lymphatic cancers are considered to be terminal and create a *fatalism bias* among many groups, even practitioners. Among cancer advocacy groups we learn that some cancers are more attractive for government funding and philanthropic fund raising efforts (see Kim, this volume). The best-known effort for cancer fund raising involves breast cancer, helped enormously by campaigns based on famous people battling a particular cancer (e.g., Betty Ford). Pancreatic cancer, less known but much more fatal, commands less attention, raises less money, and attracts less publicity (Kim, this volume).

How does cancer type affect a patient's ability to communicate within the care delivery system? First, diseases receiving greater funding will attract more focused research efforts, resulting in a richer base of information from which to advise patients. Patients will experience a wider set of options for treatment. Second, cancers with more associated information and notoriety will produce a larger base of information for patients to access as they investigate the disease on their own. Information richness brings with it both benefits and costs. Cancer patients benefit from an information base that is more diverse, mature, and seasoned from iterative claims, challenges, and ideas. Alternatively, the cost to such an information system is the sheer magnitude of the information base creating acquisition and assimilation challenges, and the number of competing ideas found in the information (see Kerr, this volume). Second, patients communicating with providers face predispositions and mindsets that result from the community of practice associated with a particular disease. For instance, with prostate cancer, "watchful waiting" has become a treatment option of choice for some providers influencing a patient's decision. Pancreatic cancer, on the other hand, is such a rapidly developing cancer that the prevailing paradigm of treatment is surgery (Whipple procedure) so long as the disease has not metastasized to an advanced stage. Third, providers view end-of-life choices differently depending on the type of cancer. With rapidly advancing cancers such as lymphoma or pancreatic cancers, many providers' proclivity is to recommend immediate hospice care, rather than suggest curative procedures. In other systems of health care delivery, particularly research centers, a tendency toward experimental options such as clinical trials may be recommended (Teeley & Bashe, 1997).

Pain Management

One of the unfortunate consequences of most cancers is the onset of pain. Over one million cancer patients in the United States experience cancer-related pain affecting both physical activity and psychosocial well being (Murphy, Morris, & Lange, 1997). The management of pain has become a controversial issue among providers, patients, health systems, and even insurance carriers (Furrow, 2001). Studies examining pain and its management among cancer patients report that upwards of 50%-70% of patients or nursing home residents are undertreated for symptoms of pain (Bernabel, Gatsonis, & Mor, 1998; Bonica, 1994). At the heart of the controversy are issues involving myths of opiate addiction, health system bias, and policy against pain management, and provider concern over legal recriminations (Furrow, 2001).

Opiates are still considered to be one of the most effective treatments for cancer pain, yet many physicians hold aversive attitudes toward opiate maintenance plans (Furrow, 2001; Hill, 1995). Although a number of factors can potentially precipitate physicians' attitudes toward pain management, and opiates in particular, two central concerns are reported most frequently: threats of legal action and ignorance of effective pain management techniques (Joranson & Gilson, 1998; Lebovits et al., 1997). Providers report that continued prescription of opiates may subject them to controlled substance abuse laws. In addition, pain management is a condition that many providers are untrained to perform adequately.

Two other system-oriented contingencies exist in the quest for pain management. One issue involves insurance coverage and reimbursement for certain types of pain management treatment. Both managed care plans and government plans (Medicare/Medicaid) impose restrictions on pain management plans, especially those involving certain drugs and protocols (Hoffman, 1998; Jost, 1998). The challenge is inducing hospitals to take a more patient-centered approach to pain management. Many hospitals have yet to embark on an organized institutional approach for pain management plans (Blau, Dalton, & Lindley, 1999).

What communication options can cancer patients exercise to encourage the cancer care delivery system to manage their pain? First, patients must be very direct and honest in their communication to their providers about pain levels and intensity (Murphy et al., 1997). The management of pain is a patient right and must be clearly articulated to the appropriate health care providers. Second, patients should communicate with their insurance providers about desired pain management plans and subsequent coverage. If adequate coverage is not forthcoming, patients should initiate appeal and grievance proceedings. Third, cancer patients should become knowledgeable about pain management options and remedies, especially as they pertain to specific sites of pain and related disease-precipitated pain symptoms. A number of online and print resources are available that prescribe alternative means of pain relief without provider input or prescription. Lastly, patients should discuss thoroughly with their providers the philosophical and practical approaches of potential hospital or in-patient care facilities regarding pain management. Patients should insist on a facility that matches their own goals for pain management.

Standards of Cancer Care

Standards of care for cancer treatment are focused on ensuring quality of care for cancer patients. The American Academy of Family Physicians (2001) endorses the Institute of Medicine Report on Ensuring Quality Cancer Care by recommending the following elements of quality care for each cancer patient:

- Experienced medical professionals make initial cancer management recommendations;
- Both the patient and provider agree upon a care plan with an outline of goals;
- Access to all resources necessary to implement the care plan;
- Access to high quality clinical trials;
- Policies requiring full disclosure of information about available treatment options;
- Systems to coordinate services; and
- Psychosocial support and compassionate care services. (p. 1)

The standard of care for cancer care is an evolutionary progression (Jacobs, 1994; McNeil, 1999) toward higher levels of treatment efficacy. Decision frameworks and guidelines associated with the standard of care are disseminated by federal agencies such as the National Cancer Institute (2001), professional societies (American Society of Clinical Oncology, 2002), clinical academic institutions (usually through scholarly journals and symposia [Aligned Management Associates, Inc., 2002]), and various other groups (Cancer Care Inc., 2001); the preponderance of information on a given standard of care for a specific cancer diagnosis tilts the regimen of treatment in a reasonably specific direction. The standard of care is driven by several factors:

1. The traditional practice of healthcare (McGuire, 2000);
2. Cancer care research (McGuire, 2000; Minsky et al., 1998);
3. Clinical trials and outcomes (Lehman & Thomas, 2001; McNeil, 1999; Rose, 2000; Siminoff, Fetting, & Abeloff, 1989);
4. Scholarly dissemination of positive and negative influences of cancer care (Carney, Eliassen, Wells, & Schwartz, 1998; Kirschbaum, 1996);
5. Government regulation and reimbursement policy (Beck, 1999);
6. Commercial reimbursement practice;
7. Quality of life and work years (Berthelot, Will, Evans, & Coyle 2000),
8. Legal liability pressures; and most importantly,
9. Patient expectations and satisfaction (Dougall, Russell, Rubin, & Ling, 2000).

The treatment of cancer as defined by the standard of care has evolved and improved dramatically since the modern era of healthcare as marked by the Flexner Report in the early 1900s. The specific diagnosis, acuity of cancer, region of the body impacted, and medical history of the patient determine what standard of care is expected and, thus, determine the alternatives and methods of treatment available to care for the patient within the jointly determined goals of care (Lunt & Jenkins, 1983) of the provider and patient. It is important to note that the standard of care is constantly stretched, usually by small increments due to new drug treatment regimens and procedures, in search of higher levels of treatment efficacy. An example of this would be federally approved clinical trials for a specific cancer diagnosis and the changes in care as a result of the trials. Standards of care are routinely published on the World Wide Web, such as the pain management standard of care for the Memorial Sloan-Kettering Cancer Center (2002).

SOCIOCULTURAL ISSUES

To decipher the communication environment associated with cancer care, the sociocultural context must be understood. The sociocultural context of the health services delivery system, health insurance, and the expectations of patients come together to form a complex fabric of standards, expectations, and outcomes encircling the cancer patient, the patient's family, and the healthcare system. Germane to these issues are the competencies associated with the social-cultural context of cancer and cancer care.

Cultural Competence of the Cancer Care Delivery System

Providers are bound within the constraints of the health delivery system. Systems enact policies and procedures that either reduce or exacerbate practice disparities in the delivery of cancer care. Health systems provide varying levels of culturally diverse staffing, interpreting services, or translation of print material, which range from appointment reminders, to provider instructions, to financing materials. Carillo, Green, and Betancourt (1999), and more recently Smedley, Stith, and Nelson (2002), suggest this "cultural competence" is the capability of a system to provide care to patients with diverse values, beliefs, and behaviors, including tailoring delivery to meet patient's social, cultural, and linguistic needs. The degree to which the system affords the provider to meet the psychographic, linguistic, and cultural needs of the patients, is the degree to which the system may be considered culturally competent.

Research on cultural disparities in the delivery of care is abundant, without regard to disease area or clinical service, even when clinical factors such as co-morbidity, age, and severity of disease is controlled for (for an in-depth review of specific disparities in the delivery of health care, we recommend Smedley, Stith, & Nelson, 2002; also Rameriz, this volume). It is also widely accepted that the disparity in delivery is strongly associated with higher morbidity and mortality rates of minority patients (Brach & Fraser, 2000). Cross, Bazron, Dennis, and Isaacs (1989) state that cultural competence is the propensity of the system, agency, or group of professionals to offer polices that match congruent behaviors and attitudes of the patients with diverse cultural backgrounds with those of the providers within the system.

Generally, in the United States, these attitudes toward cancer treatment needs are information, needs related to treatment side effects, and psychological support; however these needs are bound within a cultural population (Ali, Khalil, & Yousef, 1993). As the demographic landscape of the United States changes, identifying culturally specific attitudes toward care becomes more allusive. Of particular concern to some is the obstacle of providing necessary and legally mandated services and information, including interpreters and access to translated documentation. More recently, research supported by the Robert Wood Johnson foundation noted the significance of the linguistic barriers to non-English demographic groups. It is estimated that 20% of the Spanish-speaking population does not seek medical treatment, as a direct result of language barriers; and more than 80% of the population find it difficult to fully engage in the medical interaction with English-speaking providers (Hablamos Juntos, 2001). By the year 2030, the U.S. Census Bureau projects an astonishing increase of 358% growth in the Spanish-speaking population, likely exacerbating sociolinguistic barriers to the delivery of care. A concept frequently linked to restricted linguistic access is poverty, which is now be addressed in more detail.

Poverty's Sociolinguistic Influence

Researchers in a variety of disciplines have noted communicative disparities within the medical context between sick affluent and sick poor patients. It should be noted that the research on this subject approaches communication variables from varying operationalizations. Largely due to sociolinguistic barriers, sick poor patients are often observed as diffident participants in the provider-patient interaction (Aday, 2002; Boreham & Gibson, 1978; Waitzken, 1985). They ask fewer direct questions of providers and rely on more information volunteered by providers than more affluent patients (Cartwright, 1964). As a result, poorer patients often receive less direct information about illness and less explicit information about treatment and disease mediation. This is especially disconcerting because it is known that doctors tend to underestimate the patient's desire for information and frequently use power laden communication as a means of controlling the interaction. For example, Waitzken (1984) noted that many physicians use frequent doctor-initiated questions, interruptions, and nonverbal neglect, regardless of the patient's sociodemographic background. Bernstein (1964) suggested this disparity is due to a diffident predisposition of a patient with poor linguistic understanding of the medical terminology and medical jargon. Poorer patients typically desire as much information as more affluent patients; however, they are less likely to directly question the provider, and they rely more on nonverbal communication as a primary means of information exchange. Interestingly, although many of these disparities can be minimized by using educational coaches to train patients on proactive participation in the dyadic interaction (cf. Roter, 1977), few such coaching programs exist (Aday, 2002). Understanding the role that cultural competence of the health delivery system, and the sociolinguistic role poverty plays in the delivery of care, may ultimately aid in reducing health disparities and address future demographic changes of patients. We now turn our attention to address some systemic influences from the provider perspective.

INSTITUTIONAL/REGULATORY

In general, the healthcare delivery system is one that is highly regulated through policies, rules, and laws whose intention is to structure guidelines, criteria, and behavior for how care is administered, funded, and evaluated (Conrad & McIntush, 2003; Saunders, 2001). Adequate exposure of regulatory issues involving healthcare would consume volumes rather than pages, therefore our brief effort in this section is to identify a few salient issues involving cancer care and communication. The complexity of the institutional and regulatory environment is precipitated by the vast number of parties involved in cancer care delivery. Federal, state, local, organizational, and even professional interests are continuously being served in a quest to ensure both appropriate and affordable care. Consider the following statement from those who follow these trends:

> . . . health care continues to be subject to extensive yet ever changing regulations at both the federal and state levels. As the industry responds to these changing regulatory forces and the industry's efforts to control health care costs, the traditional roles played by providers and payers are being reconsidered and often restructured into new configurations. The restructuring of any industry as large and complex as health care sometimes brings to light conflicting laws as well as public policies that underpin the laws and regulations governing this sector of the U.S. economy. (Shaffer & Pavarini, 1997, p. 87)

We devote another section to the financing of cancer care and simply acknowledge here that paying for cancer care is an extraordinarily dynamic phenomenon that frustrates cancer patients and providers alike. Institutions such as Medicare and Medicaid, the Veterans Administration, and the managed care industry all exert complex policy and regulatory burdens for all concerned. Our interest in this section is a brief exploration of the nature and status of institutional and regulatory forces that find their way to the care delivery level.

Health Insurance Portability and Accountability Act

One of the most recent and far-reaching regulations for providers and patients is the Health Insurance Portability and Accountability Act of 1996 (HIPAA). HIPAA is intended to regulate privacy protections for patients by restricting the ways that providers, hospitals, health plans, pharmacies, and other care delivery organizations can use patients' medical information. The regulations protect medical records and other health information, regardless of the form in which the information is stored or communicated (orally, computer, paper, etc.) (HHS Press Office, 2003).

Although HIPAA is a complex law, it is one that has yet to reach a level of maturity where its full implications are known. However, the law specifies at least three communication issues that are salient for cancer patients, their providers, and care delivery organizations (HHS Press Office, 2003).

Access to medical records.   Patients will be able to inspect and copy their medical records on request, and if they find mistakes they will be able to request corrections. Those organizations holding the patient's records will have 30 days to fulfill the patient's request. This becomes an important issue for cancer patients in the sense that they can determine and track the various prognosis and treatment entries made in their records. With an ever-increasing set of provider and medical options available to cancer patients, and with greater access to medical information via the Internet, patients will be in a more informed position to assimilate and analyze all aspects of their situation, including their medical history.

Limits on use of personal medical information. HIPAA sets limits on how health plans and providers may use a patient's health information. The regulation does not restrict providers from sharing information in the conduct of cancer care. However, in other situations not related to cancer care, patient health information cannot be used, and providers and organizations may use or share only the minimum amount of information needed for a specific purpose. To ensure privacy, patients would have to sign a document releasing providers and organizations from restrictions that prevent information from being divulged to collateral organizations such as insurance companies, financial institutions, research organizations, or another organization for purposes not related to cancer care.

Confidential communications. HIPAA also stipulates that patients can request providers, cancer care organizations, and even health plans to put in place safeguards to ensure that communication with the cancer patient is confidential. If a patient does not want to communicate with a provider via email, a request can be made and honored ensuring that telephone or face-to-face contact be employed. Patients will be able to tailor their communication with providers and organizations according to their preferences.

Family Medical Leave Act

A second policy/law with substantial impact on cancer care delivery is the Family Medical Leave Act of 1993 (FMLA). FMLA requires employers to allow employees with a serious health condition to take up to 12 weeks of unpaid leave without prejudice during a 12-month period. In addition, the law stipulates that employees can use the same unpaid leave to care for an immediate family member (spouse, child, or parent) with a serious health condition. The courts have tested many aspects of FMLA in the past with varying opinions rendered (see, e.g., Sayeed, 2002). With some types of cancer that are treatment and diagnostic intensive, FMLA becomes an important tool for diverting time away from work. FMLA is a confounding issue as well. Because the ability to use the FMLA is available, there is pressure on the money earners in a family to take the time off as needed, but the tension to take time off is exacerbated with the reality and necessity of earning a wage or salary. Most families dealing with cancer have additional burdens that create the increased need for monetary support, so the FMLA on one hand allows for time off, while on the other hand reduces the family's ability to maintain or increase funds necessary to support the family during the cancer ordeal.

PAYING FOR CANCER CARE

Traditionally, there are very few methods to pay for cancer care. Access to care is associated with ability to pay for care. Access to care and the ability to pay for care are overwhelmingly associated with health insurance coverage, commercial or governmental (primarily

Medicare and Medicaid). In 2001, an estimated 14.6% of the American population, or 41.2 million people, were uninsured; in comparison, approximately 240.9 million Americans had health insurance coverage in that same year (Mills, 2002; United States Department of Commerce, 2002). Uncompensated care, that is, when health care is provided but is not reimbursed (usually from those that do not have insurance), does not routinely associate with cancer care reimbursement. The Emergency Medical Treatment and Labor Act (EMTALA), an unfunded mandate passed into law in April 1986, requires emergency departments of participating Medicare hospitals to screen and treat anyone with an emergency medical condition (Carpenter, 2001). EMTALA does not normally fit the criteria associated with cancer care. In essence, access to care highly correlates with the ability to pay for care; cancer care patients have access to care when they are either wealthy enough to afford out-of-pocket costs or have health insurance. To control costs, insurance companies, with pressure from employers and government agencies, have instituted managed care systems within the health insurance structure. Considering the vast differences in insurance vehicles, types of insurance, controls, managed care influences, the provider interpretation of reimbursement for care services, and patient expectations, considerable ambiguity and uncertainty exist surrounding cancer care from both the provider and patient sides of the equation.

Insurance and Managed Care

Insurance essentially equates to access to cancer care. However, considerable communication noise, increased ambiguity, and uncertainty exist within the payment structures of cancer care. Considering that each insurance vehicle has a standard benefits plan, that is, the list of covered services, treatments, and so on, and a set of rules that the insured, as well as the provider, must follow to ensure that care is covered (meaning that the care is reimbursable), it is understandable that for most people, insurance issues are complicated. The vast majority of people do not have a clear understanding of their own health insurance, what is covered, nor do they understand the rules that are required to execute elements of their insurance policy (American Association of Health Plans, 1998). The standard benefits plans and sets of rules vary from plan to plan, many times varying greatly within the same insurance company. Providers normally deal with dozens of different insurance vehicles of their patients in which covered items (those items listed in the standard benefits plan for each patient) vary and where the rules for reimbursement differ. These rules have become stricter over the past 20 years within the managed care structures imposed by insurance companies. Most patients do not understand the insurance package they have nor the items or services that are covered under each plan. Especially in the realm of cancer treatment, managed care (with the requirements of pre-authorization for care to ensure reimbursement for the provider) limits treatment protocols to only acceptable, evidenced-based, and standard-of-care oriented treatments.

Patients and many providers feel helpless when dealing with the complexity and bureaucracy of insurance companies and the managed care structures that those companies require. The issues related to insurance and managed care are vast, yet the fact remains that unless the patient and provider giving cancer care understand the patient's insurance vehicle, covered services, rules, and how the rules must be applied, then increased ambiguity and uncertainty create additional tension and noise during the cancer care process.

CANCER CARE DELIVERY SYSTEMS

Provider Privileging

Provider privileges determine what diagnostic tools, diagnoses, and treatments are within the scope of practice of a provider. Privileging of individual providers of care is a medical staff self-governance process that is influenced by the standard of care, as well as:

1. education, training and experience of the provider (Cohen et al., 1996; Fenton, 1988);
2. board certification of the provider;
3. staff and facility resources available to support specific privileges (Haylock, 1993);
4. demand for those specific services derived from those privileges;
5. the provider's performance (patient outcomes and efficacy) and competence with respect to those privileges (Carr, 1996; Fenton, 1988); and
6. government regulations and policy (Lumb & Oskvig, 1998; Ross, 1999).

Both of these dynamic issues, the standard of care and individual provider privileges, create a provider and facility-specific list of diagnostic tools, diagnoses, and treatments available to care for cancer patients. The responsible physician is accountable to the medical staff of the facility to be consistent with his or her scope of practice as delineated in their privileges and deliver care within the boundaries established by the standard of care. Privileging deals with mostly technical aspects of care but should also weigh the provider's ability to deliver a caring persona (bedside manner) to patients (Burton & Parker, 1997) in the overall scope of practice decision. Formal training in communication skills is usually not considered in the privileging process; this is a systemic issue because most physicians are not formally trained in communication strategies and skills (Baile et al., 1997). Provider privileging is a case-by-case process at the microlevel and a dynamic system at the macrolevel; updates on privileging trends and issues can be found at www.credentialinfo.com/new/news-arc.cfm.

Together, the standard of care coupled with individual provider privileges determines the specific and unique situation at each institution for each provider of care. The complexity increases for each patient diagnosed with cancer because each person presents to the healthcare system with specific and sometimes unique issues as well. To reduce the potential of low efficacy, at most institutions, a provider team model is embraced and encouraged. Even in organizations where the team approach for cancer care is not highly prized, a team, informal as it may be, is used to focus effort for the benefit of the patient.

Cancer Care Teams

"At the outset, the concept of team care was suggested not as a panacea but perhaps as a better approach to acquiring help in areas of expertise not held by the physician" (Brady, 1987, p. 797). There is a difference between parallel patient care activities (Dumpe & Ulreich, 2001) and team care activities; the focus here is on team care. The team of care orients around the patient and delivers multidimensional care to increase efficacy and well-being for the patient. The most important team members are the patient and their family. The care delivery team is interdisciplinary (Larsen, Neverett, & Larsen, 2001), consisting of the nursing staff, physician(s), ancillary staff of the facility, others such as social workers, counselors, and spiritual advisors such as pastors or priests. In most cancer care institutions, the nursing staff has the most contact with cancer patients; "Nurses play a key role in creating a positive experience for patients and families in a variety of cancer care services" (Haylock, 1993, p. 73). Nurses tend to be the team collaborating agents and biggest patient advocates (Larsen et al., 2001). The key issue is determining the formality of team orientation at the provider organization. The care team is not static but rather dynamic as patient needs present; for example, the pain service team can be used as adjunct to the primary care team (Coyle, 1995). In most cancer care institutions, teamwork is fostered and advocated in the delivery of care: team members are free to contribute to the discussion of delivery of care options and are encouraged to seek assistance (and at times permission) to alter the care plan based on patient specific deviations from expected outcomes.

Teams of care should enhance communication (Brady, 1987). Communication is influenced positively when the patient and the patient's family are assimilated in the care team as the most important players and presented with information, the sequence of treatment, alternatives, and expectations. The medical team must explain the list of services and support available to the patient and to the patient's family to enhance communication. The medical care team must have a clear understanding of each of their roles and responsibilities in the care process (given that the responsible physician is ultimately accountable for patient care) to extend clear communication and understanding to the patient (Scholes & Vaughan, 2002). Clear communication of diagnosis, alternatives, and expectations from the care team to the patient and their family is critical. Although clear communication is the goal, many patients continue to face ambiguity and uncertainty surrounding their situation because the provider and care team have not focused on patient understanding of their specific situation (Chan, 1997). Clear understanding is necessary for the patient and his or her family to be contributing members of the care team in which the focus is on quality patient outcomes.

The patient and family must be involved in team care decision making (Schain, 1980), and this is especially true for parents of pediatric cancer patients (Overbay, 1996). It is imperative that medical team members understand the process of cancer care and as a group attend training, such as understanding the psychosocial oncology issues of the patient (James, Jones, Rodin, & Catton, 2001), and jointly prepare, such as in preparing patients for cytotoxic chemotherapy (Ellis et al., 1993), to communicate well with the patient and their families. Ultimately teams of care must possess collective competencies in communication, collaboration, coaching, facilitation, leadership (to include knowing when to let others lead), as change agents (Dumpe & Ulreich, 2001), assertiveness, conflict management, delegation, and motivation (Walczak & Absolon, 2001). Care teams must also have the tools and resources to function effectively. Documentation and coordination are key to successful team care; automated documentation systems enable teams to develop and implement dynamic interdisciplinary care plans (Smith & Smith, 2002).

Gearing the patient and the family to become members of the care team is a critical component of care considering the physical, psychosocial, emotional, and spiritual dimensions of care. This issue moves beyond simple patient consent and basic information dissemination to the patient, although these are required, to targeting patients understanding in their situation and their responsibilities of the care process (Oliver, Turrell, Olszewski, & Willson, 1995).

Medical care team research and evaluation has mostly concentrated on improved communication and collaboration, whereas evaluation and teamwork improvement in other areas such as cross-learning and team learning have received less focus; the question to resolve is will improving team learning improve communication within the total care team (including the patient and his or her family) (Scholes & Vaughan, 2002). As the medical care team leader, the physician responsible for cancer patient care usually has received little formal training in difficult communication situations pertaining to cancer care of the patient and family. Interactive workshops addressing communication strategies for the physician (and the entire care team) have shown promise but require additional evaluation at this time (Baile et al., 1997).

Teams of care link directly back to the standard of care and privileging of providers; team members are privileged or credentialed to provide a specific set of care services within the treatment boundaries set by the responsible physician as that physician delivers care within the confines of the standard of care. Credentialing and privileging are essential for building quality provider care teams (Lumb & Oskvig, 1998). Privileging and credentialing of team members creates specific tasks for the delivery of care, reducing ambiguity and uncertainty in communication and in the delivery of care.

Clinical Trials System

It is estimated that fewer than 25% of eligible patients ever participate in clinical trials (Cheson, 1991; Sadler, 2001; Taylor et al., 1994). Historically, clinical trials have been criticized for the homogeneity of their subject pools (Eckenwiler, 1999), economic cost (Dreher, 1998), and, occasionally, institutional conflict of interest (Barnes & Florencio, 2002). Partly in response to the criticism, and to encourage more participation in clinical trials, the National Cancer Institute (NCI) developed its Cancer Clinical Trials Education Program (CCTEP), a program that facilitates patient education about the advantages and risks associated with participation in clinical trials.

Despite best intentions, misunderstanding of the purpose of the trial and fear frequently plague participation in mainstream medical trials. Especially in oncology research, there exists a significant call to increase patient's understanding of the disease and participation in treatment; frequently this is translated into encouraging patient participation in clinical trials. Most clinical research is classified into three phases, with earlier phases representing more speculative research (Sadler, 2001). For the most part, oncology trials are encouraged for patients who have exhausted all other means of proven treatment. This is especially true for patients who participate in early (Phase I) research, as opposed to later Phase II or III research, when treatment effects are better understood. Consequently, the typical enrollment in clinical trials are individuals who have significantly less likelihood for responding to treatments, which are frequently toxic and biomedically aggressive (King, 2000). A misconception common to patients is the unrealistic expectation that a clinical trial is "cutting edge" research and, therefore, a certainty for cure (Kadushin, 2000). As Guttman (1997) noted, the language used to describe medical interactions has a way of shaping the patient's understanding of truth. As such, the language used to encourage or discourage patients from participating in clinical trials creates the individual's expectations for cure. When presented with the potential to be one of the "first people" to receive a new treatment, patients often assume unrealistic optimism. Consequently, due to the nature of clinical trials, patients are not always mindful of both the benefits and the risks associated with participation in clinical trials.

Another significant factor facing patient's perceptions of clinical trials is fear. Frequently, patients are instructed that they must not be enrolled in other types of treatments, or subscribed to other types of drugs (Sadler, 2001). As a result, patients may report concern about being given a placebo, or being placed in a control group, away from traditionally accepted forms of treatment. This fear of not receiving treatment may discourage a patient from participating in experimental research.

Conversely, fear may also be a reason why people elect to choose to participate in clinical trials. For example, Blakeslee (1992) noted the increased anxiety of people who were exposed to inflated statistics from the American Cancer Society designed to encourage women to adopt preventative measures. Some individuals, especially ones with high anxiety, may view the clinical trial as their "last hope" for aggressive treatment, the fear of disease progression motivating their decision to participate in early Phase (I or II) research.

Participation in clinical studies typically has significantly greater personal inconveniences, such as time commitments, lifestyle restrictions, transportation challenges, as well as differing medical risks, such as drug side effects (Holden, Rosenberg, Barker, Tuhrim, & Brenner, 1993; Kadushin, 2000; Williams & Boykin, 1999). It is also known that traditional medical establishments and nontraditional healing centers are at odds with what is considered clinical research (Dreher, 1998). For some, the dialogue between established institutions (such as the NCI) and holistic or non-Western practices creates a confusing political discourse, frequently competing with patient ideology. It is for these reasons that the decision to participate in the trial or not, coupled with the complexity of the procedures themselves, make understanding the clinical trial from the patient's perspective significantly complex (for additional discussion of clinical trials, see Albrecht et al. chapter in this volume).

IMPLICATIONS

The aforementioned environmental influences on the delivery of cancer care may have significant affects on communication. Addressing concepts such as cultural competence and sociolinguistic obstacles associated with poverty tend to encourage provider-patient communication environments, where collaborative information exchange is encouraged. Addressing these influences on the delivery of cancer care may aid in the reduction of health disparities between providers and patients of different cultures, facilitate communication between patients and health care staff, and address future demographic trends of increasing diversity.

The utilization of Standard of Care and Privileging aids in the reduction of potential noise and uncertainty by limiting the universe of treatment options. Although we note that alternatives to the standard of care (potential clinical trials, etc.) can increase ambiguity, uncertainty, and noise. Standards of care and privileging are relatively stable, with expected options, sequencing of care, and outcomes to reduce uncertainty and ambiguity by recognizing that the responsible physician is ultimately accountable and assumes the role of primary decision maker with the patient in the process of care.

A team orientation to the delivery of care provides multidimensional information and care for the cancer patient. We expect this ultimately increases the accuracy of the communication and its timeliness. Further, we expect a team orientation also increases the potential of patient understanding. If the medical team is not properly aligned, there is potential for noise and ambiguity and increased uncertainty in the delivery of care.

We have provided identification and understanding of some of the influences on the delivery of care, which is merely the first step in modeling a complicated communicative interaction. Surely there are others. As health communication researchers uncover more systemic influences in the delivery of care, researchers may begin to sketch the relationships and significance of the multitude of influences that directly or indirectly impact communication in the delivery of cancer care.

REFERENCES

Aday, L. A. (2002). *At risk in America: The health and health care needs of vulnerable populations in the United States* (2nd ed.). Hoboken, NJ: Jossey-Bass.

Ali, N. S., Khalil, H. Z., & Yousef, W. (1993). A comparison of American and Egyptian cancer patients' attitudes and unmet needs. *Cancer Nursing, 16*, 193-203.

Aligned Management Associates Inc. (2002). Innovative solutions for prostate cancer care: Symposium overview. URL: http://www.amainc.com/prostate_overview.html. Retrieved: October 21, 2002.

American Academy of Family Physicians (2001). Cancer care: Ensuring Quality; Recommendation No. 4. URL: http://www.aafp.org/x6635.xml. Retrieved: October 24, 2002.

American Association of Health Plans (1998). *Healthcare decisions: A common sense guide to choosing a health plan.* Available from: 1129 20th Street, N.W., Suite 600, Washington, D.C. 20036-3421. Excerpts from Arthur Miller [videotape].

American Society of Clinical Oncology (2002). Tamoxifen still recommended as breast cancer standard of care. *Behind the Cancer Headlines,* May 20, 2002. URL: http://www.mabcie.com/May_20,_2002_breast_cancer.html. Retrieved: October 21, 2002.

Baile, W. F., Lenzi, R., Kudelka, A., Maguire, P., Novack, D., Goldstein, M., Myers, E. G., & Bast, R. C. (1997). Improving physician-patient communication in cancer care: Outcome of a workshop for oncologists. *Journal of Cancer Education, 12*(3), 166-173.

Barnes, M., & Florencio, P. S. (2002). Financial conflicts of interest in human subjects research: The problem of institutional conflicts. *Journal of Law, Medicine & Ethics, 30*(3), 390. Retrieved October 18, 2003, from Questia database, http://www.questia.com.

Beck, S. L. (1999). Health policy, health services, and cancer pain management in the new South Africa. *Journal of Pain and Symptom Management, 17*(1), 16-26.

Bernabel, R., Gatsonis, C., & Mor, V. (1998). Management of pain in elderly patients with cancer. *JAMA, 279*, 1877-1882.

Bernstein, B. (1964). Social class, speech systems and psycho-therapy. *British Journal of Sociology, 15*, 54-64.

Berthelot, J.-M., Will, B. P., Evans, W. K., & Coyle, D. (2000). Decision framework for chemotherapeutic interventions for metastatic non-small-cell lung cancer. *Journal of the National Cancer Institute, 92*, 1321-1329.

Blakeslee, S. (1992, March 15). Faulty math heightens fears of breast cancer. *The New York Times.*

Blau, W., Dalton, J., & Lindley, C. (1999). Organization of hospital-based acute pain management programs. *Hospital-Based Pain Management, 92*, 465-466.

Bonica, J. (1994). *Effective pain management for cancer patients.* St. Paul, MN: SIMS Deltec.

Brach, C., & Fraser, I. (2000). Can cultural competency reduce racial and ethnic health disparities? A review and conceptual model. *Medical Care Research and Review, 57*, 181-217.

Boreham, P., & Gibson, D. (1978). The informative process in private medical consultations: A preliminary investigation. *Social Science and Medicine, 12*, 409-416.

Brady, M. L. (1987). Psychological interactions for women with breast disease. *Obstetrics and Gynecological Clinics of North America, 14*(3), 797-816.

Burton, M. V., & Parker, R. W. (1997). Psychological aspects of cancer surgery: Surgeons' attitudes and opinions. *Psycho-Oncology, 6*(1). 47-64.

Cancer Care Inc. (2001). Managing your cancer. Retrieved October 21, 2002, from http://www.cancer-care.org.

Carillo, J. E., Green, A. R., & Betancourt, J. R. (1999). Cross-cultural primary care: A patient-based approach. *Annals of Internal Medicine, 130*, 829-834.

Carney, P. A., Eliassen, M. S., Wells, W. A., & Schwartz, W. G. (1998). Can we improve breast pathology reporting practices? A community-based breast pathology quality improvement program in New Hampshire. *Journal of Community Health, 23*(2), 85-98.

Carpenter, Dave (2001). Our overburdened ERs. *Hospitals & Health Networks, 75*(3), 44.

Carr, V. F. (1996). Service chief recommendations in performance-based clinical privileging. *Military Medicine, 161*(5), 277-279.

Cartright, A. (1964). *Human relations and hospital care.* London: Routledge and Kegan Paul.

Chan, A. (1997). Communicating with patients with advanced cancer. *Journal of Palliative Care, 13*(3), 29-33.

Cheson, B. D. (1991). Cancer clinical trials: Clinical trials programs. *Seminars in Oncology Nursing, 7*, 235-242.

Cohen, M.R., Anderson, R.W., Attilio, R. M., Green, L., Muller, R. J., & Pruemer, J. M. (1996). Preventing medication errors in cancer chemotherapy. *American Journal of Health-System Pharmacy, 53*(7), 737-746.

Conrad, C., & McIntush, H. (2003). Organizational rhetoric and healthcare policymaking. In In T. Thompson et al. (Eds.), *Handbook of health communication* (pp. 403-422). Mahwah, NJ: Erlbaum.

Coyle, N. (1995). Supportive care program, pain service, Memorial Sloan-Kettering Cancer Center. *Support Care in Cancer, 3*, 161-163.

Cross, T.L., Bazron, B.J., Dennis, K.W., & Isaacs, M.R. (1989). *Towards a culturally competent system of care: A monograph on effective services for minority children who are severely emotionally disturbed.* Washington, DC: CASSP Technical Assistance Center, Georgetown University.

Dougall, A., Russell, A., Rubin, G., & Ling, J. (2000). Rethinking patient satisfaction: Patient experiences of an open access flexible sigmoidoscopy service. *Social Science and Medicine, 50*(1), 53-62.

Dreher, H. (1998, January-February). Cancer and the politics of meaning. *Tikkun, 13.* Retrieved October 18, 2003, from Questia database, http://www.questia.com.

Dumpe, M., & Ulreich, S. (2001). Moving from parallel play to team play. *Seminars for Nurse Managers, 9*(2), 85-89.

Eckenwiler, L. A. (1999). Pursuing reform in clinical research: Lessons from women's experience. *Journal of Law, Medicine & Ethics, 27*(2), 158. Retrieved October 18, 2003, from Questia database, http://www.questia.com.

Ellis, C., Evans, B. D., Mak, D., Mitchell, P., Melville, P., Stone, C., Thompson, P., & Harvey, V. (1993). Patient assessment of a combined medical and nursing preparation to cytotoxic chemotherapy. *Supportive Care in Cancer, 1*(4), 209-213.

Fenton, H. R. (1988). Physicians' rights as hospital staff members. *Hospital Physician, 24*(4), 36-38, 40-41, 44.

Furrow, B. (2001). Pain management and provider liability: No more excuses. *Journal of Law, Medicine & Ethics, 29*(1). Retrieved October 7, 2005, from Infotrack databaseb (Article A75086652).

Guttman, N. (1997). Ethical dilemmas in health campaigns. *Health Communication, 9*(2), 155-190.

Hablamos Juntos. (2001). Press conference announcing how language barriers hinder access and delivery of quality care. Retrieved August 13, 2003, from http://www.hablamosjuntos.org/mediacenter/press_conference.asp.

Haylock, P. J. (1993). Oncology nursing in the small community hospital. *Oncology, 7*(9), 73-82.

HHS Press Office. (2003). *Fact sheet: Protecting the privacy of patients' health information.* Washington, DC: US Department of Health and Human Services. Accessed October 8, 2003, from www.hhs.gov.news/facts/privacy.

Hill, C. (1995). When will adequate pain treatment be the norm? *JAMA, 274,* 1881.

Hoffmann, D. (1998). Pain management and palliative care in the era of managed care: Issues for health insurers. *Journal of Law, Medicine & Ethics, 26,* 267.

Holden, G., Rosenberg, G., Barker, K., Tuhrim, S., & Brenner, B. (1993). The recruitment of research participants: A review. *Social Work in Health Care, 19,* 1-44.

Jacobs, C. (1994). Head and neck cancer in 1994: A change in the standard of care. *Journal of the National Cancer Institute, 86,* 250-252.

James, J., Jones, J. M., Rodin, G., & Catton, P. (2001). Can assessment of psychosocial orientation assist continuing education program development in psychosocial oncology? *Journal of Cancer Education, 16,* 24-28.

Joranson, D., & Gilson, A. (1998). Regulatory barriers to pain management. *Seminars in Oncology Nursing, 14,* 158.

Jost, T. (1998). Public financing of pain management: Leaky umbrellas and ragged safety nets. *Journal of Law, Medicine & Ethics, 26,* 290.

Kadushin, G. (2001). Clinical trials: A wider lens 2. *Health and Social Work, 26*(3), 203.

King, N. M. (2000). Defining and describing benefit appropriately in clinical trials. *Journal of Law, Medicine & Ethics, 28(4),* 332. Retrieved October 18, 2003, from Questia database, http://www.questia.com.

Kirschbaum, M. (1996). The development, implementation and evaluation of guidelines for the management of breast cancer related lymphoedema. *European Journal of Cancer Care, 5,* 246-251.

Lammers, J., Duggan, A., & Barbour, J. (2003). Organizational forms of the provision of health care: An institutional perspective. In T. Thompson et al. (Eds.), *Handbook of health communication* (pp. 319-346). Mahwah, NJ: Erlbaum.

Larsen, L.S., Neverett, S.G., & Larsen, R.F. (2001). Clinical nurse specialist as facilitator of interdisciplinary collaborative program for adult sickle cell population. *Clinical Nurse Specialist, 15,* 15-22.

Lebovits, A., Florence, I., & Bathina, R. (1997). Pain knowledge and attitudes of healthcare providers: Practice characteristic differences. *Clinical Journal of Pain, 13,* 237-243.

Lehman, M., & Thomas, G. (2001). Is concurrent chemotherapy and radiotherapy the new standard of care for locally advanced cervical cancer? *International Journal of Gynecological Cancer, 11*(2), 87-99.

Lumb, E. W., & Oskvig, R. M. (1998). Multidisciplinary credentialing and privileging: A unified approach. *Journal of Nursing Care Quality, 12*(4), 36-43.

Lunt, B., & Jenkins, J. (1983). Goal-setting in terminal care: A method of recording treatment aims and priorities. *Journal of Advanced Nursing, 8,* 495-505.

McGuire, W. P. (2000). Confirmation of the "old" standard of care for ovarian cancer and a challenge. *Journal of the National Cancer Institute, 92,* 674-675.

McNeil, C. (1999). New standard of care for cervical cancer sets stage for next questions. *Journal of the National Cancer Institute, 91,* 500-501.

Memorial Sloan-Kettering Cancer Center (2002). The standard of care for the patient with pain. Pain Standard Committee. Retrieved October 21, 2002, from http://www.cityofhope.org/prc/web/html/standard%20of%20care-Memorial%20Sloan.asp.

Mills, R. (2002). United States Department of Commerce Health Insurance Coverage: 2001. United States Census Bureau, September.

Minsky, B. D., Coia, L., Haller, D.G., Hoffman, J., John, M., Landry, J., Pisansky, T. M., Willet, C., Mahon, I., Owen, J., Berkey, B., Katz, A., & Hanks, G. (1998). Radiation therapy for rectosigmoid and rectal cancer: Results of the 1992-1994 Patterns of Care Process Survey. *Journal of Clinical Oncology, 16,* 2542-2547.

Murphy, G., Morris, L., & Lange, D. (1997). *Informed decisions: The complete book of cancer diagnosis, treatment, and recovery.* New York: Viking.

National Cancer Institute (2001). Digest page: NCI clinical announcement on cervical cancer. Cancer.gov. Retrieved: October 21, 2002, from http://www.nci.nih.gov/clinicaltrials/digestpage/cervical-cancer-announcement.html.

Oliver, I. N., Turrell, S. J., Olszewski, N. A., & Willson, K. J. (1995). Impact of an information and consent form on patients having chemotherapy. *The Medical Journal of Australia, 162*(2), 82-83.

Overbay, J. D. (1996). Parental participation in treatment decisions for pediatric oncology ICU patients. *Dimensions of Critical Care Nursing, 15*(1), 16-24.

Rose, P.G. (2000). Chemoradiotherapy: The new standard care for invasive cervical cancer. *Drugs, 60,* 1239-1244.

Ross, E. C. (1999). Regulating managed care: Interest group competition for control and behavioral health care. *Journal of Health Politics, Policy, and Law, 24,* 599-625.

Roter, D. L. (1977). Patient participation in the patient-provider interaction: The effects of patient question asking on the quality of interaction satisfaction and compliance. *Health Education Monographs, 5,* 281-315.

Sadler, G. R. (2001). A call to action: Patients' access to clinical trials. *Health and Social Work, 26*(3), 196.

Saunders, S. (2001). System care management: Purpose, structure, and function. In N. Weeder & W. Peebles-Wilkins (Eds.), *Managed care services: Policy, programs, and research* (pp. 97-116). New York: Oxford University Press.

Sayeed, H. (2002). FMLA: Department of Labor overstepped authority. *Journal of Law, Medicine, & Ethics, 30,* 462-465.

Schain, W. S. (1980). Patients' rights in decision making: The case for personalism versus paternalism in health care. *Cancer, 46,* 1035-1041.

Scholes, J., & Vaughan, B. (2002). Cross-boundary working: Implications for the multiprofessional team. *Journal of Clinical Nursing, 11,* 399-408.

Shaffer, A. D., & Pavarini, P. A. (1997). Resolving conflicting laws and policy in integrated delivery systems development. *Journal of Law and Health, 12*(1), 85-120.

Siminoff, L. A., Fetting, J. H., & Abeloff, M. D. (1989). Doctor-patient communication about breast cancer adjuvant therapy. *Journal of Clinical Oncology, 7,* 1192-1200.

Smedley, B. D., Stith, A. Y., & Nelson, A. R. (Eds.). (2002). *Unequal treatment: Confronting racial & ethnic disparities in health.* Washington, DC: National Academy Press.

Smith, K., & Smith, V. (2002). Successful interdisciplinary documentation through nursing interventions classification. *Seminars for Nurse Managers, 10*(2), 100-104.

Street, R. (2003). Communication in medical encounters: An ecological perspective. In T. Thompson et al. (Eds.), *Handbook of health communication* (pp. 63-89). Mahwah, NJ: Erlbaum.

Sutcliffe, K. (2001). Organizational environmental and organizational information processing. In F. Jablin & L. Putnam (Eds.), *The new handbook of organizational communication* (pp. 197-230). Thousand Oaks, CA: Sage.

Taylor, K. M., Feldstein, M. L., Skeel, R. T., Pandya, K. J., Ng, P., & Carbone, P. P. (1994). Fundamental dilemmas of the randomized clinical trial process: Results of a survey of the 1,737 Eastern Cooperative Oncology Group investigators. *Journal of Clinical Oncology, 12,* 1796-1805.

Teeley, P., & Bashe, P. (1997). *The complete cancer survival guide.* New York: Doubleday.

United States Department of Commerce (2002). Health insurance in America: Numbers of Americans with and without health insurance rises, Census Bureau reports. Economics and Statistics Administration, Bureau of the Census, Washington DC. Retrieved on December 5, 2002, from http://www.census.gov/Press-Release/www/2002/cb02-127.html.

Waitzkin, H. (1984). Doctor-patient communication: Clinical implications of social scientific research. *Journal of the American Medical Association, 252,* 2441-2446.

Waitzkin, H. (1985). Information giving in medical care. *Journal of Health and Social Behavior, 26,* 81-101.

Walczak, M. B., & Absolon, P. L. (2001). Essentials for effective communication in oncology nursing: Assertiveness, conflict management, delegation, and motivation. *Journal for Nurses in Staff Development, 17*(3), 159-162.

Williams, J. K., & Boykin, F. (1999). The role of social work in HIV/AIDS clinical trials. *Social Work in Health Care, 29*, 35-56.

8 | Public Advocacy For Cancer Care

History, Background, and Rationale For Advocacy

Paula Kim
Translating Research Across Communities (TRAC)

The role of public advocacy directed toward cancer has dramatically changed the landscape for the better, and has helped to significantly improve cancer research and care in the United States.

One of the first and most effective advocates for increased public funding for cancer research was philanthropist Mary Woodard Lasker. Lasker was a true champion of medical research and made her case for federal funding by warning, "If you think health is expensive, try disease!" Her vision set the stage for cancer advocates to follow as she founded the Citizens Committee for the Conquest of Cancer (Lasker Foundation, 2002) and, along with Benno Schmidt (NCI, 2003b), became the leading proponents of the National Cancer Act, signed into law by President Nixon in 1971. The act grew out of a Senate resolution that tasked a group of scientists and cancer advocates with developing a legislative plan for a national program. Texas Senator Ralph W. Yarborough spearheaded the effort and the report of the Yarborough Commission became the framework for the National Cancer Act of 1971.

The purpose of the act was to "enlarge the authorities of the National Cancer Institute [NCI] and the National Institutes of Health [NIH] in order to advance the national effort against cancer." It was distinctive in many ways, and in particular, it created a National Cancer Program to be coordinated by the director of the NCI. The NCI director is appointed by the President of the United States, and most notable was the annual budget estimate to be submitted directly to the president, "bypassing" the traditional channels of the (NIH) and the Department of Health and Human Services customarily required of other NIH Institute submissions to the president or to Congress (NCI, 2003f). As a result of the 1971 National Cancer Act, the NCI is the only agency with this special authority. The first "Bypass Budget" was submitted to the president in 1973.

The Bypass Budget is a professional judgment budget that outlines what is required to move cancer research forward, translate research into evidence-based interventions, and move these interventions into use for public benefit. It outlines the NCI's vision, goals, progress, and plans. Along with the NCI, many advocacy organizations and research institutions use the strategies outlined in the document much like points on a compass as references for planning and prioritizing within their own division or organization. Each year, cancer advocacy organizations actively advocate to the president and the Congress for full funding of the NCI Bypass Budget amount. Despite these efforts and including the recent steps by Congress to double the budget at the NIH, the NCI Bypass Budget amount has only been fully funded by Congress twice since 1973, with the most recent time being 1984 (NCI, 2001d).

The process of developing the NCI budget and strategies is an enormous one. One of the more challenging aspects of developing the nation's strategy to combat cancer is the challenge of developing a long-term strategy in the context of an annual budget cycle. The NCI Office of Science Planning and Assessment coordinates, develops, and produces the annual Bypass Budget document, which is published as "The Nation's Investment in Cancer Research." This document is developed internally at the NCI and the NCI is now working to develop more effective methods of including input from advocacy organizations on topics and priority areas as outlined within the budget proposal. This interactive process with the advocacy community generally begins 1 year in advance of when the budget is submitted to the president.

Cancer advocates witnessed the accomplishments of the AIDS movement and could readily identify with the need to demand more in the form of money for research, insurance coverage, and key patient care issues. There was no question that political action fueled by grassroots movements were the key to progress.

About the same time that the 1971 National Cancer Act was signed into law, organized cancer advocacy efforts aimed at disease-specific cancer, primarily breast cancer and childhood cancers, got into the advocacy movement. Modest growth of advocacy groups continued on through the 1980s and the 1990s ushered in a virtual explosion of disease-specific cancer advocacy groups. The 1990s growth in cancer advocacy was fueled by successes in increased cancer research funding for the NCI and disease-specific funding within the NCI. The advocacy group's organizational ability to rapidly grow in both size and effectiveness was enhanced by major technology advancements such as the Internet and fax machines.

Beginning in 1998 and ending in fiscal year 2003, there was an unprecedented doubling of the NIH budget by the Congress. Advocacy groups were instrumental in helping to achieve these budget increases.

These budget increases have led to an infusion of greatly needed appropriations for cancer research, but this recent 5-year upturn in funding is at risk of losing a great deal of momentum gained because the budget outlook for the foreseeable future looks very dim. The current Congress and the president have moved in the direction of flat or minimally increasing budgets. These changes will severely restrict the research opportunities for new programs and early career investigators, it is devastating for research and in particular for the many cancers still without robust research programs. In 1990, the NCI's budget was nearly $1.7 billion (NCI, 2001d) and in 2002, the NCI's budget had grown to more than $3.7 billion (NCI,

2001e). Would the NCI budget have grown to the same degree without the push by advocacy organizations? Probably not, as there are many competing priorities that the Congress must decide from when slicing up the federal budget each year. By law the NCI cannot advocate to the Congress for its budget. This heightens the importance of advocacy organizations and individuals working together to ensure that the needs of cancer research are heard on Capitol Hill. Is the 2005 NCI annual budget of $4.878 billion enough? The simple answer is, no, not even close. For example, the U.S. Congress has chosen to direct more money per month to rebuild Iraq, than it directs for an entire year's budget for cancer research in America. The demands of the disease and the burden it places on the American public requires a much greater investment than our public policymakers have been willing to make to date. The American people need to let policymakers know loud and clear that cancer research is a priority.

With the number of cancer survivors growing, along with the baby-boomer generation coming into the time when it is at greatest risk of contracting cancer, the importance of public advocacy for cancer care cannot be overstated nor underestimated.

There is a great responsibility and obligation for the federal lawmakers to allocate ample appropriations to effectively provide the research community with the tools and resources to control, manage and ultimately cure cancer. There is added obligation to ensure that all Americans have equal access to affordable quality care and treatment. These are obligations currently not being met sufficiently. Cancer advocacy organizations and voting constituents in a lawmaker's home district are a very active presence every day, reminding our elected officials of the importance of these responsibilities.

There is an equal responsibility for the federal agencies vested with these appropriations to do a better job to proactively prioritize, strategize, and manage the research programs to ensure that all cancers, particularly the most lethal and historically overlooked and underfunded cancers are actively and appropriately included in the game plan. This strategic planning must be done in unison with specific programs aimed at responding to disease and research area specific needs and Congressional concerns. If one looks at Fig. 8.1, the "NCI Overview 1996-2004 Funding for Top Five Cancers in Mortality," it is very clear that the NCI failed in some of its responsibility, most notably, to sufficiently prioritize the research needs of cancer across the board irrespective of whether or not a particular type of cancer has the constituent size and or political capability to influence research appropriations through Congressional resources. The purpose of the funding illustration is not to pit one disease type against another, this is not what advocates want, but rather to highlight the challenge being faced which is the need to prioritize and achieve some sense of parity when the playing field is not level. Funding levels are one of the key yardsticks that advocates use to measure progress.

Federal and state agencies also have the responsibility to develop and direct programs that move research from discovery through the development phase and then to ensure that these scientific discoveries are disseminated and delivered into the communities for patient benefit. The scientific community that is the recipient and end user of these appropriations has a tremendous responsibility to conduct research that seeks to answer valid scientific questions and move science forward innovatively for patient benefit and true scientific progress as opposed to scientific projects aimed at seizing a research opportunity for which one is ill-prepared or one that adds to a resume for tenure or career advancement but has little if no potential scientific or patient benefit.

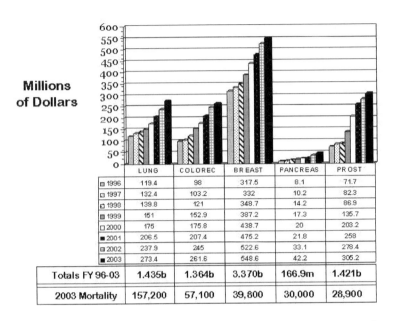

The chart above corresponds to the following data table:

	LUNG	COLOREC	BREAST	PANCREAS	PROST
1996	119.4	98	317.5	8.1	71.7
1997	132.4	103.2	332	10.2	82.3
1998	139.8	121	348.7	14.2	86.9
1999	151	152.9	387.2	17.3	135.7
2000	175	175.8	438.7	20	203.2
2001	206.5	207.4	475.2	21.8	258
2002	237.9	245	522.6	33.1	278.4
2003	273.4	261.6	548.6	42.2	305.2
Totals FY 96-03	1.435b	1.364b	3.370b	166.9m	1.421b
2003 Mortality	157,200	57,100	39,800	30,000	28,900

FIGURE 8.1. National Cancer Institute overview 1996 to 2004. Funding for top five cancers in mortality. (Copyright © Pancreatic Cancer Action Network. Source: NCI Facts Book/ ACS Facts and Figures.)

The clinical community charged with applying research discoveries and caring for patients must stay actively engaged in the continuous learning and educational process to maintain the highest level of expertise and state-of-the-art knowledge in the rapidly changing world of treatment and caring for cancer patients. The clinicians and patients will benefit when there is improved patient–health professional communication and interaction. Hospitals, clinics, and academic centers are beginning to understand the need to offer multi-disciplinary team approaches that provide cancer patients and their loved ones with more user-friendly environments and assistance with the cancer patient experience. There are some cancer centers and settings that provide above average patient- and research-related services and outreach to cancer patients, however it is unfortunate that these are the exception rather than the rule. Many cancer advocacy organizations seek to actively work with cancer centers to develop their support and outreach programs and further collaborative efforts are greatly encouraged.

The private sector shares in the responsibility of actively working to provide accessible and affordable quality care and treatments for all cancer patients. There is a continuing need for greater investment by the biotechnology and drug development companies in the oncology market, in particular the orphan cancers that lack the market size that is attractive to industry investments and attention. There is also a continuing and growing need to ensure that Americans have access to and the ability to afford adequate health care insurance to cover the costs of screening for and being treated for cancer. A diagnosis of cancer for an uninsured person should not mean financial hardship on top of dealing with the disease. Future generations stand to benefit greatly from the combined efforts of those working to improve cancer outcomes and treatment. Cancer patients have a responsibility to empower themselves with knowledge and support so they can work as a team with their healthcare professionals to make informed decisions about their treatment and care (O'Hair, Villagran, Wittenberg, Brown, Hall, Ferguson, & Doty, 2003) and to be diligent and compliant with follow-up and treatment management and surveillance steps. Many advocacy organizations provide valuable patient services that help empower the patients in this way.

There is great potential in lessening the number of people afflicted by many types of cancer by taking advantage of already known and proven strategies. As simple as this sounds, many people are either unwilling or unable to modify their behavior or lifestyle or are squeamish about early diagnostic tests and methods. The typical person who is healthy and asymptomatic and those people at high risk have a less well-known but important responsibility to follow recommended behavioral and screening guidelines to minimize one's risk of getting cancer and to participate in research studies that can unlock the many unknown mysteries of how, why, and when one develops cancer. All of the research and effective treatments are of much less impact and value unless and until enough people take notice and actively utilize the scientific technology and progress that is being made available to them.

These examples are shared as reminders of what we must all be mindful of as our respective communities work toward our common goal of curing cancer and in the words of NCI Director Dr. Andrew von Eschenbach, "eliminating the death and suffering due to cancer." Each one of us shares in some way personally or professionally, the responsibility of eliminating cancer.

Advocacy organizations work to be a "watchdog" in all of these areas as they seek to maintain and preserve the best interests of the patient community. There is a move toward improved interaction and communication in these areas and it is a move that is welcomed by all. We are at a time in the world of cancer that is being referred to by many as an "inflection" point. The cancer inflection point is a major convergence of scientific opportunity and need that point to important challenges in the future. Opportunities lie in several distinct, but complementary areas:

- Building on existing scientific discovery
- Cutting edge technology
- The mapping of the human genome and genetic based medicine
- The move from seek-and-destroy type cancer treatments to find-and-control type treatments
- More cancer survivors than any time in history
- The era of the Internet-savvy, empowered patient
- Creating the necessary infrastructures to support and optimize research

The need and opportunity for improvement is apparent because many cancers are still without early detection, a cure, or effective treatments; too many people, including the minority and underserved, continue to suffer from a lack of access to care; and more than 1.3 million Americans will be diagnosed with cancer in 2005 (ACS, 2005). There is an urgent need for greater collaboration, coordination, communication, and outreach between all sectors, including private industry, public agencies, researchers, and community healthcare professionals, to drive progress for patients.

The opportunities, needs, and challenges are much the same for the scientific world as they are for cancer advocacy, except for different vantage points. We are all working toward the same goal, that of directly improving the system and the outcomes for improved patient benefit. One of the most daunting challenges is unifying all sectors, as well as harnessing the mindset, human and fiscal resources to make it all happen.

In 1998, 22.3 million adults in the United States searched for online medical information. Cancer, in addition to being one of the most feared diseases, was one of the most requested topics (NCI, 2001i). A February 17, 1999 Harris Poll showed that cancer accounted for 15% of the diseases that generated the greatest use of the web, and in addition, 32% of web pages referenced were those containing information for patient advocacy or support groups (Marconi, 2002).

ADVOCACY FUNCTION, IMPLEMENTATION, FUNDING/FUNDRAISING AND EDUCATION-RELATED ACTIVITIES

Although many cancers, such as breast, prostate, and childhood cancers, have seen a welcomed decline in mortality rates and an improved scientific progress, there is still much work to do, as there are yet many cancers, including pancreatic, esophageal, lung, and liver cancers, that have no early detection, a severe lack of effective treatments, and no cure. These cancers continue to be the most lethal and have had no appreciable decrease in mortality rates whatsoever. A large part of this lack of progress can be directly attributed to the insufficient research funding for these cancers

The role of public advocacy for cancer care is essential and proven. It is encouraging and timely that, in addition to well-established disease-specific advocacy organizations, there are new advocacy organizations that continue to emerge for lesser known cancers and that advocacy organizations exist for nearly all forms of cancer. There are a variety of reasons as to how and why advocacy groups are established. Often, cancer advocacy organizations have founder roots from someone who is a cancer survivor or someone who has been personally affected by a loved one having a particular type of cancer. The one common thread is the recognition of unmet needs for a particular cancer and the motivation to fill those needs. Advocacy organizations are generally set apart from one another by their mission, constituencies, and basis of funding support. Each has its own goals and objectives and most often is aimed in some way toward eliminating cancer and providing support in the form of research funding and personal patient-based support.

Cancer advocacy organizations lend full support to cancer patients by providing patient education and services, working to increase the amount of research funding, and working to minimize obstacles so as to ensure the fruits of research are translated out into the community for the greatest patient benefit. Cancer advocacy organizations are crucial links between the patient community and the rest of the entire cancer universe made up of researchers, clinicians, health providers, payers, government agencies, and private industry. Many cancer advocacy organizations directly fund research as well as advocate for increased research funding and some do both.

Cancer Advocacy organizations generally have increased research funding as a top priority, along with improving the outcomes, quality of care, treatment, and survivorship for the patient along the continuum. Many organizations provide patient-based programs specifically designed for the support and information needs of their unique constituencies. With increasing burdens of health care coverage and costs combined with an aging population that is living with and surviving cancer longer, these groups are working to influence issues such as health policy, survivorship issues, practice and treatment guidelines, and job discrimination.

Interaction and communication between advocacy organizations and those seeking information such as patients, caregivers, and health professionals has been greatly enhanced by the fast-moving technology of computers and other electronic forms of communication. There is still, however, a digital divide that must be dealt with. There continue to be many underserved and rural populations who do not have access to these new forms of technology and communication.

Support and information is provided through a variety of methods. Some of the more frequently used methods include web-based, telephone, and in-person support meetings and online chatrooms.

The new technologies and application of scientific discovery bring the need to develop new methods of handling and managing the fruits of these discoveries. Changes in practice and care that emerge are not as well translated and applied into the community settings as would be optimal. In addition to practice and treatment changes, there are patient-based issues such as patient privacy, genetic testing, electronic records, and reimbursement policies that cannot keep pace with the fast-moving science that all require constant information management and dedicated resources on the part of proactive advocacy organizations who seek to provide the most up-to-date information and support for their constituents.

As we move into the 21st century, cancer continues to be a major health problem and the need for credible and objective information such as what can be found from many of the established and qualified cancer advocacy organizations becomes ever more vital. In 2005, it was estimated that 1.3 million Americans would be diagnosed with cancer and 570,280 Americans would die from cancer. It was also estimated that there were more than 8.9 million Americans living with and surviving cancer (ACS, 2005).

The cancer researchers engaged in patient-based research are generally aware of the role of cancer advocates in affecting research funding increases, providing research and clinical trials information to the cancer patient community, and providing important patient-based services, not to mention being some of the largest sources of nongovernmental research funding that exists. Community physicians, basic and lab scientists, and health care professionals involved in nonpatient-related research, are aware of, to a varying and lesser degree, the work of cancer advocacy organizations and their missions. Improving existing relationships and interactive ventures between researchers and cancer advocacy organizations, as well as developing interaction where none currently exists, would cast a much broader net of collaborative capability that can more effectively translate and deliver the discoveries into the community.

Advances in scientific discovery heavily rely on the private sector to move scientific advances along the path to commercialized use and benefit for the patient. Many of the more perceptive pharmaceutical and biotechnology companies work closely with advocacy organizations in effective programs that include research and educational-based meetings, workshops, interaction on clinical trials design, public policy issues, and patient-based issues such as expanded access.

These relationships between the private industry sector and advocacy organizations are important ones that require both parties to maintain an objective ethical balance as they work toward the common goal of improving the journey and outcome for the cancer patient.

EXAMPLES OF EFFECTIVE ADVOCACY, PATIENT SERVICES, CHARACTERISTICS

Funding for cancer research is one key aspect to scientific discovery. There is an axiom that says, "Science follows money, money creates opportunity, opportunity brings discovery and discovery brings money." As has been demonstrated in other diseases, adequate or inadequate funding lays the groundwork for advancements in all aspects of cancer research, care, and treatment. In addition to advocacy efforts aimed at increasing research funding, there are also important needs that revolve around public policy, regulations, and issues such as reimbursement and coverage.

Professional societies representing the various sectors and disciplines within the cancer research community take on an active and important role in keeping the concerns and voices of the research and clinical professionals in the forefront rather than on the back burner. The American Association for Cancer Research, The American Society for Clinical Oncology and the Oncology Nursing Society have the largest memberships representing cancer research and clinical professionals. Many of the professional societies have begun to include representatives from patient-based and disease-specific advocacy organizations as active participants in their programs. This is a wonderful advance in collaborative efforts from which everyone benefits particularly as these programs grow and strengthen

Following are a few examples of disease-specific advocacy efforts from both ends of the spectrum that illustrate the need and the importance of focused advocacy efforts.

In 1991, a group of breast cancer and cancer organizations joined together to form the National Breast Cancer Coalition (NBCC). Beginning with an October 1991 nationwide letter campaign to Congress and the White House, the new advocacy movement mobilized the nation's grassroots in political action efforts to accelerate breast cancer research funding, and give patients and survivors "a seat at the table"—increased involvement in medical and policy decision making. By 1992, the active and visible breast cancer advocacy community had stimulated both significant media interest and substantial Congressional commitments to fund the cause.

The NBCC helped to initiate an unprecedented multi-million dollar breast cancer research project within the Department of Defense (DOD, 2004) that, from 1992 to 2002 received almost $1.68 billion of appropriations supporting more than 3,650 awards (NBCC, 2002).

A significant accomplishment of the DOD program has been the integration and acceptance of breast cancer patient advocates who are involved in every step of the review process. Designed as a keystone component of the DOD program from its outset, integration of advocates as an integral part of the peer review and decision-making process was without precedent at other federal cancer research funding agencies, and continues to be highly regarded. Since 1992, the DOD disease research program has been expanded to include ovarian, prostate, and chronic myelogenous cancers. The impact and influence of breast cancer advocacy has also resulted in the expansion of research budgets at the NCI as well. The NCI budget for breast cancer research alone expanded from $90.2 million in 1991 to $566 million in 2004 (MULTI, 2005; NCI, 2004j).

Breast cancer advocacy and its impact on research funding is a successful and dramatic example of a well-focused grassroots advocacy effort. Their ability to influence the process has been hand in hand with the growth of the number of people and organizations involved in the breast cancer movement.

At the other end of the spectrum is pancreatic cancer, the fourth leading cause of cancer death and the cancer with the highest mortality rate. The NCI Progress Review Group Report (2001h) states;

> pancreatic cancer has been understudied in both basic research laboratories and the clinic. In terms of total research dollars, total numbers of researchers who are highly focused on this disease, pancreatic cancer lags significantly behind all of the most common tumors, despite the latter's more favorable survival rates . . . available data suggests that fewer than ten principal investigators have multiple grants or a primary career focus on pancreatic cancer. (p. 9)

In 1999, federal research funding for pancreatic cancer was the lowest of all major cancers at $17.3 million (NCI, 2001h). There was no national advocacy organization focused on pancreatic cancer and therefore, no voice to represent the needs of pancreatic cancer or to provide sorely needed patient education and services.

The Pancreatic Cancer Action Network (PanCAN) was established in 1999 as the first national patient-based advocacy organization for pancreatic cancer. Prior to 1999, there were no public advocacy efforts for pancreatic cancer with the federal agencies. The leadership of PanCAN knew from observing the experience of others that research advocacy was a critical area that needed immediate attention. PanCAN actively waded into the cancer advocacy public policy world and has effected unprecedented change in the research funding landscape for pancreatic cancer.

Through PanCAN's (2003) focused public policy efforts, federal research appropriations funding for pancreatic cancer grew from $ 17.5 million in 1999 to $ 52.7 million in 2004. This was an increase of 201%. However, the illustration (Fig. 8.1) of NCI funding for the top five cancers in mortality shows that despite these increases, pancreatic cancer research is still very under funded.

The shortage of pancreatic cancer researchers is a serious problem. In an attempt to enhance the NCI's funding investments and increase the number of investigators focused on pancreatic cancer, PanCAN's direct research advocacy program provides multiple career development awards to young investigators to firmly establish their research careers in pancreatic cancer. PanCAN's advocating for federal research appropriations and directly funding research is their one–two combination of research advocacy that has proven to be a very effective means of increasing research and attention in a very overlooked disease.

As the sole national resource with trained and dedicated staff for their pancreatic cancer patient services program, PanCAN is extremely sensitive and responsive to the concerns and needs of all its constituents. PanCAN has developed Patient and Liaison Services (PALS), a comprehensive program of education, guidance, and one-on-one services for patients and health care professionals that includes the most comprehensive and up-to-date database of public and private pancreatic cancer clinical trials. The PALS program is entering its fourth year and has grown to necessitate four well-qualified PALS Associates providing one-on-one guidance and navigation for patients, caregivers, and health care professionals. PALS Associates are handling more than 200 new patient inquiries and phone calls per month and sending out more than 300 patient information packets each month as well.

Both of these examples offer snapshots of effective cancer advocacy efforts for disease specific causes. The point is not about one cancer versus another or advocating for one type of cancer research funding at the expense of another. The take-home message is that the cancer research and patients communities benefit from focused public advocacy efforts. Cancer advocacy organizations are key catalysts for increased research resources, a committed national cancer program, and the joining of public and private enterprise for advancing science.

In addition to disease-specific efforts, there are there are efforts focused on broad-based research advocacy, public policy, and the big picture areas of funding for the health institutes. Translating Research Across Communities (TRAC), National Coalition for Cancer Research (NCCR), One Voice Against Coalition (OVAC), Cancer Leadership Council, Friends of Cancer Research, and Research Advocacy Network (RAN) are notable examples.

In addition to research funding, cancer advocates play key roles in helping to shape the future of NCI research programs in unmet areas. An example of this is the cancer advocates voicing the need for NCI to scientifically address the growing needs of the survivor community. In response to these and other efforts, the NCI in 1996, established the first Office of Cancer Survivorship (NCI, 2001g)

There are many organizations that provide patient support services based on a volunteer, peer-type program. Two longstanding examples of volunteer, peer-based support are the American Cancer Society's (ACS) "Reach to Recovery" program in place for more than 30 years (ACS, 2003) and the 24-hour Y-ME National Breast Cancer Hotline staffed by trained peer counselors who are breast cancer survivors. The program now includes translation into more than 140 languages (Y-Me, 2003).

Access to cancer care and treatments can be a result of geographic obstacles as well as man made ones. The man-made ones usually come in the form of insurance denials, job discrimination, and debt crisis resulting from the costs of treatment. The Patient Advocate Foundation (PAF) is a national organization that provides professional case managers and attorneys specializing in mediation, negotiation, and education, and advocates on behalf of patients experiencing difficulty in access to care, job retention and debt management (PAF, 2003).

Cancer Care and the National Coalition for Cancer Survivorship (NCCS) are two well-established advocacy organizations working on behalf of all types of cancer. More recently, the Lance Armstrong Foundation has become actively involved with many survivor and young adult issues. Each group provides specific programs and services for the cancer patient. Cancer Care provides financial information resources as well as direct financial assistance through a grants program (Cancer Care, 2003). Through an active public policy program, the NCCS strives to assure quality cancer care for all Americans (NCCS, 2003).

Advocacy organizations bring many positive influences to both the patient and professional communities. Disease-specific groups often help deliver important messages to their respective communities about the importance of following the guidelines for recommended screening and early detection methods such as mammograms for the early detection of breast cancer, prostate-specific antigen testing for prostate cancer, and pap smears for early detection of cervical cancer. These awareness and education programs are important tools to assist in greater patient compliance and ultimately improved ability to stop cancers before they start.

RESEARCH-RELATED ACTIVITIES/AGENCY INVOLVEMENT

There does not seem to be much doubt about the value and importance of advocacy participation in the eyes of many both public and private. Public agencies see the benefits of advocacy organizations as credible and effective partners representing the patient community.

The NCI, the Food and Drug Administration (FDA) and other federal agencies provide various opportunities, programs, and committees for advocacy involvement. Advocacy involvement in federal agencies is an area that is still evolving and has much room for growth. At times, there are acknowledged differences that exist between advocates and agencies as to the optimal role of cancer advocates and the extent to which they have a seat at the table as an opportunity to participate in planning and decision-making processes. The NIH and the NCI provide a variety of opportunities for advocacy involvement. The primary avenues where public advocates are involved are federally chartered advisory boards, advocacy programs, ad hoc committees and working groups. The six key federally chartered advisory boards of the NCI include the following.

The President's Cancer Panel-PCP is a three-member panel appointed by the President of the United States to a 3-year term. Their charge is to monitor the development and execution of the activities of the NCI, and report directly to the president. At least two members of the panel are distinguished scientists or physicians and the remaining member is a layperson advocate. The PCP came about as part of the 1971 National Cancer Act (NCI, 2001a).

The Board of Scientific Advisors (BSA) is a 35-member board appointed by the NCI director to a 5-year term. The BSA provides scientific advice on a wide variety of matters concerning scientific program policy, progress, and future direction of the NCI's extramural research programs, and concept review of extramural program initiatives. The BSA is comprised of knowledgeable authorities from a variety of scientific disciplines and currently includes two layperson advocates (NCI, 2001a).

The National Cancer Advisory Board (NCAB) is an 18-member board appointed to a 6-year term by the president. It also includes 12 nonvoting ex officio members representing various agencies and offices within the Department of Health and Human Services. Up to six members can be representatives from the general public. The NCAB advises the Secretary of the Department of Health and Human Services, and the director of the NCI about activities of the NCI including reviewing and recommending grants and cooperative agreements (NCI, 2001a).

The Board of Scientific Counselors (BSC) is a 60-member board appointed by the NCI director to a 5-year term. The BSC advises the directors of the intramural division of the NCI, the NCI director and deputy director on a wide variety of matters concerning scientific program policy such as the progress and future direction of research programs of each Division. The members are knowledgeable authorities representing the various scientific disciplines and currently include one layperson advocate (NCI, 2001A).

The NCI, under the leadership of its former Director, Dr. Richard Klausner, established the Director's Consumer Liaison Group (DCLG) in 1997. The goal was to bring the wisdom and insight of those whose lives were affected by cancer to NCI research efforts. The DCLG held its first meeting in 1997 and in 1998 became a federally chartered advisory committee. It was the first, and remains the only, advisory committee to NCI consisting entirely of cancer consumer advocates (NCI 2001a, 2001c).

The DCLG is comprised of 15 members who represent the diversity of those whose lives are affected by cancer. The Director of the NCI appoints the members to 4-year terms. According to its charter, the DCLG assists in developing and establishing processes and criteria for identifying appropriate consumer advocates to serve on a variety of NCI program and policy advisory committees; serves as a primary forum to discuss issues and concerns and exchange viewpoints that are important to the broad development of NCI program and research priorities; and provides recommendations to the director, the NCI in response to specific advice and requests from the director and the NCI, and to the needs of the cancer advocacy community; and establishes and maintains strong collaborations between NCI and this community to reach common goals.

The DCLG differs from the role of the NCAB, BSA, and BSC in that, as a group, it does evaluate or review grants, concepts and scientific programs for the NCI. However, its members participate on many NCI committees and workgroups such as NCI Listens and Learns, the Central Institutional Review Board, the Survivorship Knowledge Exchange Group, and the Cancer Outcomes Measurement Working Group. The role of the DCLG is continuing to evolve and there is a process currently in place that is working to refine and optimally develop the DCLG's role within the NCI.

In 2000, the NCI worked closely with the DCLG to create the Consumer Advocates in Research Related Activities (CARRA) program. The program was created to establish a systematic way to include readily available and qualified consumer advocates participating in the daily activities of the NCI. Examples of CARRA activities include grant review, NCI Web site content and navigation, focus groups, workshops, and editorial boards. The CARRA program grew out of the recognition that advocates were being invited to participate in activities within the NCI, where there was no organized method of developing best practices, identifying advocates, tracking participation, and measuring results. The program has been introduced throughout the NCI, has approximately 200 advocates who are each selected for a 3-year term, and in the first years has seen a steady rise in the numbers of requests for advocate participation in NCI activities (NCI, 2001c).

In 2001, the FDA established the Cancer Drug Development Patient Consultant Program. The FDA originally intended to select 10 patient consultants. The level of response and caliber of the applicants was greater than the FDA had expected, and it chose to select 23 disease-specific patient consultants to serve in the program. This was a decision widely applauded within the advocacy community (FDA, 2003). Because cancer drugs are approved by disease-specific indications and cancers are not one-size-fits-all, there is great variability in patient attitudes, response rates, and disease management. Cancer advocates are, by and large, very motivated to become knowledgeable about all of the elements, needs, and characteristics of the cancer they represent and bring valuable insight and expertise to the issues faced by the FDA and drug companies in the development of new cancer treatment drugs. Cancer advocates support the need to develop safe and effective treatments and continuously seek active roles in that process.

The FDA program goal is to incorporate the perspective of patient advocates into the drug development process including pre-approval and the clinical trial phase of cancer drug development. The FDA intends to provide cancer patient advocates an opportunity to participate in the FDA drug review process and provide advice to the FDA and to the drug sponsor on topics such as clinical trial design, endpoint determination, expanded access protocol development, and clinical trial patient-recruitment strategies. The program provides background and training to patient consultants on topics such as FDA overview, the drug review process, and the patient consultant's obligations under the conflict of interest and confidentiality regulations.

Conceptually, the FDA patient consultant program goals are quite consistent with goals of the advocacy community, however, in the case of cancers of lesser incidence for which the active advocacy organizations that can provide well-qualified patient consultants are far and few between, the current application of government conflict of interest rules essentially precludes the participation of many of the most qualified patient advocates for a particular disease. This inherent limitation truly negates the immense potential of the program. This is unfortunate as it is generally the lesser incidence cancers that suffer the greatest, due to a lack of effective treatments. It is therefore critical that the patient voice is a part of the approval process in all cancers, particularly those of lesser incidence. The FDA patient consultant program is extremely important and essential to the drug development process. The program would greatly benefit from exploring options that would address the conflict of interest challenges for the lesser incidence cancers, within a construct to afford maximum participation from the most qualified participants for optimal effectiveness that does not compromise the integrity of the science.

Clinical trials are the stepping stones to scientific change and progress. They are the driver of new drug, device, and treatment regimens for all patient-related issues. There is great interest on the part of advocacy organizations to ensure that clinical trials are meaningful, well designed, and impeccably conducted resulting in research that improves patient benefit based on results that are valid, credible, and objective.

As the regulatory burdens have been steadily increasing they have placed even greater demands on the clinical research community as they seek to answer important scientific questions as well as comply with strict regulations such as the newly enacted in April 2003 Health Insurance Portability and Accountability Act guidelines.

Willing and qualified patient advocates partner in the clinical trials process on many fronts. Some key areas include input on clinical trial design, including the patient informed consent form and serving on the Institutional Review Boards, the independent review committees charged with reviewing and approving a clinical trial design at each trial site location. Advocacy organizations also work to educate patients and caregivers about the facts of clinical trial participation and the importance of donating specimens for research.

In the United States, we have the remarkable privilege of advocating publicly for just about any cause we choose. Public advocacy for cancer as we know it, is merely a dream in the eye of cancer patients in most all other countries across the world.

Great strides have been made in scientific progress and patient care owing to the synergy created when advocates, researchers and the agencies share common goals. The challenge lies in creating synergy when there is none and no one is motivated to create any. We must find ways to harness the singular focus of individual goals that will exponentially leverage way beyond the vision of any one advocacy or scientific idea. The sectors of advocates, researchers, agencies, and private industry each need to develop greater unity and collaboration within their own communities and across communities.

Big problems like cancer require big thinking and big steps because despite great progress in many areas, there are still too many unanswered scientific questions and too many people dying from cancer. It will take the will and unity of many to make the progress the patient community desperately needs.

REFERENCES

American Cancer Society. (2002). *Cancer Facts and Figures 2002*. Atlanta, Ga.
American Cancer Society. (2003). Reach to recovery. Atlanta, GA. Accessed April 6, 2003, from http://www.cancer.org/ docroot/ESN/content/ESN_3_1x_Reach_to_Recovery_5.asp.

American Cancer Society. (2005). *Cancer Facts and Figures 2005*. Atlanta, GA.

Cancer Care. (2003). Financial needs. New York. Accessed April 6, 2003, from http:// www.cancer-care.org/ FinancialNeeds/FinancialNeedsmain.cfm.

Department of Defense. (2004) Fact sheet: Breast cancer. Ft. Detrick, MD. Accessed April 21, 2004, from http://cdmrp. army.mil/pubs/factsheets/bcrpfactsheet.htm.

Food and Drug Administration. (2003). FDA Cancer drug development patient consultant program. Rockville, MD. Accessed April 6, 2003, from http://www.fda.gov/oashi/cancer/pconback.html.

Lasker Foundation. (2002). Lasker history. Accessed February 21, 2003, from http://www.laskerfoundation.org/media/history.html.

Marconi, J. (2002). E-health: Navigating the internet for health information. *Healthcare Information and Management Systems Society.* Available at http://www.hipaadvisory.com/action/ehealth/himss.pdf

MULTI National Monitor. (2005). *The Breast Cancer Epidemic*. Accessed 2003, from Multinationalmonitor.org/hyper/issues/1991/11/allina.html

National Breast Cancer Coalition. (2002). History, goals and accomplishments. Bethesda, MD. Accessed February 21, 2003, from http://www.natlbcc.org/bin/index.asp?strid=22&depid =1&btnid=1.

National Cancer Institute. (2003a). Advisory boards and groups. Bethesda, MD. Accessed April 6, 2003, from http://deainfo. nci.nih.gov/ADVISORY/boards.htm.

National Cancer Institute. (2003b). Closing in on cancer. Bethesda, MD. Accessed April 6, 2003, from http://press2.nci.nih.gov/sciencebehind/cioc/molecular/molecularframe.htm.

National Cancer Institute. (2001c). *NCI DCLG FY 2001 Annual Report, 1.* Bethesda, MD.

National Cancer Institute. (2001d). *NCI Fact Book 2001 H-1-3.* Bethesda, MD.

National Cancer Institute. (2001e). NCI FY 2001 Appropriation cancer and AIDS. Bethesda, MD. Accessed April 6, 2003, from http://www3.cancer.gov/admin/fmb/2001appropriation.pdf.

National Cancer Institute. (2003f). The 1971 National Cancer Act. Bethesda, MD. Accessed April 6, 2003, from http://rex.nci. nih. gov/massmedia/CANCER_RESRCH_WEBSITE/1971.html.

National Cancer Institute. (2001g). *Office of cancer survivorship.* Bethesda, MD. Accessed April 30, 2004, from http://dccps.nci.nih. gov/ocs/history.html.

National Cancer Institute. (2001h). *Pancreatic cancer: An agenda for action, report of the Pancreatic Cancer Progress Review Group, 1.* Bethesda, MD.

National Cancer Institute. (2003i). Plans and priorities. Bethesda, MD. Available at http://2001.cancer. gov/communications.htm. Accessed February 20, 2003.

National Cancer Institute. (2001j). *NCI Fact Book 2004* (p. viii). Bethesda, MD.

National Coalition for Cancer Survivorship. (NCCS). (2003). Mission. Accessed April 6, 2003, from http://www.cansearch.org/ about/mission.html.

O'Hair, D., Villagran, M., Wittenberg, E., Brown, K., Hall, T., Ferguson, M., & Doty, T. (2003). Cancer survivorship and agency model (CSAM): Implications for patient choice, decision making, and influence. *Health Communication, 15,* 193-202.

Pancreatic Cancer Action Network. (2003). About the organization. Accessed April 6, 2003, from http://www.pancan. org/1about/pancan.html#bg.

Patient Advocate Foundation. (2003). Patient advocate foundation. Accessed April 6, 2003, from http://www.patientadvocate.org/.

Y-Me (2003). Y-Me milestones. Accessed April 6, 2003, from http://www.y-me.org/about_yme/milestones.php.

III

SELF, IDENTITY, AND SUPPORT

9 | Patient Communication Processes

An Agency–Identity Model For Cancer Care

Melinda Morris Villagran
George Mason University

Laura Jones Fox
Texas State University—San Marcos

H. Dan O'Hair
University of Oklahoma

The diagnosis of cancer is considered to be the one of the most traumatic events that an individual will ever experience (Kahana & Kahana, 2001; Mills & Sullivan, 1999). The affective challenges that cancer victims undergo when they are initially diagnosed are exacerbated as they suddenly face a number of critical decisions with which they have little familiarity (types of treatment, lifestyle changes, etc.). Many newly diagnosed cancer patients immediately begin to assess the nature of their self-identity with analyses ranging from thoughts of biological degradation ("How could my body do this to me?") to destiny ("Will I possibly be able to get through this?") to transformations in self ("Losing my breast to cancer makes me feel that I'm no longer a woman").

Shifts in identity can have particular effects on medical care decision making. Some patients will take on a renewed persona that focuses on goals of remission and becoming cancer-free. Many others become depressed and involve themselves in the care process in a much less assertive manner. The fear, dread, and terror that accompany the diagnostic message are

We gratefully acknowledge Jean Richey for her thoughtful insights on an earlier version of this manuscript.

generated by multiple factors, most importantly those that are (a) situated in conceptions of self and (b) those perceived through interactions with others' social construction of reality. A greater emphasis on communication processes related to cancer care may be a patient's best weapon against the assault on identity that is perpetuated by a cancer diagnosis. Communication becomes more salient as cognitive, affective, and behavioral responses to a cancer diagnosis become additional barriers for the patient to overcome.

THE MANY FACES OF IDENTITY

> Three blind men each feel an elephant and claim that their explanation of the animal is correct. The first blind man, feeling only the elephant's tail, insists the elephant is a rope. The second blind man, feeling only the elephant's trunk, contends that it is a snake. The third blind man, touching a leg, contends that it is a tree. As they argue over whether it is a rope, a snake, or a tree, the elephant walks away. . . . The lesson at hand is that we all need to be mindful when telling each other what we think identity is and how it should be understood. (Cotè & Levine, 2002, pp. 11-12)

Agency is a state of actualization that empowers the individual to have choice, and if desired, exert control over the environment (O'Hair et al., 2003). Structure regulates participation in organizations (Grenier, 1988), such as health care. Although institutions use both structure and agency to sustain themselves (Craib, 1992; Stohl & Cheney, 2001), a continuing issue among some social scientists is the extent to which the power to act within institutions is best explained as a function of social structures on the one hand, or an individual's internal drive on the other. This conflict, termed the *structure–agency debate* (Cotè & Levine, 2002), has important implications for the role of identity in cancer care. Identity plays an indispensable role in the health care of cancer patients (Harwood & Sparks, 2003), and after a cancer diagnosis, the identity of a patient undergoes significant changes based on the patient's own perceived powerfulness, or powerlessness, to participate in subsequent processes of decision making, reconstitution of relationships, and survivorship.

Although psychologists might focus on the cognitive processes involved in dealing with, and managing, a cancer diagnosis, sociologists might prefer to examine the normative health care structures and their effects on patients (Cotè & Levine, 2002). A communication perspective on this issue, however, dictates that agency among cancer patients is realized and negotiated in each interaction (O'Hair et al., 2003). Although the capacity for agency might be a cognitive or structural issue, the enactment of agency only occurs through communication.

Stohl and Cheney (2001) described participation in organizations, such as those that deliver cancer care, as being comprised of both structural and cognitive elements, but rooted firmly in a series of interactions that seek to complete specific goals. Moreover, Stohl and Cheney (2001, p. 369) noted the following:

> Agency entails a sense of being, efficacy, and the feeling that an individual can or does make a difference (Giddens, 1984). Agency captures the notion of the self as originator of action, a source of messages, a force to be reckoned with. In dialectical tension with structure,

agency is one of the central concepts of social theory; its implications for communication are important in that they implicate the ideas of free will and one's capacity to make a difference within a social setting. (Whalen & Cheney, 1991)

An "agentic identity" (Cote & Levine, 2002) is socially constructed through interaction, based on a patient's conceptions of self and the structure of their health delivery options. Each interpersonal relationship, each social and cultural interaction, must be negotiated through communication by the agentic patient. McPhee (1985) described how the "very existence of Structure is dependent on its communication in a formal, explicit, authoritative way . . . " (p. 160). Similarly, agentic identity is only constituted through communication in a manner that empowers the patient to act on his or her own behalf as a co-equal partner in his or her care. Communication is not merely a vehicle for the implementation for agency, but rather the basis of co-creation of an agentic identity after a cancer diagnosis. Agentic patients have the opportunity and responsibility to analyze the context and available options for care, and make decisions that best serve their own heath care needs. Agency, then, opens the door of opportunity for choice within the patient–health care context.

The Hindu folk tale of the elephant serves to underscore the importance of examining the interconnectedness of structure, agency, and identity not just from the standpoint of cognition, or from the standpoint of institutional structure, but rather based on the interactions in which cancer patients derive their new identity. Like the elephant, identity may appear differently based on perspective, and an examination of multiple perspectives helps illuminate the whole picture. The path to cancer survivorship involves agency in every aspect of a patient's life.

AGENCY–IDENTITY THEORY

It is our premise that cancer patients should have maximum opportunity for realizing and executing processes of agency in their cancer care (see O'Hair et al., 2003). Just as the body is physically attacked by cancer and cancer treatments, the self is attacked by a diagnosis of cancer. The assault on identity that is perpetuated by a cancer diagnosis may be combated through concerted actions such as empowerment and advocacy initiatives. Through processes of communication, the need for agency in cancer care moves to the central core of a patient's identity creating a new agentic self. Just as cancer permeates the biological self, agency must permeate all aspects of the socially constructed self. In order to arrive at a place where agency can be maximized, cancer patients must recontextualize their identity as co-equal participants in their own health care. In this process, patients have greater voice in how they choose to experience cancer, how their care will be approached and managed, and how having cancer affects their social and personal relationships.

This approach is partly based on a long tradition of identity research (Berger & Luckmann, 1966; Erikson, 1964; Giddens, 1991; Goffman, 1959; Mead, 1934; Richey, 2003; Richey & Brown, this volume); partly on Stohl and Cheney's (2001) description of participation in organizations, including dimensions of structure, identity, power, and agency; and in part in response to the consumer model of health care that became popular in the late 1960s (Reeder, 1972). Agency in cancer care must be examined as a function of all three of these domains to fully explore the self-identity of the patient and his or her relative ability to navigate changes in identity and perceived power after a diagnosis of cancer. As a patient's new agentic identity emerges, the patient alters the process and becomes a force in his or hers own care and experience of cancer survivorship.

THEORETICAL APPROACHES TO INDIVIDUAL IDENTITY

The long tradition of concern with self and identity began in ancient times with Socrates, Plato, and Aristotle (Gioia, 1998). From that time to the present, scholars from many disciplines have considered the nature of identity and its definition. A general finding of these writings is that identity "constitutes what is somehow core to my being, what comprises the consistently traceable thread that is me over time, and what somehow distinguishes me idiosyncratically from a myriad of other people" (Gioia, 1998, p. 19). Giddens (1991) described identity as "not a distinctive trait, or even collection of traits, possessed by the individual. It is the self as reflexively understood by the person in terms of his or her biography" (p. 53).

Erikson (1963, 1968, 1974, 1975) described identity formation over the life span in terms of three central concerns: ego identity, personal identity, and social identity. *Ego identity* is a perception of sameness and stability within oneself over time (Cotè & Levine, 2002). It includes such concepts as personality, self-concept, cognition, emotion, and behavioral control (Erikson, 1974). *Personal identity* is more of an interpersonal concept, based on experiences, primary relationships, and interactions with others (Cotè & Levine, 2002). Finally, Erikson's notion of *social identity* is the realm of identity that is most impacted by cultural and social norms. Cotè and Levine (2002) stated that this is the level at which institutional interactions are most relevant because of the prescribed nature of power and structure in organization.

Richey (2003) explained that self-identity is comprised of three systems of self that are set in a sociocultural environment. The first system, the *experiential or existential self,* is a state of being including personality and personal experiences. The *relational self* (Gergen, 1991, 1999; Wood, 2000), represents how a person is situated in his or hers various personal relationships (Richey, 2003). The third system of self, the *cultural self,* represents how a person views him or herself based on cultural influences. This aspect of self includes such concepts as gender, race, ethnicity, age, sexuality, ability, and status (Richey, 2003). The interconnectedness of the three systems of self creates a space at the center where an ongoing emergence of the self occurs (Richey, 2003).

Tajfel and Turner's (1986) social identity theory (SIT) proposes that group affiliations affect our identity. SIT maintains that self-identity is comprised of a personal identity and a social identity. Tajfel (1982) stated that *social identity* is "that part of the individual's self-concept which derives from their knowledge of their membership in a *social* group (or groups) together with the value and emotional significance attached to that membership" (p. 2). In this approach personal identity and social identity function together to create an individual's self concept. Moreover, societal perceptions of the groups with which we are affiliated either positively or negatively affect our identity. Table 10.1 offers a sampling of concepts related to the levels of identity.

TABLE 10.1
A Sampling of Concepts Within the Levels of Identity

COMMUNICATION AND AGENCY/IDENTITY	CONCEPTS WITHIN SELF
Intrapersonal aspects of identity	Information processing Decision making Capacity for agency Personality traits Emotional needs Behavioral responses Self-concept
Interpersonal aspects of identity	Family relationships Intimate relationships Friendships Co-worker relationships Computer-mediated support groups Impression management
Sociocultural aspects of identity	Gender Ethnicity Age Sexuality Ability Social status Group affiliation

Adapted from Richey (2003) and Erikson (1969, 1974).

CHRONOLOGY OF EMERGING AGENTIC IDENTITY

From the first moment of diagnosis, cancer patients begin to question their self-concept (Colyer, 1996; Flannigan, 2000; Pedro, 2001), and the anxiety associated with their uncertain future (treatment, suffering, death) becomes a preoccupation. Simultaneously, cancer victims are confronted with the social stigma associated with cancer (Colyer, 1996; Dakof & Taylor, 1990; Flannigan, 2000). The stigma of cancer is perpetuated on cancer victims from both internal forces (their own perception that cancer is malevolent) as well as external cultural norms regarding the indignity of cancer (Pedro, 2001). As self-identity becomes conflicted, and ownership of stigma and emotional suffering interact, cancer patients may go into denial as a means of coping (Gattellari, Butow, Tattersall, Dunn, & MacLeod, 1999). Denial has a tendency then to occlude the relationship between the cancer patient and health care providers (Gattellari et al., 1999).

These psychological and emotional conditions resulting from a cancer diagnosis often produce a state of crisis or "shock," not unlike the feelings associated with cultural shock. Culture shock is the "anxiety that results from losing all of our familiar signs and symbols of social intercourse" (Oberg, 1960, p. 177), and can substantially affect communication competence and produce distorted self-reflections based on interactions with others (Zaharna, 1989). A state of shock has a tendency to cause cancer victims to elevate their level of self-awareness to extreme levels (Adler, 1975). This state of shock also excites the affect system that contributes to cancer victims questioning their own self-concept (Flannigan, 2000).

Identity is additionally affected when emotional processes are heightened. Cancer patients' highly anxious cognitive and affective conditions are further taxed as they deal with a sometimes frustrating and complex health care delivery system. Patients who experience the ill effects of diminished decision-making capacity due to cognitive distractions and emotional stress are disadvantaged in two ways: (a) the capacity to make their own decisions is contaminated, and (b) their ability to objectively judge the validity of the recommendations of health care providers is compromised (O'Hair et al., 2003). Communication processes play an important role during those times that patients must interact with the health care system in order to make essential decisions about their cancer care.

Another factor that suggests the need for greater emphasis on communication processes involves the role of advocacy via the patient's social support network, particularly family members. Similar to the feelings and emotions experienced by patients, family members and significant others are under substantial cognitive and emotional duress, leaving them ill-equipped to assume counseling, decision making, and other support roles for the cancer patient. Family members and significant others who make active attempts at advocacy for the cancer patient have met with varying levels of success (Greene, Hoffman, Charon, & Adelman, 1987; Haug, 1994; Kahana & Kahana, 2001; Spiegel, 1997). Finally, even in the absence of affective arousal, cancer patients face a myriad of contexts, relationships, and ultimately decisions that are likely to create substantial cognitive load and uncertainty (Brashers, 2001; Pedro, 2001).

It is relatively easy to observe the tumultuous journey that cancer patients face on the path to survivorship. Obviously, contexts and decisions become even more salient and acute with rapidly progressing cancers (pancreatic, lymphoma, brain) or those that become metastatic. Communication processes play a central role in unpacking the complexities of identity brought about through the diagnosis of cancer.

FROM VICTIM TO AGENT: THE EMERGING IDENTITY OF THE CANCER PATIENT

After a diagnosis of cancer, previous conceptions of self-identity are transformed as individuals assume new identities as cancer victims, cancer patients, or cancer survivors (Harwood & Sparks, 2003). The cancer patient's reality moves immediately to the *now* (Richey, 2003), as now is the time of choice in terms of self-identity, in terms of care options, in terms of the dynamic process of illness and survivorship. There no longer exists a buffer of time; the now of the lived moment is all the individual has to endorse choice and action in hopes of a positive and healthy outcome. Now is the time for agency.

The lived reality of the cancer patient is determined by whether the patient feels empowered to make decisions in the face of substantial cognitive and emotional strain. Agency enables the cancer patient to act. It offers individuals an opportunity to conceptualize cancer as a process where a strengthened sense of self impacts the whole experience, from diagnosis to survivorship (O'Hair et al., 2003). Agency promotes greater communication between cancer patients and others including family members, support systems, and health care professionals. The use of effective health communication not only supports successful cancer survivorship, it can also improve quality of life throughout the experience (Kreps, 2003). All previous characteristics of identity are transformed in an "agentic" (Cotè & Levine, 2002), empowered manner to deal with the changes in cognition, emotion, relationships, and social and cultural status of the patient. An agentic identity allows the cancer patient maximum participation in their health care. Agentic identity cannot eliminate cancer from a person's life, but it can significantly alter the manner in which a person experiences cancer. Figure 10.1 depicts the postdiagnosis transformation of identity on the biological, intrapersonal, interpersonal, and sociocultural levels.

Biological Aspects of Identity

The influence of cancer on perceptions of identity originates as a biological concern. Biological changes after a cancer diagnosis eliminate a "fixed identity " and require a "robust but dynamic conception of identity that continually adapts to a turbulent environment" (Eisenberg, 2001, p. 539). Biological advantages that were previously taken for granted can no longer be assumed as previous conceptions of self are altered. For example, cancer patients might now actually consider their kidneys, their lymphatic system, or their lack of a second breast or arm as their identity is transformed.

Agentic identity in cancer care begins within what Eisenberg (2001) referred to as the "surround," where the biological self encircles the core identity of a person. An inseparable link between the mind and the body (Lakoff & Johnson, 1999) is especially apparent as the biological reality of cancer impacts the self. Thus, discussions of identity in cancer care must

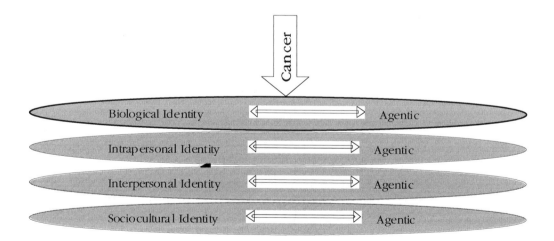

FIGURE 9.1. Model of Agentic Identity Transformation

include a distinct notice of the effects of cancer on biological changes, as for perhaps the first time, a patient's identity is affected by thoughts of previously normative bodily functioning.

Once faced with a cancer diagnosis, seemingly healthy people must contend with the failures of their physical body. Not only does the disease itself create physical changes to patients' bodies, the treatments often leave them feeling weak and vulnerable. For example, anemia is a harrowing side effect associated with chemotherapy, especially in older adults. Anemia is often associated with dramatically decreased energy levels, loss of independence, and a decreased quality of life (Hood, 2003). This diminished capacity, resulting from the actual disease or the treatment options, can leave cancer victims detached from their former identities.

A second example is that of a sudden loss of a limb or body part that can dramatically transform cancer patients' lives and relationships with those close to them. It can be a difficult process for a female breast cancer patient who has had her breast removed to feel attractive and sexually desirable. Cancer patients often find it difficult to cope with altered sexual health (Darrow, Speyer, Marcus, Ter Maat, & Krome, 1998). When this biological norm is disrupted, women may feel less attractive and less feminine, leaving their sexual relationships vulnerable after a mastectomy (Steinberg, Juliano, & Wise, 1985). It has also been reported that such biological changes do alter the victim's sexual relationships, leaving these patients vulnerable and isolated. By approaching the altered cultural norm with a sense of agency, breast cancer survivors are empowered to regain their sense of self through open communication with a partner.

Intrapersonal Aspects of Identity

Intrapersonal aspects of an individual's identity are created over time. Erikson described the "Ego Identity" (Cotè & Levine, 2002, p. 93) as the personal experiences of a person from his or her own perspective. The ego identity encompasses our personality traits associated with agency in behavioral, affective, and cognitive domains (Erikson, 1968, 1974). Erikson's notion of an "identity crisis," which came from victims of World War II, is appropriate when considering the same type of trauma a cancer patient might face (Cotè & Levine, 2002).

Cancer attacks cognition, which creates a sense of disconnect from one's previous conception of self. Early writings on the topic describe this as a distinction between me and I (James, 1948; Mead, 1934), or the "looking-glass self" (Cooley, 1902). Previous perceptions of physicality and consciousness are displaced as cancer assumes a central role in the physical and cognitive self. As the cancer patient's cognitive identity is affected by cancer diagnosis, the capacity for agency becomes reality. The patient's cognitive reality in cancer care moves the need to be an agent for oneself to the central core of self-identity. This process enhances patient's concepts within self, such as capacity for agency, decision making, behavioral responses, emotional needs, information processing, and personality traits.

The capacity for agency becomes a vital aspect of the intrapersonal identity. The self as a once "organized set of cognitive schema" (Cotè & Levine, 2002, p. 21) must be reordered to deal with emotions and behavior focused on objectively assessing the best course of action for care. Being conscious of the ability to take action in all aspects of life allows the patient to feel reconnected with his or her physical and emotional environment, which in turn can lead to greater awareness and adjustment to the illness. The ability to relate to others is negotiated as the agentic identity takes an active role in verbal and nonverbal exchanges regarding the health care and leads to a strengthened self-concept.

As a cancer patient takes on an agentic cognitive identity and becomes responsible for decisions made in treatment, his or her sense of identity is strengthened. Decision making is squarely in the court of cognition. The ability to choose among viable options leads to improved adjustment, attitudes toward the future, beliefs about coping and physical and psychological functioning (Morris & Ingham, 1988). Brody (1980) described how patients with a positive self-concept tend to be more independent, more willing to make assertions about their own goals and expectations, and more willing to articulate their values in clinical decision making.

Behavioral response can also be altered by the cancer experience. A damaged ability to communicate can have harmful affects on the person's sense of identity, leaving the patient at the mercy of health care providers to dictate the next course of action. The agentic patient manages interactions, feels a greater sense of choice within the cancer treatment process, and takes an active role in the treatment process by openly expressing questions, concerns, and preferred treatment options. This allows for more active participation on the part of the patient, which can result in more controlled behavioral responses and a sense of ownership over the disease (McWilliam, Brown, & Stewart, 2000). Creating an agentic identity allows the cancer patient to take control of the relationships in his or her life and can empower and give the patient the strength to focus on goals of remission.

Cancer creates an emotional drain that can potentially lead to withdrawal from social networks. Communication with others becomes restricted as cancer patients turn to concealment in hopes of protecting themselves and others from the emotional suffering (Northouse & Northouse, 1987). Moreover, depression from chronic illness puts extreme strain on cancer patients and their support networks (Dunkel-Schetter & Bennett, 1990). Agency in the cognitive sense, is taking an active role in relating to others the feelings one is having no matter how emotionally draining this process might be.

By taking control of the information processing and re-establishing personality traits, a new agentic identity can allow one to regain the sense of control over life as well as maintain vital relationships with others. Taking control of the intrapersonal aspects of one's being allows further comprehension of what is happening during the cancer process, while helping the patient re-establish the personality that once existed. This will allow for more information sharing and relationship building throughout the cancer treatment, which can result in a greater sense of control and mastery over the illness (McWilliam et al., 2000). As agency moves to the central core of a patient's cognitive identity, greater potentiality for personal growth and development throughout survivorship exists.

Interpersonal Aspects of Identity

Interpersonal identity, which has been depicted as "an interpersonal tool" for understanding self (Baumeister, 1998, p. 700), relates directly to the primary personal relationships in life, such as those experienced in family, intimate friendship, and co-worker relationships. Personal relationships present throughout life are considered a unique joining of two separate entities (Richey, 2003). When cancer diagnosis occurs, the personal relationships in a patient's life become vitally important. However, people who are sick often isolate themselves from others and feel they are unable to pursue normal social relations because of their illness (Cockerham, 2004). Distancing is one of the most common coping mechanisms for cancer patients (Dunkel-Schetter, Feinstein, Taylor, & Falke, 1992). As the cancer diagnosis attacks the interpersonal identity of the patient, the need for agency becomes heightened. Relationships are necessary for the reflection of identity in relation to others and the creation of an agentic identity leads to greater control of those relationships.

Agentic identity can have a positive affect on the interpersonal aspects of a cancer patient's relationships and can lead to greater healthy outcomes and a more positive outlook. By taking the initiative and the decision-making role, the sense of alienation and distancing from the relationships in the patient's life can be minimized (Brody, 1980). When patients are diagnosed with cancer, an interpersonal agentic identity gives them the power to decide when and where, or if, they tell the people in their lives and what type of social support they desire. Agentic identity and social support are dependent on the type of relationships with the patients. Agency is taking an active role in deciding whether and when to tell family, friends, and co-workers about the cancer diagnosis. It also means becoming a co-equal partner in one's health care.

First, an interpersonal agentic identity during the cancer process gives these patients the ability to discuss the disease, treatment, and their emotions with their family. The agentic identity provides patients with the power to choose how they will tell family members, allowing them to be an active participant in the relationship. Supportive communication is an important element that allows cancer patients to adjust to the losses associated with the disease (Robinson & Turner, 2003). By actively seeking this support from family members and taking the lead role in sharing information about the disease with them, the relationship will be strengthened and health benefits will occur.

In some cases, family members and spouses are reluctant to talk about the disease openly leaving potential room for patients to feel isolated. Typically, the initial phase of cancer is the most difficult for families (Northouse & Northouse, 1987). However, with an agentic identity at the core of patients' communicative process, patients can become the leader of the interaction within their interpersonal relationships. This open communication between family members and the cancer patient can lead to lower emotional duress and a greater sense of adjustment for both the patient and the family (Lichtman, Taylor, & Wood, 1987).

Family members also play a vital role in attaining and coping with cancer care. Family represents a social experience that influences how an individual perceives his or her health situation. Prevailing opinion strongly suggests the proper place of external advocacy within the patient–family–significant other subsystem (Lichtman et al., 1987). Beyond the role of external advocate, family members and significant others are eligible candidates for advocacy training and counseling as they become willing to assert rights for the patient and serve as a source of support.

Next, an interpersonal agentic identity allows the patient to take the initiative in the disclosure of information about the disease to friends. By putting the initiative in the hands of the patient, an agentic identity gives the cancer victim a greater sense of ownership and can result in a more positive view of self. Support from friends is closely associated with a patient's adjustment to the disease (Albrecht & Goldsmith, 2003). When a patient takes on the role of agent and becomes responsible for seeking and establishing this source of support from friends, the patient assumes the leadership role for recovery and survivorship. Social support is not only a communication behavior innate in ordinary social structures, it has a profound effect on the physical and mental well-being of cancer patients (Albrecht & Goldsmith, 2003).

The established friendships in a cancer patient's life become vital after initial diagnosis. A health-enhancing social encounter not only functions as a means of helping the patient adjust to cancer, but with the new agentic identity at the core of the patient's communication in interpersonal relationships, it can increase the perception of personal control and the sense of achievement toward improved heath outcomes (Albrecht, Burleson, & Goldsmith, 1994). This type of face-to-face interaction between close friends allows the cancer patient to take control of his or her needs by determining how and when to rely on pre-existing supportive friendships.

Cancer patients might also desire to turn to unfamiliar groups and make "new" friends in their effort to compensate for threats to their self-identity and the stigmas associated with having cancer. Often, the type of social support desired is not the typical face-to-face interaction between existing friends or family members. Computer-mediated communication (CMC) provides a robust arena for social support to gain potential coping strategies related to illness (Wright, 1999). Agentic identity gives cancer patients the control to decide what type of support is appropriate for them and allows them to initiate the action in the most suitable manner. This may result in seeking support and emotional reassurance outside of their pre-existing social networks. Patients might desire to remain anonymous as they express their doubts and fear about cancer.

CMC gives patients independence to reveal their own emotions without being an emotional burden to loved ones and close friends (Robinson & Turner, 2003). A major advantage to computer-mediated support allows patients to participate in supportive communication any time they choose and often times without leaving the comforts of their own home (Weinberg & Schmale, 1996). An agentic interpersonal identity is critical in allowing these patients to seek the social help and reach out to the friends most beneficial to their fight against cancer.

In addition, an interpersonal agentic identity allows cancer patients to approach co-workers and supervisors about their disease in their own time and manner. Sharing information about a potentially life-threatening disease in the workplace can be frightening. Cancer diagnosis is often the beginning of a long period of medical treatments and side effects as well as a great deal of uncertainty in the lives of these patients. By moving agency to the center of one's interpersonal identity, these patients become responsible for who and when they tell members of their work environment about their disease.

Sociocultural Aspects of Identity

Social identity is rooted within a specific cultural belief system and ideology. It is not surprising that an individual's social location often guides the perceptual process or signals the perspective from which one's place in society and the total society is viewed (Cockerham, 2004). The cultural self depicts an aspect of self-identity, which is nurtured, shaped, and influenced by the normative values, social practices, and symbolic interactions that exist within a particular the society (Richey, 2003; Richey & Brown, this volume). Moreover, the individual interpretations of a certain situation can easily be connected to the environment in which the individual is situated. However, culture becomes a defining point of identity based on perceived ability to act within the framework of a specific culture.

The capacity for agency is interpreted partly by how individuals view themselves in relation to the beliefs of their socially constructed culture. After diagnosis, cancer patients directly or indirectly enter a new cultural world of illness. Individuals must deal with the difficulty of resuming normal roles and adjusting their activities and attitudes to such an evasive health disorder (Cockerham, 2004). However, agency can assist patients as they manage to maintain relatively normal patterns of cultural roles in which they define themselves. Normative values embedded in individuals' cultural identity affect their approach to agency in cancer care. A cancer patient's gender, age, ethnicity, and social status may all be approached with a sense of agency.

Gender is an identity-defining, social, and symbolic creation that can be attacked by cancer diagnosis. The meaning of gender is cultivated in social values and beliefs (Wall & Kristjanson, 2005). Cancer diagnosis often disrupts the gender roles society sets out and can damage a patient's identity by threatening to destroy conceptions of male or female roles. Agency gives patients the power to control their own gender identity by giving them the strength to maintain the specific roles personally desired or predetermined by society.

Although feelings of femininity or masculinity can be adversely affected by surgical treatments for cancer such as a mastectomy (Hall, 1997), supportive relationships before and after the cancer episode are strongly associated with positive patient adjustment (Lichtman et al., 1987). A sense of agency can cultivate supportive relationships and lead to greater adjustment and health outcomes. Supportive relationships before and after the cancer episode are strongly associated with positive patient adjustment (Lichtman et al., 1987). A sense of agency can cultivate supportive relationships and lead to greater adjustment and health outcomes.

Second, age plays a large role in how people define themselves and deal with cancer diagnosis. Cancer is a disease that is increasingly affecting an older population. Roughly 55% of cancer cases occur in individuals age 55 or older (Sparks, 2003). The social construction of frailty and aging often lead to diminished views of the value and status of older adults (Taylor, 1994), and the stigma of cancer only adds to this burden.

The older adult with cancer often lacks a great deal of experience with the cancer culture and is at the greatest disadvantage to uncovering the mystery of living with cancer (Sparks, 2003). However, younger, more knowledgeable patients tend to reject the idea of the authoritarian physician and demand a more active role in the decision-making process (Haug & Lavin, 1981). Agency provides all cancer patients, especially older patients, with the ability to increase and control the information-seeking process, allowing them to learn more about cancer and how it affects them and their loved ones.

A cancer patient's sense of agency is enacted through the communicative process and functions to redefine the cultural roles associated with age through increased communication with others, especially physicians and health care providers. Increased communication with loved ones and supportive figures can allow older cancer victims to continue to age successfully.

Next, cancer can disrupt patients' identity in relation to their ethnicity. Ethnicity can impact patients' view of medical institutions and illness and can lead to a negative self-view when diagnosed with cancer. Their behaviors and views of illness and medicine can be directly linked to their social relationships and ethnic orientation (Cockerham, 2004). Research has noted that racial and cultural disparities in access to quality health services exists and contribute to cultural inequalities in health status (LaVeist & Nuru-Jeter, 2002). Agency can give a cancer patient the power to overcome aversions and skepticism of the medical community that are imbedded in the specific ethnic culture.

Finally, the social status of cancer patients affects whether they feel empowered to act as an agent in their own care. Race and ethnicity may interact with poverty to interfere with life opportunities, as racism, discrimination, and prejudice create disparities between people of color and White Americans in terms of economic power, political influence, civil rights, and access to resources (Murry, Smith, & Hill, 2001). Social status is considered the most important overall factor when dealing with quality of health care and has emerged as a determining factor in both providing and receiving medical information (Link & Phelan, 1995). In other words, members of cultural groups who feel powerless in society may also feel powerless in their own health care.

Patients from lower socioeconomic status tend to be more passive in response to health care, whereas middle and upper class patients are more likely to negotiate health care and involve themselves in the decision-making process (Cockerham, 2004). In light of this circumstance, agency is way for cancer patients from all levels of society to take control of their illness. Agency strengthens the communicative process with health care providers and allows patients to take responsibility for information seeking and treatment options. As agents, patients can demand the personal attention and treatment they deserve.

As culture continues to shape the identity of individuals through socially constructed values and beliefs, a sense of agency at the central core of the communicative process can help cancer patients make the adjustment to the unknown cancer culture less difficult. Agency can help cancer patients answer the lingering question of, "Who am I now that I have cancer?" Information seeking can assist patients in the struggle to feel normal again and maintain a positive sense of self (Darrow et al., 1998). Agency gives cancer victims the power to take the information seeking process into their own hands and make positive changes in the way cancer affects their individual roles.

AGENCY–IDENTITY THEORY AND ILLNESS

Although thus far we have discussed agency–identity theory related directly to the cancer context, this approach has utility for all communication related to illness because of the potential damage illness causes to the identity of ill individuals. Even illnesses that may be invisible to the unknowing outsider have the ability to threaten the established identity of people of all ages (Kundrat & Nussbaum, 2003). Illness disrupts and threatens the order and meaning by which people make sense out of their lives (Freund & McGuire, 1999). The overwhelming, uncontrollable, and unpredictable feeling that follows diagnosis of illness often paralyzes people's ability to act and manage their lives in a previously normative manner (Freund & McGuire, 1999). Illness, in this sense, is a peril to an individual's ability to plan for the future and control the activities of daily life.

Responses to illness that affect social identity may include a sense of agency on the part of the ill person. Agency-identity theory suggests that the decision-making process of the intrapersonal, interpersonal, and sociocultural self all benefit from an agency approach to health communication. Because agency in communication translates to an empowered "originator of action, a source of messages" (Stohl & Cheney, 2001, p. 369), acting as an agent or advocate for oneself is useful in every realm of identity. Heightened emotions caused by illness, language choices, and perceptions of physical and cognitive abilities are all areas where agency can take place. Each word choice, each interaction, each relationship can be an opportunity to enact agency-identity. Illness of any kind can create a barrier to agency that must be consciously addressed in all psychosocial decision making.

SUMMARY AND CONCLUSION

Patients' communication processes in the cancer care interaction are impacted by the biological, intrapersonal, interpersonal, and sociocultural levels of identity. Biological changes that occur throughout the cancer diagnosis and treatment process create new challenges for maintaining or redefining conceptions of the biological self. Intrapersonal identity is interlinked with a cancer patient's ability to cope with the shock of identity transformation occurring in response to cancer. Continuity in interpersonal communication in romantic, family, co-worker, and social relationships is achieved through exploration and embodiment of agentic identity. Sociocultural norms prescribe general patterns for the cancer experience, but the agentic identity approach allows for individual decision making in this process.

The agency-identity model for cancer care elevates the patient from a powerless position of *receiving* care, to a more empowered role of active agent in their own care. Although numerous scholars have discussed levels of identity and their potential meanings, the agency-identity approach to cancer care contextualizes the study of identity as a vital part of health communication. Health communication scholars and practitioners interested in a patient-centered approach to care must consider the multidimensional role of agency-identity in every level of the cancer care process.

REFERENCES

Adler, P. (1975). The transnational experience: An alternative view of culture shock. *Journal of Humanistic Psychology, 15*, 13-23.

Albrecht, T. L., Burleson, B. R., & Goldsmith, D. J. (1994). Supportive communication. In M. L. Knapp & G. R. Miller (Eds.), *Handbook of interpersonal communication* (rev. ed., pp. 419-449). Newbury Park, CA: Sage.

Albrecht, T. L., & Goldsmith, D. J. (2003). Social support, social networks, and health. In T. L. Thompson (Ed.), *Handbook of health communication* (pp. 263-284). Mahwah, NJ: Erlbaum.

Baumeister, R. F. (1998). The self. In D. T. Gilbert, S. T. Fiske, & G. Lindzey (Eds.), *The handbook of social psychology* (4th ed., pp. 680-740). New York: McGraw-Hill.

Berger, P.L., & Luckmann, T. (1966). *The social construction of reality: A treatise in the sociology of knowledge*. Garden City, NY: Doubleday.

Brashers, D. E. (2001). Communication and uncertainty management. *Journal of Communication, 51*, 477-497.

Brody, D. S. (1980). The patient's role in clinical decision-making. *Annals of Internal Medicine, 93*, 718-722.

Cockerham, W. C. (2004). *Medical sociology* (9th ed.). Upper Saddle River, NJ: Pearson.

Colyer, H. (1996). Women's experience of living with cancer. *Journal of Advanced Nursing, 23*, 496-501.

Cooley, C. H. (1902). *Human nature and the social order*. New York: Scribner's.

Cotè, J. E., & Levine, C. G. (2002). *Identity formation, agency and culture: A social psychological synthesis*. Mahwah, NJ: Erlbaum.

Craib, K.J. (1992). *Modern social theory; From Parsons to Habermas*. London: Prentice-Hall.

Dakof, G., & Taylor, S. (1990). Victim's perception of social support. What is helpful and from whom? *Journal of Personality and Social Psychology, 58*, 80-89.

Darrow, S. L., Speyer, J., Marcus, A. C., Ter Maat, J., & Krome, D. (1998). Coping with cancer: The impact of the cancer information service on patients and significant others. *Journal of Health Communication, 3*, 86-96.

Duck, S. (1994). *Meaningful relationships: Talking, sense, and relating*. Thousand Oaks, CA: Sage.

Dunkel-Schetter, C., & Bennett, T. L. (1990). Differentiating the cognitive and behavioral aspects of social support. In B. R. Sarason, I. G. Sarason, & G. R. Pierce (Eds.), *Social support: An interactional view*. New York: Wiley.

Dunkel-Schetter, C., Feinstein, L. G., Taylor, S. E., & Falke, R. L. (1992). Patterns of coping with cancer. *Health Psychology, 11*, 79-87.

Dunphy, J. E. (1976). Annual discourse: On caring for the patient with cancer. *New England Journal of Medicine, 295*, 313-319.

Eisenberg, E. M. (2001) Building a mystery: Toward a new theory of communication and identity. *Journal of Communication, 51*, 534-552.

Erikson, E. H. (1963). *Childhood and society* (2nd ed.). New York: Norton.

Erikson, E. H. (1964). *Insight and responsibility*. New York: Norton.

Erikson, E. H. (1968). *Identity: Youth and crisis*. New York: Norton.

Erikson, E. H. (1969). *Ghandi's truth*. New York: Norton.

Erikson, E. H. (1974). *Dimensions of a new identity*. New York: Norton.

Erikson, E. H. (1975). *Life history and the historical moment*. New York: Norton.

Flannigan, J. (2000). Social perceptions of cancer and their impacts: Implications for nursing practice arising from the literature. *Journal of Advanced Nursing, 32*, 740-749.

Freund, P. E., & McGuire, M. B. (1999). *Health, illness, and the social body* (3rd ed.). Englewood Cliffs, NJ: Prentice-Hall.

Gattellari, M., Butow, P. N., Tattersall, M. H., Dunn, S. M., MacLeod, C. A. (1999). Misunderstanding in cancer patients: Why shoot the messenger? *Annals of Oncology, 10*, 39-46.

Gergen, K. J. (1991). *The saturated self: Dilemmas of identity in contemporary life*. New York: Basic Books.

Gergen, K. J. (1999). *An invitation to social construction*. Thousand Oaks, CA: Sage.

Giddens, A. (1984). *The constitution of society*. Berkeley: University of California Press.

Giddens, A. (1991). *Modernity and self-identity: Self and society in the late modern stage*. Stanford, CA: Stanford University Press.

Gioia, D. (1998). From individual to organizational identity. In D. A. Whetton & P.C. Godfrey (Eds.), *Identity in organizations: Building theory through conversations* (pp. 17-31). Thousand Oaks, CA: Sage

Goffman, E. (1959). *The presentation of self in everyday life*. Garden City, NY: Doubleday.

Greene, M. G., Hoffman, S. S., Charon, R., & Adelman, R. (1987). Psychosocial concerns in the medical encounter: A comparison of the interactions of doctors with their old and young patients. *The Gerontologist, 27*, 164-168.

Grenier, G. (1988). *Inhuman relations: Quality circles and anti-unionism in American industry*. Philadelphia, PA: Temple University Press.

Hall, L. (1997). Re-figuring marked bodies on the borders: Breast cancer and femininity. *International Journal of Sexuality and Gender Studies, 2*, 101-121.

Harwood, J., & Sparks, L. (2003). Social identity and health: An intergroup communication approach to cancer. *Health Communication, 15*, 145-160.

Haug, M., & Lavin, B. (1981). Practitioner or patient—who's in charge? *Journal of Health and Social Behavior, 22*, 212-229.

Haug, M. E. (1994). Elderly patients, caregivers, and physicians: Theory and research on health care triads. *Journal of Health and Social Behavior, 35*, 1-12.

Hood, L. E. (2003). Chemotherapy in the elderly: Supportive measures for chemotherapy-induced myelotoxicity. *Clinical Journal of Oncology Nursing, 7*, 185-191.

James, W. (1948). *Psychology*. Cleveland, OH: World Publishing.

Kahana, E., & Kahana, B. (2001). *Health care partnership model of doctor-patient communication in cancer prevention and care among the aged*. Paper presented at the Consumer/Provider Research Symposium, Health Communication and Informatics Research Branch, Behavioral Research

Program, Division of Cancer Control and Population Sciences, National Cancer Institute, Bethesda, MD.

Kreps, G. L. (2003). The impact of communication on cancer risk, incidence, morbidity, mortality, and quality of life. *Heath Communication, 15,* 161-169.

Kundrat, A. L., & Nussbaum, J. F. (2003). The impact of invisible illness on identity and contextual age across the life span. *Health Communication, 15,* 331-366.

Lakoff, G., & Johnson, M. (1999). *Philosophy in the flesh: The embodied mind and its challenge to Western thought.* New York: Basic Books.

LaVeist, T. A., & Nuru-Jeter, A. (2002). Is doctor-patient race concordance associated with greater satisfaction with care? *Journal of Health and Social Behavior, 43,* 296-306.

Lichtman, R. R., Taylor, S. E., & Wood, J. V. (1987). Social support and marital adjustment after breast cancer. *Journal of Psychosocial Oncology, 5,* 47-74.

Link, B. G. & Phelan, J. (1995). Social conditions as fundamental causes of disease. In W. C. Cockerham & M. Glasser (Eds.), *Readings in medical sociology* (2nd ed., pp. 3-17). Upper Saddle River, NJ: Prentice-Hall.

McPhee, R. D. (1985) Formal structure and organizational communication. In R. D. McPhee & P. K. Tompkins (Eds.), *Organizational communication: Traditional themes and new directions* (pp. 149-178). Thousand Oaks, CA: Sage.

McWilliam, C.L., Brown, J. B., & Stewart, M. (2000). Breast cancer patients' experiences of patient–doctor communication: A working relationship. *Patient Education and Counseling, 39,* 191-204.

Mead, G. H. (1934). *Mind, self and society from the standpoint of a social behaviorist.* Chicago: The University of Chicago Press.

Mills, M. E., & Sullivan, K. (1999). The importance of information giving for patients newly diagnosed with cancer: A review of the literature. *Journal of Clinical Nursing, 8,* 631-642.

Morris, J., & Ingham, R. (1988). Choice of surgery for early breast cancer: Psychosocial considerations. *Social Science and Medicine, 27,* 1257-1262.

Murry, V. M., Smith, E. P., & Hill, N. E. (2001). Race, ethnicity, and culture in studies of families in context. *Journal of Marriage & the Family, 63,* 911-115.

Northouse, P.G., & Northouse, L.L. (1987). Communication and cancer: Issues confronting patients, health professionals, and family members. *Journal of Psychosocial Oncology, 5*(3), 17-46.

Oberg, K. (1960). Cultural shock: Adjustment to new cultural environments. *Practical Anthropology, 7,* 170-179.

O'Hair, D., Villagran, M. M., Wittenberg, E., Brown, K., Ferguson, M., Hall, H. T., & Doty, T. (2003). Cancer survivorship and agency model: Implications for patient choice, decision making, and influence. *Health Communication, 15,* 193-202.

Pedro, L. W. (2001). Quality of life for long-term survivors of cancer: Influencing variables. *Cancer Nursing, 24,* 1-11.

Reeder, L. G. (1972). The patient–client as a consumer: Some observations on the changing professional–client relationship. *Journal of Health and Social Behavior, 13,* 406-412.

Richey, J. A. (2003). Women in Alaska constructing the recovered self: A narrative approach to understanding long-term recovery from alcohol dependence and/or abuse. Unpublished doctoral dissertation, University of Alaska, Fairbanks.

Robinson, J. D., & Turner, J. (2003). Impersonal, interpersonal, and hyperpersonal social support: Cancer and older adults. *Health Communication, 15,* 227-234.

Sparks, L. (2003). An introduction to cancer communication and aging: Theoretical and research insights. *Health Communication, 15,* 123-131.

Spiegel, D. (1997). Psychosocial aspects of breast cancer treatment. *Seminars in Oncology, 24,* S1-36-S1-47.

Steinberg, M. D., Juliano, M. A., & Wise, L. (1985). Psychological outcome of lumpectomy versus mastectomy in the treatment of breast cancer. *American Journal of Psychiatry, 142,* 34-39.

Stohl, C., & Cheney, G. (2001). Participatory processes/paradoxical practices: Communication and the dilemmas of organizational democracy. *Management Communication Quarterly, 14,* 349-407.

Tajfel, H. (1982). *Social identity and intergroup relations.* New York: Cambridge University Press.

Taijel, H., & Turner, J. C. (1986). The social identity theory of intergroup behavior. In S. Worchel & W. G. Austin (Eds.), *Psychology of intergroup relations* (pp. 7-24). Chicago: Nelson-Hall.

Taylor, B. (1994). Frailty, language, and elderly identity: Interpretive and critical perspectives on the aging subject. In M. L. Hummert, J. M. Wiemann, & J. F. Nussbaum (Eds.), *Interpersonal communication in older adulthood: Interdisciplinary theory and research* (pp. 185-208). Thousand Oaks, CA: Sage.

Wall, D., & Kristjanson, L. (2005). Men, culture and hegemonic masculinity: Understanding the experience of prostate cancer. *Nursing Inquiry, 12,* 87-97.

Weinberg, N., & Schmale, J. (1996). Online help: Cancer patients participate in a computer-mediated support group. *Health & Social Work, 21,* 24-32.

Whalen, S., & Cheney, G. (1991). Contemporary social theory and its implications for rhetorical and communication theory. *Quarterly Journal of Speech, 77,* 467-479.

Wood, J. T. (2000). *Relational communication: Continuity and change in personal relationships* (2nd ed.). Belmont, CA: Wadsworth.

Wright, K. B. (1999). Computer-mediated support groups: An examination of relationships among social-support, perceived stress, and coping strategies. *Communication Quarterly, 47,* 402-414.

Zaharna, R. (1989). Self-shock: The double-binding challenge of identity. *International Journal of Intercultural Relations, 13,* 501-525.

10 Cancer, Communication, and The Social Construction Of Self

Modeling the Construction Of Self in Survivorship

Jean Richey
University of Alaska Southeast

Jin Brown
University of Alaska Fairbanks

Recent years of health communication scholarship have demonstrated emphatically that communication is of central significance to the cancer patient in a variety of ways. The National Cancer Institute (2001) states that: "Communication is central to effective, quality cancer care, from primary prevention to survivorship and end of life issues" (p. 1). The quality of the interaction between physician and patient impacts compliance as well as recovery from both diagnosis and treatment (Anderson & Urban, 1999; Gattellari, Butow, & Tattersall, 2001; Krupat et al. 2000, Mishel, 1999). Interaction between the cancer patient and her or his primary caregivers is a determinant of the quality of life experienced by the patient whether the disease is life-threatening or surmountable (Anderson & Urban, 1999; Bakker, Fitch, Gray, Reed, & Bennett, 2001; Jenkins, Fallowfield, & Saul, 2001; Roberts, Cox, Reintgen, Baile, & Gibertini, 1994). Yet, for all the many communication studies that address these important interactions, there is little consideration of the person with cancer as a growing experience of the life world. Ultimately, the decisions that make a patient a survivor or a victim, a fighter or one who relinquishes the necessary hope, while influenced by physician interaction, are produced by choices of the patient. Studies are continually being done to explain the cancer patient overcoming the fears and hardships of experiencing the disease (Deadman, Leinster,

Owens, Dewey, & Slade, 2001; Maguire, 1999; Siminoff, Ravdin, Colabianchi, & Saunders-Sturm, 2000); yet communication scholarship is just beginning to address matters of self and identity in understanding these experiences.

One way of addressing concepts related to the person experiencing cancer is to consider the matter of survivorship. Chapter 9 (this volume) suggests that the matter of "agency" may be cultivated and/or enhanced in the cancer patient by offering the patient the most timely and significant information and access to the best options so that the individual experiencing cancer will be able to make the most optimal choices for surviving. The matter of agency in this conception, as in most traditional social science models, focuses on a psychological view of the self as an individual; as a compendium of state and/or trait structure, with a "will" or an agentive ability existing on a range of possibility. Agency, then, as an orchestration around the cancer patient, offers the potential of strengthening the patient's will making the best choices for survival.

This view of self incorporates our generally accepted social scientific and cultural assumptions. If, however, we consider setting aside the monolithic structure of psychological individualism that has guided Western concepts of self over the last millennium, there exists another perspective from which to base knowledge production about the self. Much has already been written taking the view that the self is a social construction (Gergen, 1991, 1994a, 2001; Harré, 1995, 2002a, Harré & Gillett, 1994). This perspective requires that the central disciplinary approach must necessarily be communication in that social construction claims human realities are created, maintained, and transformed in communication (Deetz, 1982). We learn all that we learn in regard to our embodied presence in the world in relational contact (Gergen, 1994b; Gergen & Gergen, 1993). Simply, from this view, the self is essentially a social entity.

The social constructionist movement in sociology, psychology, and communication has provided a frame of conceptualization that has been usefully extended to incorporate all of what we have called human science into the epistemology of constructionism (Crotty, 1998). Although the grounds for discussing the self as a product of social construction are well established, it is a useful exercise in discussing the lived experience of the cancer patient, to provide a model, that can specify the process as systematic. Establishing a model of the social construction of self can lead to further research in understanding the relationship between a patient's ongoing interpretation of self and the lived experience of diagnosis and life with cancer.

The model of self in lived experience offered here (Richey, 2003) was developed in graduate classes and research to address recovery from addiction. Locating meaning as the product of interpreted experience, created in communicative social interaction, provides a basis for discussing a socially constructed self, emergent within a constitutive framework of intersubjectivity (Deetz, 1982; Gergen, 1994b). The notion of intersubjectivity, of intersubjective interpretations, grounds lived experience within networks of social relationships and existing cultural perspectives or standpoints. The model of the emergent self attempts to conceptualize the foundational process of social self-construction, wherein the development of self and one's continuous restructuring (reconstruction) as a self are contextually embedded in the ongoing, shared locus of lived communicative experience. As a matter of course, any contextualization of self, we believe, can be explored within the framework of choice that is the ongoing creation of the emergent self.

If we take self to be a first product of interpretative processes (Neisser, 1976), a first result of socially constructing the meanings (interpretations) in which we live, we accept an understanding that centralizes the person as a composite individuation of his or her lived experience, which is necessarily at once social experience, and cultural experience. This emergent production of self is conceived in the model as always being in a state of becoming. Human life, that is, takes place at the nexus of being and becoming with choice as both the nature and the impetus of the process. We move, moment to moment, through the results of choices we just made as well as choices we have made often enough to be perceived as giving stability to products of our decision making. Human beings experience life as coherent even given the recognizable potential for momentary revolution. The self is one reality; one product of our ongoing, communicative social construction activities.

If communication is the alembic in which human realities are continuously formed and reformed, then self is a product of social interaction, contextually constituted within an intersubjective framework of communication. Another way of stating this is that communication is fundamental to the developmental process of the emergent self in that it is constitutive of the self. There seems here an essential consonance between this view and the use of the concept of "agency" as defined by O'Hair et al. (2003) within an "organizational model of patient communication." In the Cancer Survivorship and Agency Model (CSAM), agency is viewed within an essentially mixed frame of psychological and social concepts. The perspective of constructionist science both clarifies the concept of agency and eliminates the confusion of mixing psychological and sociological views. Taken as a discursive construct, agency considers the social grounding of advocacy and empowerment, as outlined in the CSAM, and subsumes the individuation of the concepts of uncertainty and problem integration into discursive processes, rejecting the psychological ground in the sense advocated by Gergen (1994b, 1999, 2001), Harré (1995, 2000, 2002a), and Harré and Gillett (1994).

A COMMUNICATION MODEL: THE SOCIAL CONSTRUCTION OF THE EMERGENT SELF AS AGENT IN RECOVERY

The ongoing, interactive human social process of communication occurs at the dynamic intersections between one's experience of self, one's social interactions, and one's situated cultural identity. The premise of this perspective suggests that the becoming *self* emerges continuously and contextually, over time, within an ongoing sociocultural environment through the intersubjective interpretive framework of self as being. The self here is conceived as an ongoing process of social construction (Edwards, 1997; Gergen, 1991, 1994d, 1999, 2001; Gergen & Gergen, 1993; Harré, 1983, 1989, 2000, 2002a; Harré & Gillett, 1994; Lorber, 1997; McLeod, 1997; McNamee & Gergen, 1999).

The model suggested in Fig. 10.1 is comprised of three interwoven systems of self, which are embedded in a physical and sociocultural matrix: (a) the *experiential or existential self* (i.e., the self we take into any interactive moment), (b) the *relational self* (the aspects of the experiential self that reflect prior, *in situ* decision-making products of communicative action), and (c) the *cultural self* (the aspects of one's experiential self that reflect broader, contextual decision making and its products). One's personal experience of embodiment and capacity for the construction of personality and sociality through one's shared cultural symbolicity, and the ability to act on choices constitute the *experiential self*—a radically transient state of being in the world.

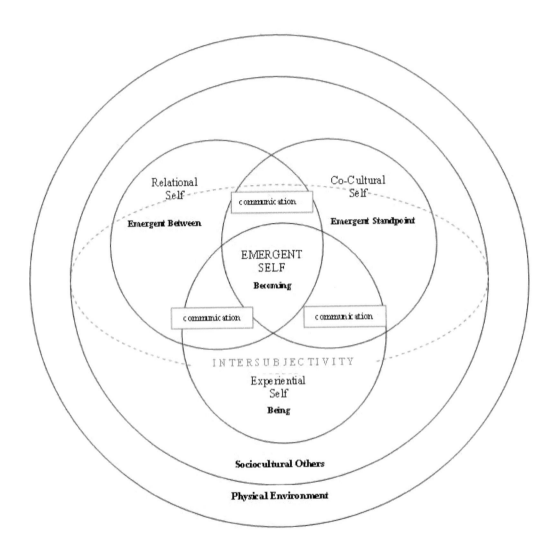

FIGURE 10.1. Modeling the social construction of the emergent self.

The second system of self, the *relational self* (Gergen, 1991, 1994b, 1999; Wood, 2000), represents how we experience ourselves enmeshed in our various personal relationships. The third system of self, the *cultural self*, represents knowledge of self in the context of one's sociocultural perspectives or our experienced standpoints (Hartsock, 1997a, 1997b; Kramarae, 1981, 1996; Orbe, 1998; Stoetzler & Yuval-Davis, 2002; Wood, 1996b), which include contexts such as gender, race, ethnicity, age, sexuality, ability, and status. The overlapping or interconnectedness of the three systems of the model creates a space at the center for an ongoing emergence of the self in the moment or in the *now* of that lived moment, which can be considered as the human condition: *being in a state of continuous becoming*.

The matter of focusing on the experiential *now* is clarified by framing the concept in a social interaction (e.g., health behavior) perspective because the present moment, with others either physically or cognitively present, is the only place where choice and action can be enjoined for potential change. As Simmel (1950) noted, interaction is the place where "being and conceiving make their mysterious unity empirically felt" (p. 309). The communication that occurs at all conjunctures within the system of the emergent self as well as between self and sociocultural others is the process by which humans construct and share intersubjective meaning and co-construct lived realities. Intersubjectivity grounds the whole human interactive system, integrating aspects of the three main dimensions of the conscious self. Thus, communication, as the alembic in which the experiential self participates in acts of symbolicity and thereby transmutes itself, according to context and the significances noted in the participation of the relational and sociocultural dimensions of self, intersubjectively conceived, incorporates the potential of integrating advocacy and manifesting empowerment. A model of a human system without this ability to reconstruct self in intersubjective discourse is inconceivable.

To conceive the human condition as one of intersubjective embodiment allows the concepts of uncertainty and problematic integration to become less nebulous and to ground them in the constitutive locus of becoming as a socially constructing process. Outside of our own experience, that is, cancer and its diagnosis remains a cultural and relational experience. When one must reconstruct self as the person having cancer, all such relational and cultural information with which previous, less involved selves were constructed necessarily undergo significant transformation. When embodiment is thus radically altered, the embodied self, too, must radically change. "Cancer as a wake-up call" is how one research respondent perceives it (Gibbs & Franks, 2002, p. 158). Choosing from potential courses of action and possible conceptions of self becomes a radically conscious process. Health empowerment, for instance, is transformed from social potential (a matter in which others attempt to clear the way for a positive construction; a positive future of the patient) to a radically constructive choice. One cannot be empowered by others, but one can choose to engage in the discursive interaction that opens empowered decision making; that constructs an empowered self. Advocacy too is a social choice intended to allow the person experiencing cancer to participate in a reconstituting dialogue. In both cases, the self that emerges from diagnostic and postdiagnostic discourse is a product of choices made from moment to moment by the person experiencing cancer in co-construction of the socially shared realities of the disease with health care personnel and immediate relational others.

Agency, then, as Harré (1995) made clear, is not a psychological concept connected to some abstract designation such as "will power." One cannot "not" have agency so defined. Agency must be understood as an ongoing product of communication between the person with cancer and her or his immediate social and medical relationships in light of chronologically earlier cultural and relational "selves" constructed in interaction regarding the nature of "having" cancer. Our ability to act as a self with cancer will be understood by both self and other as a product of choice. The association of cancer and death in our culture can mean that our choice will be to become a self "dying of cancer." Conversely, the plethora of examples of persons surviving and leading productive lives can mean that our choice will be to construct self, to act, as a survivor. Or we can choose to be "recovering" from cancer. Importantly, as a discipline, Communication must understand how such choices are made by the afflicted in order to teach the path toward fostering the most positive choices for self and other in constitutive processes.

THE MODEL'S THEORETICAL UNDERPINNINGS:
THE SOCIAL CONSTRUCTION OF REALITY

The theory of the social construction of reality (Berger & Luckmann, 1966; Bradley & Morss, 2002; Burr, 1995; Crotty, 1998; Gergen, 1994a, 1994b, 1999, 2001; Harré, 1989, 2000, 2002a, 2002b; Harré & Gillett, 1994; Pearce, 1995; Shotter, 1991, 1993; Shotter & Lannamann, 2002) is foundational to the processes described in the Emergent Self Model. In the first part of the 20th century, G. H. Mead began an academic dialogue regarding a social construal of the self. He referred to a significant aspect of personhood as a "social self" (Mead, 1934, 1968, 1982). Mead (1982) suggested that in the process of perception a person "addresses himself [*sic*] and thus becomes an object to himself [sic]. . . . The identification takes place in the social process out of which mind arises" (p. 187). Mead's notion of the self as a social entity hints at an emergent process of self in that a person involved in social interaction "becomes a self . . . who organizes his [*sic*] response by the tendencies on the part of others to respond to his [sic] act" (1968, p. 57). As Blumer (2004) made evident, Mead was troubled that in scientific discourse, "interaction is still treated as a medium in which the combined psychological and sociological factors, whatever the combination may be, operate to determine and account for what takes place in interaction" (p. 32). The centralization of communication in social construction theory corrects for this earlier disciplinary confusion.

Berger and Luckmann (1966) extended both social phenomenology and Mead's conversation regarding the social creation of self in their seminal work, *The Social Construction of Reality: A Treatise in the Sociology of Knowledge*, in which they stated:

> Identity is . . . a key element of subjective reality, and . . . stands in a dialectical relationship with society. Social processes form identity. Once crystallized, it is maintained, modified, or even reshaped by social relations. The social processes involved in both the formation and the maintenance of identity are determined by the social structure. Conversely, the identities produced by the interplay of organism, individual consciousness and social structure react upon the given social structure, maintaining it, modifying it, or even reshaping it. Societies have histories in the course of which specific identities emerge; these histories are, however, made by men [*sic*] with specific identities. (p. 173)

A reciprocal process of social and personal creation and action intrinsically related to identity formation, in a more contemporary form, continues to be a key concept in social constructionism. Gergen (1999) referred to the process of reality creation as a "communal construction" (p. 33), which suggests four underlying assumptions inherent in its structure:

1. For any state of affairs a potentially unlimited number of descriptions and explanations [interpretations] is possible.
2. Our models of description, explanation, and/or representation are derived from relationship . . . meanings are born of coordinations among persons— agreements, negotiations . . . from this standpoint, relationships stand prior to all that is intelligible.
3. As we describe, explain, or otherwise represent, so we do fashion our future . . . as our practices of language are bound within relationships, so are rela-

tionships bound within broader patterns of practice – rituals, traditions, "forms of life" . . . In a broad sense, language [symbolic interaction] is a major ingredient of our worlds of action; it constitutes social life itself.
4. Reflection on our forms of understanding is vital to our future well being. (pp. 47-49)

Gergen (1994b) centralized the notion of relationships as primary to all human development. The study of human meaning originates in "human relationship . . . it is not the individual who pre-exists the relationship and initiates the process of communication, but the conventions of relationship that enable understandings to be achieved" (p. 263). In this sense, a process of the emergent self was conceived as a template to understanding how the convergence of society, culture, and the individual create the self and how the self continuously recreates itself through interpretation in interaction with sociocultural others.

Social and human researchers have eloquently stated the case for relational and social constructionism as the premise for human reality creation and maintenance (Berger & Luckmann, 1966; Gergen, 1994a, 1994b, 1999, 2001; Schutz & Luckmann, 1973; Shotter, 1991, 1993; Shotter & Lannamann, 2002). The theoretical perspective of social constructionism locates human communication in *relationship* as the process by which human meaning is established, maintained, and changed over time. As phenomenologists have made evident (e.g., Pilotta & Mickunas, 1990), human communication is an intersubjective process. Schutz & Luckmann (1973) posit that human realities are constituted "in the world of everyday life . . . [in] a common, communicative, surrounding world . . . , [which] from the outset, my life-world [and the life-world of others] are not . . . private worlds, but, rather, are intersubjective; the fundamental structure of . . . [human] reality is that it is shared by us" (p. 4). The creation of shared, intersubjective meaning originating in human relationships is, thus, the central process in identity formation, maintenance, and change. Deetz (1982), in moving toward a clarification of the social nature of the self, says candidly, "subjectivity *is* intersubjectivity" (p. 8).

CO-CONSTRUCTION OF IDENTITY

Identity creation or the development of self is a socially co-constructed process, which emerges through human communication in a relational and social matrix. Interpersonal interaction is the arena where "reality construction, confirmation, and transformation [originate] . . . [it] . . . has a special residual capacity to support the individual and maintain identity and meaning" (Deetz, 1982, p. 2). Harré (1983) suggested that one's self-identity is temporally located within an ongoing "autobiography" (p. 31) and that one's stories of self are situated in a social environment. He continues his discussion of self-identity creation in stating, "personal identity depends upon a socially enforced theory of self by which a human being conceives a continuous coordination of point of view and point of action within the general spatio-temporal system of material beings including other people" (p. 41). Harré's notion of an ongoing autobiography corresponds to a continuous formulation of an emergent self, contextualized by relational interaction. According to Carbaugh (1996), the emergent self "is not a given in nature, but is a consequence of discursive and interactive life" (p.

6). Gergen (1994) framed relational interaction as constitutive of people's formulations of reality:

> The terms and forms by which we achieve understanding of the world and ourselves are social artifacts, products of *historically and culturally situated interchanges* among people. For constructionists, descriptions and explanations are neither driven by the world as it is, nor are they the inexorable outcome of genetic or structural propensities within the individual. Rather, they are the result of human coordination and action . . . to achieve intelligibility is to participate in a reiterative pattern of relationship, or if sufficiently extended, a tradition. It is only by virtue of sustaining some form of past relationship that we can make sense at all. (p. 49; italics added)

Jacoby and Ochs (1995) grounded identity formation in co-constructive social interaction by suggesting that there is an "interactional basis of the human construction of meaning, context, activity, and identity" (p. 175). A co-constructionist approach to human reality and the development of identity, therefore, relies on an intersubjective, dynamic process of meaning-making. Self-identity, conceptualized in a co-constructive interpretive framework, suggests that any conceptualization of self cannot be separated from relational contexts.

UNPACKING ASPECTS
OF THE EMERGENT SELF MODEL

The model of the social construction of the emergent self (Fig.10.1) is depicted in part as concentric circles representing specific human systems embedded within a cultural context in the natural world. The world of others—sociocultural others—is a continuum of co-cultural others (including cultural insiders and cultural outsiders). The model graphically represents the process of social construction regarding how each person is situated in a natural and social world. Eisenberg (2001) referred to the material and social external world of a person as the "surround" (p. 543). His perspective of the surround includes categories of human activity such as spirituality, economics, cultural values, societal rules, interpersonal values and behavior, and "biological . . . patterns that shape human development" (p. 543). The concentric circle labeled "*sociocultural others*" in the emergent self model implies a similar conceptualization of the experiential world as the surround in Eisenberg's model of the "identity process" (p. 543).

Intersubjectivity, which pervades the human interactive system, is shown in (Fig. 10.1) as an additional plane, but understood to be permeating all sociocultural activity and human meaning. A specific context of self interpretation can be overlaid onto the model, such as disease (its use here) or substance abuse (Richey, 2003), which reveals, within the emergent self-system, the constitutive, co-constructive processes established within that context through personal, social, and cultural communication. A general discussion of the components of the systems of the emergent self must be explicated first before an actual health behavior context is introduced for discussion.

FIRST SYSTEM OF THE EMERGENT SELF:
THE EXPERIENTIAL SELF AS EMBODIMENT

The originating place of self is one's experience of being in the world. We are all born "into a social world with pre-existing languages, relationships, social networks, and culturally pre-scribed patterns of behavior" (Eisenberg, 2001, p. 543). In the emergent self model, the system of self is referred to as the *experiential or existential self*. The following concepts are sub-sumed within the experiential self: (a) embodiment—consciousness of and through one's physicality and presence in the natural world, (b) agency—consciousness of one's power to choose (*interpret*) among possibilities and to act on one's choices in the world, (c) symbolicity—capacity for and reliance on symbolic interaction; language and nonverbal communication, (d) personality—capacity for the development of personal affect and behavior over time, and (e) sociality— capacity for and inclination toward relating to others. These aspects of the experiential self are individual potentialities, malleable, and developed discursively over time, tempered by the unique quality of one's ongoing physical and cognitive abilities and relationships.

Traditional concepts of a person according to Western belief systems suggest, in a Cartesian framework, that the sensory body and consciousness are somehow separate forms. Mellor and Shilling (1997) stated in their discussion of the "sensory body . . . that people's knowledge of themselves, others, and the world around them are . . . shaped by their senses . . . humans are not disembodied rationalist beings, but acquire information through their bodies" (p. 5). Lakoff and Johnson (1999), who thoroughly analyzed a new philosophy of embodiment, supported the latter view of consciousness as an aspect of embodiment because human beings "conceptualize only through the body . . . the mind is not separate from or inde-pendent of the body" (p. 555). In this sense, individual consciousness is understood as a part of a person's embodied experiential knowledge.

The concept of agency here is subsumed within the experiential self as one's ability to exercise volition in interpreting self in the world of human interaction. In discussing Mead's view as a rejection of both a psychological and a sociological explanation, Blumer (2004) stat-ed that: "To view the human act as a product of an initiating agent is to strip the self from the human being as an actor and to exclude the role of the self-process in the formation of the human act" (p. 82). This notion of agency is an integral aspect of symbolic interactionism (Mead, 1932, 1968). People, in this view, are active interpreters who choose in making deci-sions. Furthermore, human beings take communicative action interpersonally based upon their personal, experiential, yet intersubjective interpretations of their shared worlds and their interactions with others (Blumer, 2004; Lal, 1995, p. 422). According to Bandura (2001), the psychological notion of agency "refers to acts done intentionally" (p. 6). Bandura's psycho-logical concept of human agency involves intentionality, forethought, self-reactiveness, and self-reflectiveness [reflexivity] (pp. 4-11). Self-regulation and self-efficacy, which are impor-tant aspects of a psychological construal of health behavior change, are subsumed within Bandura's perspective of personal agency and the human ability to practice self-reflexivity [reflexivity] (p. 10). Intentionality, as part of the notion of human agency, refers to anticipa-tion, "what [it] . . . brings to the fore is interaction between subject and object. . . It is in and out of this interplay that meaning is born" (Crotty, 1998, p. 45). As agents in our own expe-rience, we create, maintain, and transform our realities and our selves in communicative, interpretive interaction. A capacity for symbolicity, personality, and sociality are human potentialities that develop in interaction, over time, through experience within a shared soci-ocultural environment.

SECOND SYSTEM OF THE EMERGENT SELF: THE RELATIONAL SELF

The *relational self* is the second dimension of this model of self. The communicative relation-ships referenced in the relational self, while understood to be a range, are primarily signifi-cant personal relationships such as experienced in family, intimacy, friendships, and cowork-er relationships. However, a person can develop interpretive perspectives in communication with fictitious people, such as characters in books and movies, or with public personalities beyond our interactive space. A conceptualization of the relational self encompasses the notion that every personal relationship (distinct from uneventful, casual, or one-time encounters with others) with another human being is a unique, communicative joining together of two separate entities. The other, in regard to the self, is an ongoing composite of interpretive reflection distinct to that particular relationship. As a result, the existential self is redefined and renegotiated within each separate relationship, becoming a self—saturated with other selves (Gergen, 1991). *Relational culture* is a term used here to describe this aspect of relationship as "an extensive set of definitions, values, and rules which comprise a unique-to-the-relationship world order" (Wood, 1996a, p. 13). Wood explained that the self in rela-tionship "becomes a substantially different self than the one existing prior to the relation-ship" (p. 14). Duck (1994) extended this notion in *Meaningful Relationships: Talking, Sense, and Relating*, when he stated "relationship brings together two previously independent beings and, by connecting them, creates something new from their sharing—something that presumably feeds back into each individual and affects the ways in which each thinks about [self and] the other in the future" (p. 17). The relational self is that dimension of self-defini-tion that evolves and shifts through constant interpretation in regard to each personal rela-tionship experienced.

The idea of the emergent "between" was initiated into the relational dialogue in an attempt to describe what was happening in the interactive space between people in relation-ship (Buber, 1970; Josselson, 1996). Josselson explicated this *between* as the "emergent we" in her discussion regarding mutuality and relational resonance:

> Related to, but not identical with, companionship is the emergent *we*. Here experience is enriched simply because it occurs in tandem. We feel empowered, larger than self; partici-pate in something that could not have been created alone . . . and in these comings-togeth-er, we know (together) with deep conviction that whatever it was that we made happen was not because of you or because of me, but because of *us*. (p. 159)

The concept of the *emergent we* implies an active intersubjective process of relational mutu-ality in which both relationship and selves are ongoing products. As a consequence of rela-tionship, a person's interpretation of self is in constant reconstructive motion—part as reac-tion to the distinct relational other, but also as a synergistic construction of new vistas of self-expression, self-creativity, and self-knowledge. The relational self, framed in this sense, is analogous to a chemical reaction. Selves in relational interaction are systematically and constitutively transforming through layers of interpreted representations within the alembic of discourse. Such dialogue is constitutive of both self and other in direct relation to the significance of the relationship.

THIRD SYSTEM OF THE EMERGENT SELF: THE CULTURAL SELF

Human beings are culturally embedded beings. We are born and raised in cultural settings that pre-exist our arrival. Culture, to members, is transparent; we seldom notice it unless confronted with difference. The third dimension of the emergent self, the *cultural self*, depicts an aspect of self which is nurtured, shaped, and influenced by communicating within a society's parameters of value, social practice, and symbolic interaction. Wood (2000) defined culture as "composed of intricately interconnected structures and practices that individually and collectively sustain a particular social order" (p. 104). Geertz (1973) cited a particular conceptualization of culture as:

> essentially a semiotic one . . . man [*sic*] is an animal suspended in webs of significance he [*sic*] himself [*sic*] has spun. I take culture to be those webs, and the analysis of it to be therefore not an experimental science in search of law but an interpretative one in search of meaning. (pp. 4-5)

In regard to identity construction, cultural ways of being in the world define the potential qualities from which individuation of self may emerge. One's ongoing, cultural interpretation of self is one's *individuation* of culture.

Societal roles and rules prescribe and sanction specific ways of being in the world. According to a feminist perspective, people are situated differently, socially and materially, within particular cultural settings, which allows for a particularly unique construction of a person's lived experience. Socially constructed demographics such as gender, race, ethnicity, age, sexuality, ability, and status operate as interpretive standpoints that shape people's viewpoints and influence the construction of self. The cultural self is situated in society, grounded in specified prescriptions and beliefs. How one is situated in a cultural matrix can be conceived as locating oneself in *emergent standpoints*, which initiate, foster, and mold interpretive aspects of self.

THE EMERGENT SELF: DYNAMIC NEXUS OF INTERSUBJECTIVE INTERPRETATIONS OF SELF AND OTHERS

The emergent self is grounded in the perspective of the "agency of relational selves" (Wood, 2000, p. 125), and the agency of cultural selves. Wood suggested that shifting to an orientation of the self as relational tends to negate "a view of the self as singular and constant over time and space allowing us to enlarge our understanding of personal identity. Precisely because we internalize pluralistic perspectives into our consciousness, we are continually emerging, forming, in process" (p. 125). The model of the emergent self centralizes the multiple dimensions of self as a *dynamic emergent process* rather than a static or stable product. McLeod (1997) grounded his ideas about narrative therapeutic constructions of self in stating "Polkinghorne argues that . . . [social and physical indices of the] . . . self-concept ignore the existential notion that the 'self' is not experienced as a static 'entity' but as a process of becoming" (p. 44). The emergent self is always in a state of *becoming* as we shed and/or edify our old interpretations of self by replacing them with new and/or reconstructed versions. This emergent process is embedded within the ongoing communication that occurs between the intersectionality of our experiential self within cultural and relational contexts.

SELF-NARRATION AND COMMUNICATION AS A MEANS FOR EMERGENT IDENTITY CONSTRUCTION

Gergen and Gergen (1993) argued that narrative accounts of self are "products of social interchange—possessions of the socius" (p. 18). The structure of narrative self-accounts can be understood as a person's socially constructed perceptions of self because self-narrative is always embedded in a social milieu (Richey, 2001). A person's lived experience (cultural individuation) is the basis on which narratives originate. Self-narrative (formed within intersubjective interpretation of a person's lived experience) functions as "a mirror to nature [the lived world]," which motivates storytelling (Gergen & Gergen, 1993, p. 20). The following description of the processes involved in the emergence of self situates self-constitution in sociocultural communication:

> Self-narration performs the functions of self-understanding and social conduct, making the process of self-construction a relational process rather than a solely self-realized process. The self, like the communication in which it is constituted, is social in origin. (Richey, 2001, p. 23)

Narrative therapeutic strategies, for example, challenge the individual precisely at the cognitive site where reality construction and reconstruction originate. McLeod (1997) explicated this concept in a constructionist framework:

> Classical psychoanalysis employs an image of the person as combined mechanism (the "hydraulic" model of libinal energy) and organism (the "id"). These images convert into images of therapy: a mechanism is "fixed", an organism is "healed", a computer is "re-programmed", and a person "grows." Those who have developed and espoused social constructionist approaches to therapy regard these images as inadequate and limiting. . . . They are limiting because they are images that implicitly deny the capacity of the person to be aware, to challenge existing oppressive social structures, and to be creative in developing new ways of living together. Social constructionist therapies are based in an image of the

person as a *social being*. . . . From a social constructionist perspective, any way of making sense of the self is socially constructed, and can be understood as deriving from a particular set of social, cultural and historical conditions. (p. 90)

APPLICATION OF THE EMERGENT SELF IN CANCER—RECOVERY STRATEGIES

Other forms of self-narration occur in therapeutic encounters, which function to reconstruct a person's self-concept (Gergen, 1994b, 2001; Gergen & Gergen, 1993; Lorber, 1997; McLeod, 1997; Polkinghorne, 1988; Richey, 2001; Sabat, Fath, Moghaddam, & Harré, 1999; Shotter, 1991). Shotter suggested that self-identities are "re-authored" from the perspective of "what to be" in life rather than "what to do" and "what they have been in the past, to enable them to face what they might be in the future" (p. 105). In regard to cancer, strategies for behavior change that centralize the role of narrative communication in identity reconstruction would seem to be more effective than forms of treatment that target already formed attitudes about cancer, beliefs about the disease itself, anticipated behaviors in regard to embodying the disease, or health outcomes, as the locus of health behavioral change. The emergent self model can assist in advocacy planning of strategic communication for and in that process.

The embodiment of cancer requires a new dialogue. That dialogue will involve a change in the ongoing self constitution in regard to all aspects of the emergent self. Positive change is an emergent, constructed part of the interpretive, sociocultural communicative process involved in the ongoing reconstruction of self. A social constructionist perspective of the emergent self emphatically rejects a disease model explanation for health behavior change. Instead, people's potential for positive change in health behavior is constitutively embedded and reconstructed within the systems of the emergent self model—which represents an interpretive, intersubjective process of constant self-reconstruction.

For example, anti-tobacco media campaigns in Alaska over the past decade have focused on fear appeal messages regarding smoking health outcomes. The fear appeal in anti-tobacco messages is in the showing, in graphic detail, negative health outcomes of smoking. Photographs of blackened lungs or emphysema, and cancer victims breathing through stomas are central to such messages. Concurrently in the state of Alaska, from 1990 to 1995, the incidence of cigarette smoking in adolescents spiraled upward; in particular, cigarette smoking increased by 26% among Native American/Alaska Native youth. And, recently the American Lung Association indicated Alaska Native adolescents have the highest rate of smoking in the nation—34.1% (State of Alaska, 1999). A reasonable critique of health behavior messages, framed as fear appeals, could indicate that without addressing the relationally embedded self as assailed by smoking behavior, such messages fail to engage self-change processes. Witte (1992), who included personal differences [sic, emergent self] as an integral point in her discussion of an extended parallel process model in regard to fear appeals, compares people's responses to fear through appraisals of threat and efficacy (p. 338). In this regard, people "evaluate the components of messages in relation to their prior experiences, culture, and personality characteristics . . . the same fear appeal may produce different perceptions in different people, thereby influencing subsequent outcomes" (pp. 338-339).

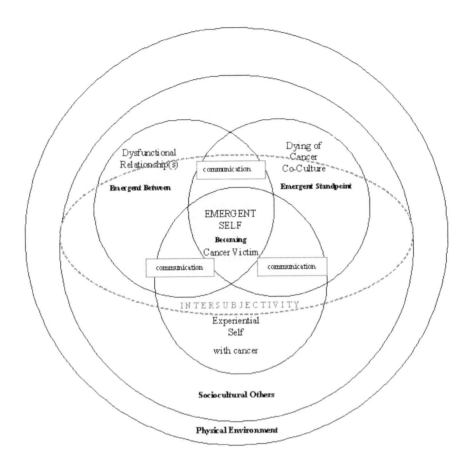

FIGURE 10.2. Emergent self as afflicted with cancer.

The conceptual framework of the emergent self obviates Witte's cognitive expectancy value approach to fear appeals, by locating the source of behavior change in social construction processes within a person's intersubjective lived experience. In this sense, for a fear appeal message to be personally effective, it should enter into the sociocultural communication system within the individual's relational and cultural interactions—the construction sites of the emergent self.

The emergent self model can be effectively applied to the common situations of developing and experiencing cancer. The representation of the model Shown in Fig. 10.2 depicts how a socially constructed process perpetuates self construal and behavior in the emergent self. The interplay of the self dimensions of communication within the model reinforces interpretations of self as *having cancer*. People with negative cultural perceptions of having cancer may tend to create and maintain the emergent self, as an afflicted self, through interaction within family and personal relationships (Beattie, 1989; Beck, 2001; Gergen, 2001; Irvine, 1999; Lorber, 1997; Schaef, 1986, 1987). In addition, one may begin to move within the dialogue of social circles with the potential of framing a self-with-cancer construal and corresponding behaviors. In order to shift one's self-interpretation toward the positive, a change

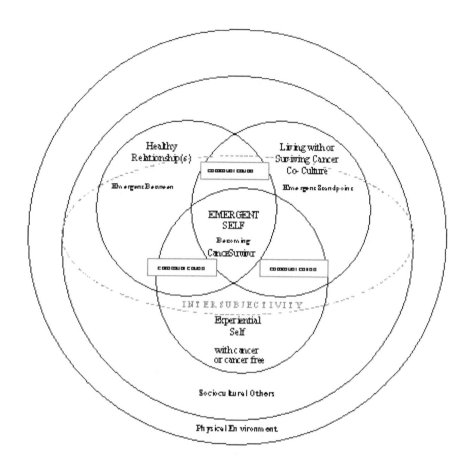

FIGURE 10.3. Emergent self as cancer survivor.

in self-knowledge must somehow be enacted through the dimensions represented in the model and interactions with relational others who aid in the construction of a more life embracing standpoint. Advocacy and empowerment, as sociocultural and relational interaction, can ground the individual choices that reconstitute self-with-cancer as a self embracing and/or celebrating life.

Health behavior interventions designed to communicatively help a person shift one or more of the self-systems tend to be more effective than interventions focused on negative health behaviors or potential health outcomes (Brown, 1995; Gergen, 1994a, 2001; McLeod, 1997; Thompson, 1992). In contrast, a *recovered self* or the reconstructed, surviving self can be effectively represented within the dimensions of this model of the social construction of the emergent self (Fig. 10.3). The emergent self is shown here as a person who actively engages in the process of positive identity reconstruction through positive and supportive interactions (Brown, 1995; Gergen, 1994b, 2001; McLeod, 1997; Miller, 1986, 1989; Sabat, et al., 1999; Thompson, 1992). The formerly afflicted person systematically and incrementally shifts intersubjective interpretations of self toward positive, health-promoting interactions in all self-systems including self-narrations (Gergen & Gergen, 1993).

SUMMARY AND CONCLUSION

A social constructionist perspective, in regard to a person's ability to change health behavior, centralizes socially and culturally situated interactions with others, as well as one's self-narrations, as constitutive to a reconstructive process of healthy change. The focus of the model suggested, the social construction of the *emergent self*, is understood as *a process of becoming*. In this respect, a person choosing to be involved in recovery from a negative health occurrence (e.g., the diagnosis of cancer), continuously reconstructs the self, through interactive interpretation, as the *recovering self*. Although there is no question that persons with cancer are not all going to recover or to choose recovery perspectives, when the self is interpreted as "in control" of one's life, that is, when the person experiencing cancer has the benefit of the most complete information possible (what the CSAM labels agency), there is an anticipated positive effect that will enhance the benefit of the treatment program and the patient's quality of life aside from eventual outcomes.

A conceptualization of the person, as constantly involved in a reconstructive process through a positive interpretation of lived experience in sociocultural interaction, posits a proactively reforming self, consciously engaged in moving toward a quality life experience. In this view, a person can be actively recovering as she or he emerges as a recovered self.

The model of the emergent self describes how communicative social construction drives a person's strategies in identity construction. The traditional framework of health behavior change understood through the disease model approach may in part describe how the recovery or remediation process works in a human body, but fails to capture the essential complexity of how an afflicted person beneficially shifts his or her attention toward a self in recovery. The constructionist explanations described here allow a more detailed understanding of the recovery process. In this sense, health belief and health behavior theories that have included notions of self-identity, self-efficacy, social interaction, and social support to describe a person's recovery process (Ajzen, 1991; Ajzen & Fishbein, 1980, 2000; Bandura, 1986, 1997, 2001; Chatham-Carpenter & DeFrancisco, 1997; Cohen, Gottlieb, & Underwood, 2000; DiClemente, 1999; Finkelstein, 1996; Lakey & Cohen, 2000; Prochaska, Redding, & Evers, 1997; Segrin, 1992, 2000; Strecher & Rosenstock, 1997; Thompson, 1992), but that have assumed a static, psychological existence of self, are provided a model that can better address the self as it exists in the self constituting moment-to-moment, interactive interpretation of lived experience. Health belief and health behavior models, with their assumptions of self-identity, are essentially subsumed within the processes of the social construction model of the emergent self. For perceptions of self beyond such conceptions (e.g., Lorber, 1997), the model of the experiential self, provided here, can help to visualize and track interactions that reconstitute self in the light of health information (e.g., diagnosis of cancer or remission). Constitutive changes in self-identity occur as an ongoing matter of *becoming* through an interpretive process of self and social interaction as described in the emergent self model: (a) the *experiential self*, (b) the *relational self*, and (c) the *cultural self*. This interactive, intersubjectively dynamic process of communication between self and others (present or imagined) is the primary process underlying all constructions of human reality and co-constructions of self-identity.

The social construction of the emergent self is a theoretical communication model that centralizes the process of human communication. A communication perspective applied to health behavior change suggests that people are sociocultural actors who interpret their reality and constructions of self through an ongoing matrix of social interaction. Communication models created from a positivistic perspective tend to compartmentalize constructs outside the framework of social interaction and apply them in an abstract, linear-sequential fashion, which is antithetical to how human beings actually construct their ongoing meanings and lived realities. The site of reality construction and identity creation takes place intersubjectively in a complex interpretive process. In this regard, strategies aimed toward health behavior change should centralize communication and the notion that self-identity is a socially constructed emergent process constituted in social communication.

REFERENCES

Ajzen, I. (1991). The theory of planned behavior. *Organizational Behavior and Human Decision Processes, 50*, 179-211.

Ajzen, I., & Fishbein, M. (1980). *Understanding attitudes and predicting social behavior*. Englewood Cliffs, NJ: Prentice-Hall.

Ajzen, I., & Fishbein, M. (2000). Attitudes and the attitude-behavior relation: Reasoned and automatic processes. In W. Stroebe & M. Hewstone (Eds.), *European review of social psychology* (pp. 1-33). New York: Wiley.

Anderson, M. R., & Urban, N. (1999). Involvement in decision-making and breast cancer survivor quality of life. *Annals of Behavioral Medicine, 21*, 201–209.

Bakker, D. A., Fitch, M. I., Gray, R., Reed, E., & Bennett, J. (2001). Patient health-care provider communication during chemotherapy treatment: The perspectives of women with breast cancer. *Patient Education and Counseling, 43*, 61–71.

Bandura, A. (1986). *Social foundations of thought and action: A social cognitive theory*. Englewood Cliffs, NJ: Prentice-Hall.

Bandura, A. (1997). *Self-efficacy: The exercise of control*. New York: Freeman.

Bandura, A. (2001). Social cognitive theory: An agentive perspective. *Annual Review of Psychology, 52*, 1-26.

Berger, P.L., & Luckmann, T. (1966). *The social construction of reality: A treatise in the sociology of knowledge*. Garden City, NY: Doubleday.

Blumer, H. (2004). *George Herbert Mead and human conduct* (T. J. Morrione, Ed.). Walnut Creek, CA: Altimira Press.

Bradley, B. S., & Morss, J. R. (2002). Social construction in a world at risk: Toward a psychology of experience. *Theory & Psychology, 12*(4), 509-531.

Brown, P. (1995). Naming and framing: The social construction of diagnosis and illness. *Journal of Health and Social Behavior*, 34-52.

Buber, M. (1970). *I and thou* (W. Kauffmann, Trans.) (3rd ed.). New York: Scribners.

Burr, V. (1995). *An introduction to social constructionism*. New York: Routledge.

Carbaugh, D. (1996). *Situating selves: The communication of social identities in American scenes*. Albany: State University of New York Press.

Chatham-Carpenter, A., & DeFrancisco, V. (1997). Pulling yourself up again: Women's choices and strategies for recovering and maintaining self-esteem. *Western Journal of Communication, 61*(2), 164-187.

Cohen, S., Gottlieb, B. H., & Underwood, L. G. (2000). Social relationships and health. In S. Cohen, L. G. Underwood, & B. H. Gottlieb (Eds.), *Social support measurement and intervention: A guide for health and social scientists*. New York: Oxford University Press.

Crotty, M. (1998). *The foundations of social research: Meaning and perspective in the research process*. Thousand Oaks, CA: Sage.

Deadman, J. M., Leinster, S. J., Owens, R. G., Dewey, M. E., & Slade, P. D. (2001). Taking responsibility for cancer treatment. *Social Science and Medicine, 53,* 669–677.

Deetz, S. (1982). Hermeneutics and research in interpersonal communication. In J. J. Pilotta (Ed.), *Interpersonal communication: Essays in phenomenology and hermeneutics* (pp. 1-13). Washington, DC: Center for Advanced Research in Phenomenology & University Press of America.

DiClemente, C. C. (1999). Motivation for change: Implications for substance abuse and treatment. *Psychological Science, 10*(3), 209-213.

Duck, S. (1994). *Meaningful relationships: Talking, sense, and relating.* Thousand Oaks, CA: Sage.

Edwards, E. (1997). *Discourse and cognition.* Thousand Oaks, CA: Sage.

Eisenberg, E. M. (2001). Building a mystery: Toward a new theory of communication and identity. *Journal of Communication, 51,* 534-552.

Finkelstein, N. (1996). Using the relational model as a context for treating pregnant and parenting chemically dependent women. In B. Underhill & D. Finnegan (Eds.), *Chemical dependency, women at risk.* New York: The Haworth Press.

Gattellari, M., Butow, P. N., & Tattersall, M. H. N. (2001). Sharing decisions in cancer care. *Social Science & Medicine, 52,* 1865–1878.

Geertz, C. (1973). *The interpretation of cultures.* New York: Basic Books.

Gergen, K. J. (1991). *The saturated self: Dilemmas of identity in contemporary life.* New York: Basic Books.

Gergen, K. J. (1994a). *Toward transformation in social knowledge.* Thousand Oaks, CA: Sage.

Gergen, K. J. (1994b). *Realities and relationships: Soundings in social construction.* Cambridge, MA: Harvard University Press.

Gergen, K. J. (1999). *An invitation to social construction.* Thousand Oaks, CA: Sage.

Gergen, K. J. (2001). *Social construction in context.* Thousand Oaks, CA: Sage.

Gergen, K. J., & Gergen, M. M. (1993). Narrative and the self as relationship. In K.J. Gergen (Ed.), *Refiguring self and psychology* (pp. 17-56). Brookfield, VT: Dartmouth.

Gibbs, R. W., & Franks, H. (2002). Embodied metaphor in women's narratives about their experiences with cancer. *Health Communication, 14*(2), 139-166.

Harré, R. (1983). Identity projects. In G. M. Breakwell (Ed.), *Threatened identities* (pp. 31-51). New York: Wiley.

Harré, R. (1989). Language games and texts of identity. In J. Shotter & K. Gergen (Eds.), *Texts of identity* (pp. 20-35). Newbury Park, CA: Sage.

Harré, R. (1995). Agentive discourse. In R. Harré & P. S. Stearns (Eds.), *Discursive psychology in practice.* Thousand Oaks: Sage.

Harré, R. (2000). Personalism in the context of a social constructionist psychology: Stern and Vygotsky. *Theory & Psychology, 10*(6), 731-748.

Harré, R. (2002a). Public sources of the personal mind: Social constructionism in context. *Theory & Psychology, 12*(5), 611-623.

Harré, R. (2002b). Social reality and the myth of social structure. *European Journal of Social Theory, 5*(1), 111-123.

Harré, R., & Gillett, G. (1994). *The discursive mind.* Thousand Oaks, CA: Sage.

Hartsock, N.C.M (1997a). The feminist standpoint: Developing the ground for a specifically feminist historical materialism. In D.T. Meyers (Ed.), *Feminist social thought: A reader* (pp. 461-483). New York: Routledge.

Hartsock, N.C.M (1997b). Standpoint theories for the next century. In S.J. Kenney & H. Kinsella (Eds.), *Politics and feminist standpoint theories* (pp. 93-102). New York: The Haworth Press

Jacoby, S., & Ochs, E. (1995). Co-construction: An introduction. *Research on Language and Social Interaction, 28*(3), 171-183.

Jenkins, V., Fallowfield, L., & Saul, J. (2001). Information needs of patients with cancer: Results from a large study in UK cancer centers. *British Journal of Cancer, 84,* 48–51.

Josselson, R. (1996). *The space between us: Exploring the dimensions of human relationships*. Thousand Oaks, CA: Sage.

Kramarae, C. (1981). *Women and men speaking: Frameworks for analysis*. Rowley, MA: Newbury House.

Kramarae, C. (1996). Classified information: Race, class, and (always) gender. In J. Wood (Ed.), *Gendered relationships* (pp. 20-38). Mountain View, CA: Mayfield.

Krupat, E., Rosenkrantz, S. L., Yeager, C. M., Barnard, K., Putnam, S. M., & Inui, T. S. (2000). The practice orientations of physicians and patients: The effect of doctor-patient congruence on satisfaction. *Patient Education and Counseling, 39*, 49–59.

Lakey, B., & Cohen, S. (2000). Social support theory and measurement. In S. Cohen, L. G. Underwood, & B. H. Gottlieb (Eds.), *Social support measurement and intervention: A guide for health and social scientists*. Oxford, UK: Oxford University Press.

Lakoff, G., & Johnson, M. (1999). *Philosophy in the flesh: The embodied mind and its challenge to Western thought*. New York: Basic Books.

Lal, B. B. (1995). Symbolic interaction theories. *American Behavioral Scientist, 38*, 421-441.

Lorber, J. (1997). *Gender and the social construction of illness*. Thousand Oaks, CA: Sage.

Maguire, P. (1999). Improving communication with cancer patients. *European Journal of Cancer, 35*, 1415–1422.

McLeod, J. (1997). *Narrative and psychotherapy*. Thousand Oaks, CA: Sage.

McNamee, S., & Gergen, K. J. (Eds.). (1999). *Relational responsibility: Resources for sustainable dialogue*. Thousand Oaks, CA: Sage.

Mead, G. H. (1934). *Mind, self and society from the standpoint of a social behaviorist*. Chicago: The University of Chicago Press.

Mead, G. H. (1968). The genesis of the self. In C. Gordon & K. J. Gergen (Eds.), *The self in social interaction, Vol. I: Classic and contemporary perspectives*. New York: Wiley.

Mead, G. H. (1982). *The individual and the social self: Unpublished work of George Herbert Mead*. Chicago: The University of Chicago Press.

Mellor, P. A., & Shilling, C. (1997). *Re-forming the body: Religion, community, and modernity*. Thousand Oaks, CA: Sage.

Miller, W. R. (1986). Haunted by the zeitgeist: Reflections on the contrasting treatment goals and concepts of alcoholics in Europe and the United States. In T. Barbor (Ed.), *Alcohol and culture: Comparative perspectives from Europe and America*. New York: New York Academy of Sciences.

Miller, W. R. (1989). Treating alcohol problems: Toward an informed eclecticism. In R. Hester & W. Miller (Eds.), *Handbook of alcoholism treatment approaches*. New York: Pergamon.

Mishel, M. H. (1999). Uncertainty in chronic illness. *Annual Review of Nursing, 17*, 269–294.

National Cancer Institute. (2001). Scientific priorities for cancer research: NCI's extraordinary opportunities. Accessed January 20, 2004, from http://2001.cancer.gov/communications.htm.

Neisser, U. (1976). *Cognition and reality: Principles and implications of cognitive psychology*. San Francisco, CA: Freeman.

O'Hair, D., Villagran, M. M., Wittenberg, K., Brown, K., Ferguson, M., Hall, H. T., & Doty, T. (2003). Cancer survivorship and agency model: Implication for patient choice, decision-making, and influence. *Health Communication, 15*, 2.

Orbe, M.P. (1998). *Constructing co-cultural theory: An explication of culture, power, and communication*. Thousand Oaks, CA: Sage.

Pearce, W. B. (1995). A sailing guide for social constructionists. In W. Leeds-Hurwitz (Ed.), *Social approaches to communication* (pp. 88-113). New York: Guilford.

Polkinghorne, D. (1988). *Narrative knowing and the human sciences*. Albany: State University of New York Press.

Prochaska, J.O., Redding, C.A., & Evers, K.E. (1997). The transtheoretial model and stages of change. In K. Glanz, F.M. Lewis, & B.K. Rimer (Eds.), *Health behavior and health education: Theory, research and practice* (pp. 60-84). San Francisco, CA: Jossey-Bass.

Richey, J. A. (2001). *Co-constructed interpersonal perceptions of self: Meaning-making in the astrological consultation.* Unpublished master's thesis, University of Alaska, Fairbanks.

Richey, J. A. (2003). *Women in Alaska constructing the recovered self: A narrative approach to understanding long-term recovery from alcohol dependence and/or abuse.* Unpublished doctoral dissertation, University of Alaska Fairbanks.

Roberts, C. S., Cox, C. E., Reintgen, D. S., Baile, W. F., & Gibertini, M. (1994). Influence of physician communication on newly diagnosed breast patients' psychologic adjustment and decision-making. *Cancer, 74,* 336–341.

Sabat, S. R., Fath, H., Moghaddam, F. M., & Harré, R. (1999). The maintenance of self-esteem: Lessons from the culture of Alzheimer's sufferers. *Culture & Psychology, 5*(1), 5-31.

Schutz, A., & Luckmann, T. (1973). *The structures of the life-world* (R. M. Zaner & H. T. Engelhardt, Jr., Trans.). Evanston, IL: Northwestern University Press.

Segrin, C. (1992). Specifying the nature of social skill deficits associated with depression. *Human Communication Research, 19,* 89-123.

Segrin, C. (2000). Poor social skills are a vulnerability factor in the development of psychosocial problems. *Human Communication Research, 26*(3), 489-514.

Shotter, J. (1991). Consultant re-authoring: The "making" and "finding" of narrative constructions. *Human Systems: The Journal of Systemic Consultation & Management, 2,* 105-119.

Shotter, J. (1993). *Conversational realities: Constructing life through language.* London: Sage.

Shotter, J., & Lannamann, J. W. (2002). The situation of social constructionism: Its "imprisonment" within the ritual of theory-criticism-and-debate. *Theory & Psychology, 12*(5), 577-609.

Siminoff, L. A., Ravdin, P., Colabianchi, N., & Saunders-Sturm, C. M. (2000). Doctor–patient communication patterns in breast cancer adjuvant therapy discussions. *Health Expectations, 3,* 26–36.

Simmel, G. (1950). *The sociology of Georg Simmel* (K.H. Wolf, Trans.). London: Collier-MacMillan Ltd.

State of Alaska, Division of Public Health, Behavioral Risk Factor Surveillance.

Stoetzler, M., & Yuval-Davis, N. (2002). Standpoint theory, situated knowledge and the situated imagination. *Feminist Theory, 3*(3), 315-333.

Strecher, V. J., & Rosenstock, I. M. (1997). The health belief model. In K. Glanz, F. M. Lewis, & B. K. Rimer (Eds.). *Health behavior and health education: Theory, research and practice* (pp. 41-59). San Francisco, CA: Jossey-Bass.

System (BRFSS). (1999). Health effects of exposure to environmental tobacco smoke: The report of the California Environmental Protection Agency. *Smoking and Tobacco Control Monographs, 10.* National Cancer Institute, NIH.

Thompson, T. L. (1992). Interpersonal communication and health care. In M. L. Knapp & G. R. Miller (Eds.), *Handbook of interpersonal communication* (2nd ed., pp. 696-725). Thousand Oaks, CA: Sage.

Witte, K. (1992). Putting the fear back into fear appeals: The extended parallel process model. *Communication Monographs, 59,* 329-349.

Wood, J. T. (1996a). Communication and relational culture. In K. M. Galvin & P. J. Cooper (Eds.), *Making connections: Readings in relational communication* (pp. 11-15). Los Angeles, CA: Roxbury.

Wood, J. T. (1996b). Standpoint theory: Social locations. In K. M. Galvin & P. J. Cooper (Eds.), *Making connections: Readings in relational communication* (pp. 36-39). Los Angeles, CA: Roxbury

Wood, J. T. (2000). *Relational communication: Continuity and change in personal relationships* (2nd ed.). Belmont, CA: Wadsworth.

11 | Becoming an Effective Advocate/Caregiver

Experiential Knowledge from Women's "Third Shift" with Cancer Patients and Other Care Receivers

Terri Babers
University of Alaska, Fairbanks

Pamela McWherter
University of Alaska, Fairbanks

Jin Brown
University of Alaska, Fairbanks

The presence of female caregivers in health care interviews and encounters is increasing, and will continue to do so as public policy and demographic trends increase the demand for unpaid care in the home (Abel, 1991; Ellis, Miller, & Given, 1989; Gerstel & Galleger, 1994). Some physicians, according to Beisecker and Moore (1994), estimate that as many as 75% of their cancer patients bring a caregiver with them to appointments. Ellingson (2000) claimed that the "vast majority of geriatric oncology patients bring a friend or relative. . . . with them to help with communication" (p. 2). Rutman (1996) suggested that the caregiver and the patient "should be recognized as a dyad by the health care team; both equally are users of the system" (p. 12). Recognition of the caregiver as an important component of the health care team has led to increasing examination of family caregiving over the last 30 years, but that research has primarily investigated the economic, psychosocial, and medical impact of caregiving on the caregiver and on society (Abel, 1991; Ellis et al., 1989).

Recognition of the increasingly triadic nature of communication within medical encounters (Gafni, Charles, & Whelan, 1998; O'Hair & McNeilis, 1993; Rutman, 1996) has only recently led to a focus expanded from an examination of dyadic interpersonal communication between the health care providers and patients (Ballard-Reisch, 1993; Gafni et al., 1998) to an investigation of communication in medical encounters that include the presence of a caregiver who often advocates for the patient and acts as an interpreter (Ellingson, 2000). Additionally, current research regarding interpersonal communication in medical encounters between health care provider and patient has noted a continuing presence of the traditional, paternalistic model of medicine (Ballard-Reisch, 1993; Gafni et al., 1998).

A review of extant literature reveals that the majority of interpersonal communication research regarding medical encounters, whether dyadic or triadic, has focused on the interpersonal communication needs and responsibilities of providers to the neglect of the needs and responsibilities of patients (Charles, Gafni,, & Whelan, 1998; Tates & Meeuwesen, 2001; Thompson, 1984). Research on dyadic communication, Kreps (1993) said, has

> centered around planning and directing relationship development in provider–patient interviews. . . . [It has] identified specific communication characteristics used by health care providers to control interview communication, and developed strategies to help health care providers establish rapport and elicit full and accurate information from health care consumers. (pp. 52-53)

There is a shift occurring away from this paternalistic model to a more participative, patient-centered model of decision making in medical encounters that is accompanied by recognition of the communication needs and responsibilities of the patient in medical decision making. There is also an increasing recognition of the presence of a third participant in medical encounters, the advocate/caregiver who often accompanies a patient to a medical visit.

Research literature pertinent to understanding the perceptions of advocate/caregivers who are involved in communication in triadic medical encounters is reviewed here, under four topic headings: (a) the shift from paternalistic to participative decision-making; (b) an overview of triadic communication in medical encounters including a description of the patients who bring companions or advocate/caregivers with them to medical encounters; (c) a description of the women who serve in the role of unpaid advocate/caregiver and the functions they perform including their "third shift" of work; and (d) a discussion of communication issues that are potentially relevant to triadic medical encounters.

SHIFT FROM PATERNALISTIC TO PARTICIPATIVE DECISION MAKING IN MEDICAL ENCOUNTERS.

In 1993, Ballard-Reisch discussed the occurrence of a paradigmatic shift from traditional, paternalistic decision making by the physician, toward participative decision making that increasingly involves the patient in the process. According to Charles et al. (1999), the paternalistic model assumed that for most illnesses there was a single best treatment and that the doctor would best understand the treatment ("Doctor knows best"). The model also assumed that the physician would be in the best position to evaluate the risks and benefits of that treatment ("Don't worry yourself so much, honey"). These assumptions, in addition to issues of status, education, income, and gender, created an expectation on the part of both patients and physicians that the physician would play the dominant communication role in the interaction. Charles et al. reported that in the 1980s those assumptions began to be challenged. It became evident that there were various treatment options for certain illnesses. Patients and doctors alike began to recognize that it was the patient and his or her family who had to live not only with the illness, but also with any lifestyle changes that might be necessary to treat or prevent illness.

There has been a concomitant movement from traditional provider-centered research toward a more patient-centered focus with emphasis on the function and participation of patients in decision making during the medical encounter. Brown, McWherter, and Leipzig (1995) identified this as "a matter of negotiated health care" (p. 266), wherein active participation and responsibility for health outcomes occurs from both, or all, persons involved in the medical encounter (see also Street & Millay, 2001; von Friederichs-Fitzwater & Gilgun, 2001). An example is the issue of compliance that traditionally focuses on the one-way communication of information and directives with the patient held accountable to the provider. Kreps and Thornton (1984) suggested "redefining the issue of compliance to a relational issue of 'co-operation' to fully take into account the interdependent communication functioning of health care provider and the consumer" (p. 55). According to Kreps (1993), primary factors in improved cooperation are the patient's understanding of the process of restoration and/or maintenance of health as well as the creation of shared responsibility on the part of the patient. Research indicates that improved cooperation (traditionally called compliance) enhances medical outcomes and occurs when participants' communication competence is improved (Brown, McWherter, & Leipzig, 1995).

Kreps (1993) stated that communication competency in medical interviews (for all participants in the interview) is the "ability to utilize interpersonal skills to elicit co-operation from, gather information from, and share health information with relevant individuals in the health care system" (p. 56) in order to fully participate in the communication interaction. Research regarding improved communication competence on the part of the patient includes ideas from a study by Beckman, Kaplan, and Frankel (1989) who suggest that increased understanding of patient negotiation and assertiveness skills, along with training to enhance those skills, may result in "creating more realistic treatment plans and goals" (p. 226) and therefore more cooperation. Greenfield et al. (1985) and Feeser and Thompson (1988) reported successful training interventions to increase patient interactions and involvement in medical interviews. McGee and Cegala (1998) extended this research to training patients for improved information exchange skills. Cegala, Socha McGee, and McNeilis (1996) explored both patients and physicians perceptions of communication competence during a medical interview. More recently, in the only study of its kind found by an extensive search, Cegala, Gade, Broz, and McClure (2002) examined "patients' and physicians' perceptions of communication competence during the medical interview . . . specifically, what behaviors constitute competent patient communication" (p. 2). Again, no research was found examining caregiver perceptions or understandings of communication competence.

TRIADIC COMMUNICATION IN MEDICAL ENCOUNTERS

Often, by necessity or for other reasons, the patient has a companion who is involved in communication between the medical professional and patient, creating a triad. The third party of the triad is referred to in various ways such as "caregiver" (Abel, 1991; Ellis et al., 1969; Rutman, 1996), "lay caregiver" (duPre, 2000), "care partner" (Miller & Zook, 1997), "companion" (Beisecker, 1989), "parent" (Parrot, 1993), and "advocate" (O'Hair & McNeilis, 1993). Caregivers, lay caregivers, family caregivers, care partners, companions, and parents are all labels for the role of people who provide unpaid, in-home care for a person who is a patient. For purposes here, the third party involved in triadic communication is referred to as the advocate/caregiver.

The advocate aspect of the concept label is important to recognize because this person is often present to advocate for the patient who is unable or unwilling to communicate or advocate effectively for him or herself during the medical encounter. It is equally important to recognize the caregiving aspect of the advocate/caregiver role because her ability to effectively communicate on behalf of or in conjunction with the patient in a triadic medical encounter is often a result of experiences in the caregiving role outside the medical setting. "Companions of cancer patients," Beisecker et al. (1996) reported, believe that they "provide support and companionship, increase patient understanding, ask questions, and furnish transportation" (cited in Ellingson, 2000, p. 4), all clearly matters requiring communication. The importance of the advocate/caregiver's communication competency in the triad may often be equal to that of the patient and the provider in a communication context.

As previously stated, the shift from a paternalistic to a participative, patient-centered model of medical interaction is accompanied by the recognition that, in many cases, communication in medical encounters is often triadic rather than dyadic (Ballard-Reisch, 1993; O'Hair & McNeilis, 1993). Patients who bring advocate/caregivers with them to medical encounters include people who have language or cultural barriers; persons with chronic, debilitating, and/or stigmatizing illnesses such as AIDS or cancer; minor children; adult children, siblings, spouses, and/or parents with mental, emotional, or physical disabilities and/or severe acute illnesses; and with increasing frequency, frail or infirm elderly people. Such people are frequently among those who require intensive caregiving, usually unpaid and outside the medical system. Public policy, privatization of care, and demographic changes (our population continues to age and the chronic nature of illness and disease continues to intensify) has created an increase in the number of people who require intensive, unpaid care.

THE FEMALE ADVOCATE/CAREGIVER
WORKS A "THIRD SHIFT"

US public policy, which seems committed to increased reliance on private, unpaid services and the shortening of federally and privately funded hospital stays, has put tremendous pressure on families to provide unpaid care for both nuclear and extended family members (Abel, 1991). For example, according to Foster and Brizius (1991), "'informal,' or unpaid caregiving by family members and friends provides 80 to 90 percent of care for the frail elderly" (p. 4). The U. S. Department of Health and Human Services has stated that, "families are to become the first line of defense in the care of the needy" (Gerstel & Gallager, 1994, p. 520). "Families are increasingly replacing skilled health care workers," said McCorkle and Pasacreta (2001) "in the delivery of complex care to their relatives with cancer despite other obligations and responsibilities that characterize their lives." (p. 37). Research demonstrates that the word *families* most often translates to mothers, wives, sisters, and adult daughters (Abel, 1991; Foster & Brizius, 1991; Gerstel & Gallager, 1994; Rutman, 1996). Usually, the advocate who accompanies a patient to a medical interview is a female family member who has the role of unpaid caregiver at home. In many, if not most cases, this woman provides the vast majority of both the visible and the "often invisible aspects of care" (Rutman, 1996, p. 2).

Visible care usually occurs in direct conjunction with formal medical care. Invisible care is that which occurs in the privacy of the home and is often unrecognized by society in general and medical professionals in particular. O'Hara (2001) claimed that "a recent study by the United Hospital Fund of New York found that if [family] caregivers were compensated at market rate, their services would cost nearly $200 billion per year" (p. 1). Invisible care provides the advocate/caregiver with intimate experience and knowledge of the patient's physical, emotional, and mental conditions as well as an understanding of the patient's lifestyle, cultural values, and beliefs that are related to health issues.

It is important to be aware of both aspects of care provided to the patient in order to understand the caregiver's qualifications to communicate as an advocate for the patient. That awareness is important to understanding why and how the advocate/caregiver's lived experience with the visible and invisible components of patient care and medical encounters matters, and why and how their perceptions of communication effectiveness and competence in medical encounters matter.

Gerstel and Gallager's (1994) research indicates that "the majority of Americans continue to believe that it is the responsibility of adult women (more than men) to provide personal and household assistance to elderly parents and in-laws, aging siblings, and adult children [as well as minor children]" (p. 519). In fact, Foster and Brizius (1991) found that 72% of informal, unpaid caregiving is provided by women. Most of these women are over the age of 57 and they provide care 7 days a week, usually in addition to paid employment and their everyday housework. Additionally, Gerstel and Gallager found that the mean number of hours spent in caregiving activities for both nuclear and extended family was more than double for wives than for husbands. About 11% to 13% of women who care for elderly parents quit their jobs. The 83% of caregivers who do not leave paid employment add more than an extra 40-hour work week to their monthly load by the care work they undertake.

It is this extra work week that Gerstel and Gallager (1994) labeled the third shift; an addition to the woman's "first shift" of paid work and the "second shift" of ordinary housework and child care as identified by Hoschild. Caregiving activities involved in the third shift of unpaid, usually invisible care

> ranges from checking periodically on an elderly person's welfare to round the clock nursing care . . . [including] . . . transportation, performing household chores, administering medicine [and other prescribed medical regimens] . . . bathing, eating, and toileting. (Foster & Brizius, 1991, p. 5)

The third shift also includes the care that takes place during the medical encounter including the (often invisible and/or unacknowledged) responsibility to negotiate for shared control with professional providers and to share or assist in decision making and paperwork with the patient (Abel, 1991). In order to understand and improve communication in triadic medical encounters, the roles, responsibilities, understandings, observations, and perceptions of the advocate/caregiver should be taken into account along with those of the patient and physician.

An examination of the research regarding communication between physicians and patients in dyadic medical encounters is valuable to understanding the communication interactions that occur in triadic encounters and is necessary because little research regarding the communication role of the advocate/caregiver is found in a search of the literature.

However, O'Hair and McNeilis, (1993) do suggest that "a different set of patterns, rules, roles, and perceptions" are created when there is a third person in addition to the patient and the medical professional present in a medical encounter (p. 62). Tates and Meeuwesen's (2001) findings regarding the doctor–parent–child medical interview show that the "interactional dynamics of a triad differ[s] fundamentally from those of a dyad . . . [and that] . . . future research should focus on the implications of a third participant's presence . . ." (p. 849). Additionally, they stated that such research should not be restricted to only the physician's perspective as has most existing research on communication in medical encounters; adding "only...by dealing with the perspectives of all three participants, can the process of mutual influence of the interactants be fully examined" (p. 850).

The intent of this chapter is to examine, from the perspective of women who work this "third shift," how each understands herself to be effective and competent in interpersonal communication with her care receiver and the professional care provider in medical encounters.

POTENTIALLY RELEVANT COMMUNICATION ISSUES

O'Hair and McNeilis (1993) suggested that some of the relevant health communication issues that should be examined regarding communication and negotiation of roles in triadic medical encounters include (a) relational agreement and/or control as relates to patient–advocate satisfaction and medical outcomes; (b) patient–advocate satisfaction as relates to medical outcomes; (c) success of medical interviews as a result of physician attitudes toward the patient and the advocate; and (d) communication behaviors of the patient, the advocate, and/or the patient advocate-dyad. This chapter considers the advocate aspect of the fourth issue identified by O'Hair and McNeilis, the communication behaviors of the advocate. The first three issues (relational control, satisfaction, and physician attitudes) appear to have a strong impact on interpersonal communication behaviors of all three participants in the interaction.

Rutman's 1996 study of female caregiving revealed negotiation issues of an equally pragmatic but more experiential nature. Using narrative analysis of focus group interviews, Rutman studied, from a feminist, interpretive perspective, feelings of powerlessness and powerfulness that caregivers experience. The feeling that their knowledge and contributions were devalued, minimized, and dismissed epitomized a general theme of caregiver powerlessness. The following synopsis of feelings expressed by participants in her focus group research regarding the role of caregiver appears to closely mirror experiences noted in the focus groups of this research.

> Caregivers felt that insufficient value had been placed on their knowledge of the care receiver. . . . Not only did they feel that their knowledge and contributions had been dismissed, they also felt that the care provided . . . was compromised because others [medical professionals] did not make use of their knowledge and experience. (Rutman, 1996, p. 5)

Additional communication themes emerged from Rutman's study, including a feeling of powerlessness experienced as a result of the lack of respect for caregivers' experiences and a lack of shared control over the decision-making process. Caregivers also revealed frustration over the lack of physician respect for patient autonomy and a "clash" (p. 4) in preferences and values of both the patient and caregiver in regard to the treatment options and plans made on their behalf by the medical professionals. In addition to frustration at

> having insufficient resources for quality care . . . [advocate/caregivers expressed frustration because] . . . situations were often socially constructed [to create] notions of rules that define how we "should" be feeling [and therefore behaving?] in any given situation . . . (pp. 7-8)

Another important communication issue of concern to advocate/caregivers as revealed in Rutman's study is the "social construction of documentary reality . . . the official record written by a higher status health care professional who, in fact, had less hands-on, day-to-day knowledge of the . . . situation than they [the caregiver] did, while their own [the caregiver's] expertise was overlooked (pp. 5-6). Caregivers expressed feelings of frustration and powerlessness because the information that professionals put in the permanent record of fact, information that becomes the official reality, often disregards, dismisses, or even contradicts and changes or eliminates the reality of the caregiver's understandings and experiences regarding the patient's health and illness.

Kreps (1993), in his summary of existing research related to communication in medical interviews, identified five relevant areas of interpersonal communication. These recurring areas are identified to enhance the success of health care in dyadic medical encounters, but they may be usefully applied to understanding interpersonal communication in triadic encounters. They address negotiation of "patterns, rules, roles, and perceptions" that occurs differently in a triadic communication than in dyadic communication (as described in O'Hair & McNeilis, 1993, p. 62) and the location of feelings of "powerlessness" and "powerfulness" (Rutman, 1996) that many advocate/caregivers experience during interactions with patients and professional providers. The five problem areas identified by Kreps are:

> 1) low levels of patient compliance . . . [possibly caused by]; 2) miscommunication and misinformation; 3) insensitivity, low levels of interpersonal respect, and attempts at relational control [on the part of the provider] . . . ; 4) unrealistic and unfulfilled patient expectations linked to cultural stereotypes . . . ; and 5) dissatisfaction with health care by both providers and consumers [patients] . . . (p. 53)

Consider, too, what Beisecker (1989, p. 61) identified as the three basic roles or communication activities provided by the advocate/caregiver: (a) a significant other, someone for the patient to rely on for emotional and physical support; (b) a surrogate parent, someone to help make decisions along with the physician; and (c) the watchdog. The watchdog role seems closely aligned with the surrogate parent role and must be carefully negotiated with both the patient and the physician because of power, autonomy, and status issues and because patterns, rules, roles, and perceptions are often changed with the addition of a third party to the medical encounter. The watchdog role includes communication responsibilities such as provision of information; elaboration and clarification of information from patient to physician and from physician to patient; questions to the physician regarding reasons for treatment, obtaining complete information regarding the illness and treatment of the patient; and providing encouragement to the patient to expand on feelings, symptoms, fears, concerns, desires, understandings, and the interrelationships of treatment, illness, and lifestyle. Consideration of these communication activities by the advocate/caregiver must also recognize experiences of expected gendered behavior in a medical encounter. As participants report, such expectations include (but certainly are not limited to) being compliant, listening to those "who know best," waiting for a secondary turn at speaking, never disputing authority, and relying on expert-others' status and education over one's own experience and intuition.

RESEARCHING ADVOCATE/CAREGIVERS

While considerable research now exists regarding patient-provider communication (Cegala et al., 2004; Cegala, Mainelti, & Post, 2001; Charles et al., 1999; Greenfield et al., 1989; Roter, 1997), an extensive search found no previous research that has examined advocate/caregivers perceptions of what communicative actions and interactions they consider to be effective during medical encounters. The issue of interpersonal communication competency or effectiveness, and the negotiation of roles in the triadic medical encounter, is here expanded and studied from the perspective of the advocate/caregiver. This research focuses on the lived experiences and perceptions that female family caregivers have about the interpersonal communication interactions that occur in triadic medical encounters.

Until recently, most research on interpersonal communication in medical contexts has used questionnaires, surveys, and closed-ended interviews, and has provided valuable social science information regarding precise, skills-based communication behaviors in medical encounters. However, such research fails to consider communication as a co-constructed process. The present human science research focuses on the personal understandings and insights of female advocate/caregivers in regard to how interpersonal communication in triadic medical encounters is co-constructed among the participants.

Experientially grounded understandings and insights are studied here from a gendered, interpretive framework, informed by the theory of the social construction of reality (Gergen, 2001), and the co-construction of identity (Gergen, 1994; Harre & Gillett, 1994; Harre & Stearns, 1995). Because advocate/caregivers are overwhelmingly female family members, who provide care to patients "invisibly" at home (du Pre, 2000; Gerstel & Gallager, 1994; Greene, Majerovitz, Adelman, & Rizzo, 1994; Rutman, 1996; Tates & Meeuwesen, 2001, a gendered, interpretive perspective helps develop a picture of the social context in which the advocate/caregiver, as a partner to and an advocate for the patient (Rutman 1996) interacts as a member of the triad described by O'Hair and McNeilis (1993).

This research design involved narrative methodology (Kvale, 1996; Polkinghorne, 1988). Narratives were gathered, by audiorecording and observation, from two focus group conversations in which advocate/caregivers shared their life experiences, in the form of interactive stories, with other advocate/caregivers in the groups. Quinn (1997) said that we may use "clues in ordinary discourse for what they tell us about shared cognition." Following contemporary convention, participants in this research are referred to as "co-researchers" in that they are, equally with the facilitator and observer, co-constructors of the interview conversations. The distinction of this study is that the focus is on the lived experiences of the advocate/caregiver and her understandings of communication effectiveness in interpersonal communication in the triadic medical encounter, rather than on the needs, responsibilities, and competencies of either the provider or the patient. Taking this research perspective, we find insights for health professionals into the unique understandings and meanings shared by female advocate/caregivers about their own lived experiences during communication in medical encounters. The current research was done primarily as thesis work (Babers, 2003), but provides rich, human science understanding that complements the extensive social science findings to date.

FINDINGS

The intent of this research was to begin to understand the experiences of female advocate/caregivers. Of particular interest are the ways in which they understand themselves to become communicatively effective on behalf of their care receivers in triadic medical encounters and to determine what, if any, are the commonalities in their experiences of becoming effective in their roles as advocate/caregivers. Co-researchers for this project were women whose care receivers were dealing with a range of health issues from cancer to autism to Alzheimer's disease.

Participants were asked to identify the kind of caregiving responsibilities they have for their care receivers. All participants identified the following activities: emotional/spiritual support, transportation, assistance with access to and understanding of information, leisure/social support, and personal care. The most frequently identified personal care activities included bathing, toileting, dressing, grooming, getting in and out of bed, and walking. Two caregivers report that they provide this kind of care work 2 to 4 hours per day, 7 days per week, and more than a few indicate spending between 5 and 8 hours per day, 7 days per week. Most of these women are not only the primary caregiver, but are in fact the only caregiver in the household. All the caregivers also have the equivalent of full-time employment outside the home.

If the participant's lived experience is the foundation of human science research, then the structure for understanding those lived experiences is built with themes that researchers identify in their reports as salient frames "emerging" from the narratives of their participants. Emergence is a result of a process of analysis that takes place continuously in every stage of narrative research (Kvale, 1994). Importantly, themes emerge from a final analysis in which the researcher becomes saturated through close inspection of audiotaped narratives and transcriptions of those narratives. Arriving at themes in this study was accomplished following the ideas of Kvale (1996), van Maanen (1990), and Wolcott (1994). Although themes are the focus of narrative research, the end product is intended to be the development of social understanding. In this case, we come to understand advocate/caregivers' perceptions of their becoming effective communicators in triadic medical encounters.

Perceptions of effectiveness begin in recognition of the many difficulties the advocate/caregiver must face in establishing a place alongside her care receiver in interaction with the medical community. Many obstacles must be overcome in regard to the advocate/caregiver and communication status.

POWER AND STATUS (PHYSICIAN "GOD COMPLEX")

Power represents control of many aspects of communication in the medical encounter and appears to subsume several subthemes. Primarily, it references the ability the physician has to make a decision to either share control of the interaction or not, share information or not, to define the topics, and ultimately, to share control of decision making with the care receiver and caregiver, or not. The theme of power is demonstrated by co-researcher statements such as, "*You're fighting an endless battle because they have the power,*" "*You do what they want, exactly and precisely,*" and "*He*[the doctor] *is dismissive and inattentive.*" Status is the socially constructed location of the interactants in a hierarchy of ability to influence. It is often based on education, income, and title. Because the perceived power and status in medical encounters is heavily weighted on the physician's end of the relational continuum, the physician has a choice whether or not to shift from a paternalistic to participative decision-making model for the interaction that he or she controls. The physician can decide to leave the room at any time (time control); to listen or not listen to the advocate/caregiver and the patient (doctor listening, or not listening, to caregiver expertise); to include or exclude the caregiver and/or patient in conversation; to make eye contact or not (doctor engagement); and to reveal or withhold information (information control).

Additionally, the doctor has control over the medical records, what is or is not entered, how the information is phrased, and whether or not it is true. The social construction of documentary reality becomes the final reality, created and maintained by those with power and status in the system. Social hierarchy metaphors and dismissive authority metaphors were used repeatedly by co-researchers revealing issues of power and status. For example, one says, "*They are the doctors looking down on us . . .*" and "*Oh yeah, oh yeah, whatever . . .*" while nonverbally demonstrating the doctor patting them on the head or behind. Almost without exception, the themes that emerged reflect some aspect of power and status and were spoken of in terms of a struggle or battle to overcome.

Advocate/caregivers talk also about how the doctor can use his or her power positively. For example, the physician has some power to advocate for caregivers and their care receivers as they work within the "system" whether it is the hospital, the insurance company, the health maintenance organization, or Workers' Compensation. A co-researcher describes what a relief it is to have a doctor "*go to bat for you . . . for the little guy, or the poor guy, or the disabled guy . . .* [a doctor who will] *rip 'um down for you! It feels great to have someone on your side, who understands your situation!*"

The matter of the physician's attitude and character appears to represent a great deal of frustration to the advocate/caregivers because of the power and status the physician holds in the medical encounter. The physician's attitude toward the caregiver and her care receiver includes among others, the issues of respect, trust, blame, honesty, motivation, engagement, time spent, and what is labeled here the God complex.

Respect includes the physician's ideas about the reliability, trustworthiness, and even the relevance of the lived experiences of the advocate/caregiver and her care receiver regarding health, illness, symptoms, lifestyle, and values. Participants' stories included words and phrases such as, *condescending, dismissive, would* or *would not listen,* and anecdotes such as Karen's that describe the doctors "*totally treating us like inanimate objects.*" Both successful and unsuccessful interactions appear to hinge to a great degree on the presence or absence of respect from the physician toward the caregiver and her care receiver. One woman, for example, describes the "*female doctor who started looking at [her care receiver] as the problem instead of her medication or her ideas. She was openly rude to us and condescending as though we didn't know what the hell we were talking about.*" Caregivers repeatedly stated that they automatically feel respect and trust for the physician until proven otherwise.

The respect physicians have toward the caregivers and care receivers leads to trust (in both directions) which the advocate/caregivers believe greatly impacts the treatment options that are presented to them. For example, an out-of-state physician "*trusted and respected*" one co-researcher enough as a caregiver to telephonically describe to her how an important procedure should occur so she could explain to a pediatrician in her own town how to accomplish the task. On the other end of the spectrum, one care receiver's physicians do not display trust and respect when they look at the kind of medication he must take for pain control and assume that "*Oh! You're an addict and you're just . . . trying to get more pills.*"

In one narrative, a participant recounts how she "*watched and watched for the feeding tube to pass.*" She reports that she stopped worrying about the failure of the feeding tube to appear in her daughter's diaper because she trusted the radiologist when he pointed to an x-ray and said "*I see it; it's right down there.*" But he hadn't seen it. Her daughter suffered terribly because he was not honest or correct about what he saw, and the woman reports that she should not have trusted him, his expertise, or his honesty.

Honesty is defined by participants here as truthful and straightforward communication; it involves completely and compassionately provided information. Participants expressed a desire to be assured that their physician is being honest and "*upfront*" with them and they report that they must be on guard because they so frequently encounter dishonesty. One tells a story she sees as demonstrating dishonesty on the part of physicians. She describes how important information was intentionally withheld in order to force the decision of the doctor's choice, one that her care receiver/husband would probably not have made if he had been given full and complete knowledge.

An extreme example of medical dishonesty and lies that become reality is the "social construction of documentary reality" (Smith, 1999). It is the power that higher status medical professionals have to construct the medical record as they see fit with no input from the lower status, but highly involved and well informed advocate/caregiver and the care receiver. One woman provides an example when she talks about how their physician "*made up her mind, she wrote things down that were wrong. Things that were lies! Outright lies that became part of the permanent record! And the record goes to Workers' Compensation . . . and it doesn't do any good to protest, because doctors' opinions are respected more than patients.*"

A doctor's respect or lack of respect for care receivers and advocate/caregivers alike can be impacted by the social construction of documentary reality. A concern that many of the advocate/caregivers expressed was the idea that they would "*look like a you-know-what,*" or "*like a jerk*" if they question doctor expertise or authority. In the experience of the co-researchers, not only can an advocate/caregiver be perceived this way, but several reported seeing medical records in which doctors have formally characterized the advocate/caregiver using words and phrases such as "*overly anxious mother,*" and "*schizoid mother, overbearing.*"

The placing of blame on the advocate/caregiver and her care receiver by the physician is also a perceived attitude that impacts the way communication occurs and who has control. For example, one woman tells the group with a great deal of intensity that her husband perceived the doctor's attitude toward his lung cancer as "*a slap in the face, that the doctor, that* [her husband] *felt it as BLAME!*" Another describes how "*suddenly I was the problem!*"

when she asked the hospital staff why she and her Aunt had been kept waiting in the emergency room for hours. Another describes how her continued insistence to hospital staff that something was wrong with her daughter was characterized as *"only making things worse."* The attitude of blame indicates a lack of respect on the part of medical professionals for the advocate/caregiver and her voice in the medical process of her care receiver. Each participant relates that this lack of respect/blame greatly impacts her ability to feel respect and/or trust for the physician in return.

The doctor's motivation is suspect by the majority of the co-researchers in this study. One co-researcher, for example, states that her experience with medical students and doctors both demonstrate that *"80% of them are in it for two reasons, money and family."* Participants also discussed how *"a doctor's ego"* is a motivator that greatly influences information flow. For example, the doctors' willingness to listen to findings co-researchers have made in their own research as one woman explains, *"we have done a lot of research . . . but [her husband] is not taken seriously."* Ego is perceived to also impact the doctor's willingness to make referrals to specialists. Several participants were forced to ask for and even insist on referral to a specialist. Co-researchers believe that doctors' willingness to listen to descriptions and understandings of the medical condition that are based in the lived experiences and intuition of care givers, especially if it is contrary to doctors' expertise, is influenced by ego.

The women also talk about their desire to assume the best motivations. *"We're assuming that they really do care, empathize . . ."* but must occasionally deal with the fact that health care providers might not empathize or feel compassion. Empathy and compassion were noted frequently by co-researchers as physician attitudes and motivations that were important to successful communication in medical encounters. Empathy and compassion represent the physician's ability and motivation to understand and respond thoughtfully and attentively to physical and emotional circumstance in which the advocate/caregivers and care receivers find themselves. One woman emphasized that *"some doctors—they really want to be there, they really want to help."*

Participants emphasized that it is vital to the effectiveness of communication in medical encounters of any kind that the doctor makes the choice to be *"engaged."* Doctor engagement means that the doctor is focused on the care receiver and the advocate/caregiver and is connected with what is happening in the interaction at the moment. It means that that he or she has left other patients and concerns outside the interaction. Co-researchers describe evidence of doctor engagement as the way *"she takes the time to make eye contact,"* *"pays attention,"* *"listens,"* and *"remembers."*

Time spent was a broad concern of all participants and defined as the amount of clock time the doctor actually takes for communication in the medical encounter. Time spent impacts the kinds and quantity of information exchange, the appearance of doctor engagement, respect, and motivation. A co-researcher describes an encounter when she was

> . . . *trying to get information out of a doctor . . . calling him down, he's standing by the door, one hand on the door knob, his pencil already in his pocket . . . I remember saying to him "I know there's other patients, and I know you have a lot to do, and that you're a very busy person . . . but we've waited to see you too. And we have a lot of questions." I'm not shy about these things. But you know, on this particular day, with this particular doctor, the problem was, it didn't help! He left anyway!*

This example, like most others, has many overlapping themes and subthemes: time, power, respect, information control, doctor engagement, and the system.

The doctor's expertise is perceived by co-researchers to include such things as medical training, knowledge about the nature and symptoms of illnesses, and her or his knowledge of potential cures for, as well as treatment and management of symptoms of those illnesses. Expertise also includes the doctor's knowledge of how best to work within the medical system. Primary themes that emerged regarding doctor expertise included the "doctor's world" and "information control."

Much of the power for the kind and amount of relational control in the medical encounter and the efforts that advocate/caregivers must make to obtain some semblance of shared control may lie in the fact that the advocate/caregiver has entered the terrain or field of the doctor's expertise (co-researchers used the word "doctor" rather than "physician" or "medical care provider" almost exclusively). The advocate/caregiver is on the physician's home turf, so to speak, as there are seldom house calls in contemporary society. She is in the arena of the physician's expertise, and her own expertise is rendered invisible; it is left at home where the majority of her caregiving activities occur. One advocate/caregiver describes how *"we're forced into* [an unfamiliar] *world with our medical need . . ."*

An aspect of being *"forced into a world"* is learning to negotiate the language and jargon of medical culture. *"I feel like I'm talking a different language here, asking questions in a different language and he can't understand what I'm trying to ask, or describe to him,"* was one description of this experience. Another co-researcher simply says they *"stuff you full of jargon."*

An additional problem that advocate/caregivers expressed regarding doctor expertise is that medical professionals do not seem aware that just because a procedure or medication is easy and routine to prescribe and to explain, does not mean it will be easy and routine to apply in the daily life of the care receiver's home. For example, the doctors appeared completely insensitive to one woman's *"twice monthly ordeal of returning to the children's hospital* [and to the fact that] . . . *I just don't think I can take this . . . nothing is happening there!"* Another example is a story a participant tells about her *"lesson"* in using the suction machine that she must use to keep her daughter's airways open, *" . . . they send you home and my lesson was, 'you just put it in and swish, swish, swish' and that's it! Well it wasn't that easy!"*

Information control refers to the choices physicians can make, by virtue of their power, status, and expertise, whether to impart full and complete information or to withhold information. *"The doctor has this idea"* one co-researcher reports, *"of where it is all going and you have no idea. And the further you, as the patient or caregiver, stay away from the total amount of information, the more your expectations are violated."* She goes on to discuss the emergency room physician who refused to provide requested information. She remembers him as an *"arrogant son-of-a you know what. He refused to answer questions such as why my son had to stay in the hospital . . . he said 'because I told you! He'll be fine! He's in good care!' And he left us there!"*

Advocate/caregivers perceive that information is withheld for many reasons: (a) the physician is paternalistically protecting the caregiver and patient and/or does not think the caregiver or patient can mentally or emotionally handle some kinds of information as in another woman's example about the *"doctor's philosophy . . . he waits for the questions. Like when you are telling your kids the facts of life, you don't want to tell them too much before they are ready";* (b) the doctor doesn't have time, *"he is in a rush . . . patients are in the other room,"* often because of time constraints from the hospital or clinic that force *"only 6 min-*

utes for each patient;" (c) the doctor's attitudes toward the advocate/caregiver and patient such as in one narrative about the advocate/caregiver's doctor describing her as *"an overbearing mother";* (d) the doctor's personal whims as when the emergency room doctor told the co-researcher *"because I say so"* when she asked why her son needed to stay in the hospital so long; (e) fear of litigation, *"they can't admit they don't know because of litigation,"* as two women stated simultaneously at one point; and (f) the *"doctor ego"* as exemplified by a co-researcher's perception that the radiologist who said he saw something in her son's x-ray that was not there did so because he did not want to admit to a mistake.

Participants express frustration over a major problematic issue with communication in medical encounters wherein choices are taken out of their own and their doctors' hands by policies of the "system." The system is the organizational bureaucracy within which doctors must often work and patients' treatment decisions are often impacted. One aspect of the system is the *"requirements of the hospital"* or clinic. For example, one participant was told by her doctor that he is *"allowed 6 minutes for each patient, booked 10 hours a day . . .* [seldom] *saw the same patient . . . had to read the history in that time."* Co-researchers refer to the system with the industrial metaphor of the *"assembly line."* Some implications of the assembly line metaphor are that all patients are alike (one woman relates that the doctors in Children's Hospital treated her and her care receiver like *"inanimate objects"*); the doctor must see as many patients as possible in as little time as possible which creates the impression that quantity is more important than quality; all the "rules" must be followed with little or no consideration for specific situations; decision making is top–down in that the administrators with no medical training often control the final medical decisions.

The system also includes HMOs, Workers' Compensation, and insurance companies. Those bureaucracies often appear to control what choices the advocate/caregiver and her care receiver can make regarding not only treatment options, the kind of medical professionals they are permitted to consult, but also which providers they can consult and how much time he or she can spend with them during a medical encounter. One usually quiet participant tells of her first experience with the concept *"preferred providers . . . OH! I just thought that was un-AMERICAN!"* Her descriptor illustrates the feeling of a loss of control and choice that is part of the average, individualistic, independent American citizen's life.

In contrast, uninformed choice is sometimes forced upon advocate/caregivers by the system. Several of the participants discussed regulations within the system that require them to make selections of medical providers, agencies to assist them with caregiving, and even medical supply houses without any kind of guidance. One offers, for example, that *". . . they tell you to pick two doctors, but no one can tell who or how to pick because of lawsuits and stuff. Finally a nice person told us [who to pick and why], the person had to whisper to me though because everybody is bound, you are in the dark about these things but you have to pick."*

There exists among advocate/caregivers the idea of a physician "God complex." This is a label for the socially constructed expectation that, as one woman says, *"the doctor knows best . . . yet they make mistakes and they are not God,"* to which another immediately responds, *"no, but some doctors THINK they are!"* These comments were generally agreed upon as evidenced by the rousing laughter and affirmative nonverbal of all co-participants. Despite the laughter drawn from the comment, the God complex is a very real and disturbing construct that has a strong impact on advocate/caregiver perceptions of communication with physicians. The God complex, then, is a theme that subsumes all the subthemes that relate to the doctor's world including the physician's power and status, the attitudes and character of the physician, and the language of the medical culture.

Participant attitudes about the physician God complex vary from bitterness to plaintive desire as suggested by their liberal use of the terms *"blind trust"* and *"blind faith in doctors."* Bitterness in their vocal tone alludes to the futility of having that kind of trust and faith in the physician's recommendations only to have their care receivers suffer irreparable damage such as the irreversible, life changing immunization injury one woman's son received. Plaintive desire to rely on the physician as all-powerful, highly trained, knowledgeable, and compassionate is demonstrated by a participant's comments about physicians, *"you love them . . . you depend on them because you have to have this trusting relationship with them,"* and *"I need that other kind of expertise, the doctor's expertise."*

POWER AND STATUS
(ADVOCATE/CAREGIVER BEING A "GOOD GIRL")

A gendered "double-bind" or dialectic tension emerges as an overarching theme in the focus group conversations. Drawing on Gregory Bateson's seminal work on schizophrenia, Watzlawick, Bavelas, and Jackson (1967) suggest the double bind is a feeling of "damned if he [*sic*] does and damned if he [*sic*] doesn't" (p. 241). It is an interactional paradox that co-researchers face in communication with doctors in triadic medical encounters as they attempt to find balance between their own expertise as advocates and caregivers and the doctors' expertise (they need to respect, trust, and rely on the doctor and need also to respect, trust, and rely on their own, often contradictory lived experiences and expertise). The paradox is revealed as the advocate/caregivers struggle for balance. First, they must find a balance between the doctors' socially constructed power, authority, and status, and their own socially constructed dependence, and powerlessness. Then they experience the need to reconcile their powerlessness and their very real need to rely on their own expertise. The double bind is demonstrated in the conflicting relational issues that arise in the communication of advocate/caregivers as they negotiate for their role as advocate for the care receiver in the triadic medical encounter. It emerges as the understanding that women, as caregivers who are advocates for their care receivers, must also act from traditional gendered positions, to act as well socialized "good girls."

Good girl behavior involves being compliant, listening to those "who know best," waiting for a turn at speaking, never disputing or questioning authority, and relying on expert others' status and education over one's own experience and intuition. For example, a co-researcher describes with regret, but no apparent bitterness, how she did what was expected, did not question the authority of the doctors or the system, and generally behaved as a *"good mom"* when she signed papers allowing her son to receive the immunization shot that resulted in his permanent learning disability. She even took him in for his next shot *"like a good mother"* despite evidence of immunization injury, and she accepted the doctor's diagnosis that her son's fever and odd behavior was *"normal"* despite her intuitive fear that it was not normal. She expresses no blame toward the doctor, only regret that she thought she was being a *"good mom"* by doing what was expected of her without question, but that she was not, after all, a *"good mom"* because she did not question what was expected of her.

A participant describes her hesitant compliance with her *"regular"* physician's referral to his new medical partner. She says, *"I felt a little uncomfortable but I also very much trusted my regular physician.*" The new doctor treated her concerns dismissively and while she continued to express her intuitive uneasiness, she complied without question. In retrospect, she says she sees it as a lesson learned.

Another woman tells how she was poorly trained to use the suction machine to keep her daughter's airways open. If she did not use it properly, she risked her daughter's life; yet she didn't want to "*bother the nurses . . . here I am again, calling in the middle of the night.*" She tells the story with self-derision, as though she isn't sure which behavior is worse, to bother the nurses, or to be worried about bothering the nurses.

A co-researcher describes sitting like a good girl in the hospital hallways, outwardly patient but agonizingly impatient on the inside. She says she was "*waiting for whatever answers they had. I kept seeing them in the halls. . . . They* [the doctors] *are laughing and walking up and own the halls and it's like, you know, life is going on for them but my life is at a standstill! They just seem to be dragging it out and dragging it out.*" She reports that her mother (acting as advocate/caregiver for her even as she acted as caregiver for her baby) finally asked one of the doctors, "*why are you TORTURING her this way?*" She tells us he seemed surprised that there was even a problem, but he did finally talk to her.

Another paradox associated with "good girl" behavior is the advocate/caregivers' expressed desire to please and apparent sense of responsibility for the emotional well being of the doctor that conflicts with their perceived responsibility to advocate for their care receiver. Each of the advocate/caregivers addressed some version of this double bind related to emotional care work. Some examples are: "*you don't want to tick them off*" by asking too many questions; "*you don't want to bother them*" by calling too many times; "*don't want to hurt their feelings*" by seeking a second opinion or by explaining something you have learned in your own research; "*they might think you don't trust them*" if you tape the encounter or obtain advice from other sources; "*we really like our doctor and don't want to hurt her feelings*" so one hesitates to go to a specialist when one believes one is getting inadequate care; "*you don't want to make them angry*" by reminding them that "*you have been waiting for hours;*" "*you don't want to embarrass him*" by reminding him that one's care receiver is allergic to the medicine he intends to use; and "*you feel like you are imposing but at the same time you really need their help.*"

An older participant refers to this "*uncomfortable shield that is with me in my journey with* [her daughter]. *I feel like it is my job to make them* [the doctors and nurses] *more comfortable, to make them more at ease with her . . . I think it is uncomfortable to confront a doctor. There is weirdness about that.*" Despite the weirdness, she reports that she has learned to confront.

Advocate/caregivers perceive that their reputations and identities as either a "good girl" or "not a good girl" are socially constructed in the context of medical encounters. One co-researcher expressed irritation, for example, that she was identified as "*an anxious mom;*" another actually saw herself characterized in the permanent documentary record as an "*overbearing, schizoid mother.*" Advocate/caregivers spoke of how "*you want them to like you.*" In frustration, they repeatedly mention how the doctors "*make you feel a fool,*" or "*you'll feel like a you-know-what,*" and how "*you run the risk of being a real jerk*" when communicating in a persistent manner in the doctors' world, up against their expertise and power. Advocate/caregivers are aware of the double bind that is socially constructed in medical encounters and learn to actively resist it. For example, one reports "*I trust people and I tend to be a people pleaser . . . but not as much now, not after* [her daughter's illness] *. . . I have a little fire in me.*"

One participant recalls the reluctant but empowering words of her pediatrician following an emergency situation that had a positive outcome only because she resisted his characterization as an overbearing, worried mother who was contributing to her daughter's problems by persisting in her attempts to *"make them listen."* He told her *"98% of the time you're going to be wrong when you're up against us* [the doctors]*, but it's worth it for you to push . . . just in case THIS time is that two percent."*

EMPOWERMENT

Although "empowerment" may have become a somewhat cliched concept in the 1990s, it is a word used repeatedly and spoken with intensity by co-researchers in both focus groups. It represents the strength and competency end of a power and status continuum and is often used in conjunction with strategies the caregivers and patients have developed to overcome the negative effects of the power and status of the physician. In many cases, such strategies force a more participative interaction, with shared control of the communication and the decision-making. One woman perceives that she *"was empowered by reading or hearing statistics about how many people are dying every year at the mistakes of medicine."* Another describes being *"empowered by support from friends and the agency,"* and yet another says that for her *"the first step was to know myself and do a lot of reading . . . just get myself educated."*

The most frequently used metaphor in both focus groups was a war metaphor. Co-researchers used war metaphors when they spoke of their attempts to empower themselves despite the power and attitudes of physicians. Examples of this expressed dialectic include: *"I think the best weapon we have is education,"* *" . . . my best defense was . . . ,"* *" . . . best ammunition . . . ,"* and *" . . . divide and conquer . . . "*

Empowerment was also revealed as a theme through the metaphor of gift giving from physician to the caregiver, as though acknowledging that physicians have ownership of medical information and can choose to dispense, or withhold it. Examples are: *"I was empowered by respect from the doctor,"* *" . . . he and his staff spent a great deal of time . . . answering questions and providing information . . . it was very empowering."* In a third example, a woman speaks of *"getting from A to B in this education, empowerment process."*

THE CAREGIVER'S EXPERTISE

One woman summarizes the intensity of belief that all co-researchers share, in the importance of respecting their own expertise: *"we have to be respected as the experts on our children, not just lip service. It has to fully happen. Our expertise is a very valid area of communication."* The advocate/caregivers' expertise comes directly from knowledge and wisdom gained through their third shift of work. It is developed in the context of work they do providing both visible and invisible care, the physical, emotional, and spiritual care work for their care receiver. When they talk about expertise, advocate/caregivers are speaking of the knowledge and understandings gained by their day-to-day responsibilities and their lived experiences of the wellness, illness, values, and lifestyles of their care receivers. Their expertise includes: understanding the values and lifestyle of their care receiver, their instincts and intuition, and the education they have pursued regarding the health and illness of their care receiver through both formal and informal channels.

Each of the advocate/caregivers who participated in this research identified "emotional and spiritual support" and "personal care" for their care receiver as activities in which they participate on a daily basis; they are intrinsic components of their third shift of labor. The advocate/caregiver is familiar with the lifestyle, culture, and the value system of the care receiver in a way that no medical professional can be. They are often responsible, but are not always successful in their attempts to explain and defend (e.g., advocate for) their care receiver's personal values system and their autonomy as human beings with the right to make their own choices. For example, a woman tells the poignant story of her husband's final days as he died of lung cancer and how the doctors talked [her husband] and her into a decision without fully informing them of the consequences. They "*separated us, and you know, 'divide and conquer,' they caught him at a vulnerable moment . . . so they essentially robbed [him] of his value system.*" With visible regret she continued that "*it was my understanding that he wanted to freeze to death underneath a spruce tree and the last thing he wanted to do was go on a respirator! He was robbed!*"

Another co-researcher complains of how unaware and unconcerned doctors seem to be about the impact that a sudden, unilateral decision to change prescriptions has on both advocate/caregivers and their care receivers. Doctors, all participants agreed, apparently have no idea how physically and emotionally demanding and even painful the waiting period for new side effects to subside can be and how exhausting it is to establish new medical regimens in the home.

Caregivers also speak of the attention that must be paid to the intuitive component of their expertise; their "*gut instinct*" about what is going on despite the medical knowledge and training they may be missing. As example, one participant knew instinctively her son was having seizures after his immunization shot, but she paid attention to the doctor's expertise instead of attending to her own expertise, which came in the form of intuition; therefore "*nothing was done for him.*" When advocate/caregivers speak about their own expertise, they are addressing their knowledge of the values and the lifestyle of their care receiver. They say repeatedly and emphatically, "*We have to be listened to from that perspective.*" Their knowledge is knowledge of the particular, the mundane, quotidian experience of being there.

Using the dialectic or war metaphor, advocate/caregivers discuss education as a weapon to develop their expertise beyond personal experiences with the wellness and illness of their care receivers and beyond information dispensed or not dispensed by their physicians. Although the war metaphor is predominant in the research conversations regarding strategies for communication in triadic medical encounters, Beisecker's (1989, p. 61) characterization of the advocate/caregiver's role of "watchdog" appears consonant as a description of their perceived role in triadic medical encounters. The "*strategies*" and "*tactics*" that advocate/caregivers report using, to construct successful communication in medical encounters, were linked to the theme of empowerment by the identities, attitudes, and behaviors they develop toward themselves, the doctor, and their care receiver and toward their respective roles in the encounters.

Strategies here are linked to perceptions of competency in communication; the interpersonal interactions advocate/caregivers initiate to make communication work. Kreps (1993) stated that communication competency in medical interviews (for all participants in the interview) is the "ability to utilize interpersonal skills to elicit co-operation from, gather information from, and share health information with relevant individuals in the health care system" (p. 56) and to participate more fully in the communication interaction. The strategies identified in both focus group conversations to construct successful encounters included proactive behaviors such as walking away, educating herself, documentation, protecting the care receiver's autonomy, and persistence in communication.

The first strategy many of the co-researchers discuss is *"walking away"* from medical encounters. It is a strategy that comes from strength and competency in that the advocate/caregiver recognizes, often because of doctor attitude and power issues, communication in the medical encounter will not likely improve and the best way for her to advocate for her care receiver is to *"move on to a different doctor."* One participant's first comments about medical encounters describe her *"attitude* [about a doctor that she] *can't communicate with. . . . If I'm around a doctor who I don't feel is listening, I just say 'see you later' . . . so, I kind of avoid the problem right off the bat."* Another says, *"If I am working with a person within the medical community who does not respect* [my knowledge and expertise], *recognize it, AND accept it, because that is the really important thing, then I have to move on to someone else."* However, as another woman states when discussing the responsibility that caregivers have to change doctors, *"Unfortunately, sometimes you don't have that option"* because choices may be limited by location and/or the system.

Advocate/caregivers used "investment" as a metaphor to describe the tension that arises over *"not knowing WHEN to change doctors."* One explains that when her husband was dying of lung cancer, they did not want to call in specialists because they had *"invested so much in him* [the doctor], *to save my husband's life! You invest all your thoughts and hopes and actions toward this one doctor . . ."* The emotional labor and time involved in re-investing, in developing a new relationship with a new physician, appears to interfere occasionally with decision making about changing doctors. A further part of the discussion addressed how, as advocate/caregivers, it is often easy to second guess oneself, to doubt one's instincts, or to have one's own instincts in conflict. The caregiver feels a need or responsibility to change doctors, but is *"not to a place emotionally where you feel like you ought to . . . you know, maybe this next thing will work."*

Co-researchers describe education as a *"weapon"* they use to access the doctor's arena of expertise; a tool that allows them to come closer to *"speaking the same language"* that is spoken in the doctor's world, and to level the metaphorical battle field. Advocate/caregivers speak of education as *"the best weapon,"* *"my best defense,"* and *"the ammunition"* they use to construct successful communication in medical encounters. Such education is obtained through several avenues including the obvious tactic of question asking in the medical encounter.

Often, because of time constraints and/or many of the physician attitude issues discussed earlier, advocate/caregivers find it necessary to research their care receiver's condition and potential treatments on their own. The co-researchers report that they have learned to educate themselves in multiple ways: by reading articles from popular magazines and newspapers, through internet research, in dialogue with support groups both on the internet and face to face, by attending to television documentaries, by seeking second opinions, and in conversation with friends and family. One co-researcher tells the participants that she was able to educate herself by becoming familiar with the medical jargon, a feat she accomplished by *"hanging around Intensive Care, where you start to pick up some of the lingo. They will talk to you in their own lingo."* She perceived that once she could *"talk their language"* the doctors began to pay attention to her questions and she *"could keep them talking and get more information."* Advocate/caregivers report that they also educate themselves through resource agencies, research foundations, and alternative health sources such as naturopathic physicians, doctors of osteopathy, and chiropractors.

One broadly experienced participant says that the advocate/caregiver must pay attention, educate herself about the treatments she allows, and read the fine print in documents before she signs them. She says, *"you really do need to know your family history . . ."* She emphasizes that it is the advocate/caregiver's responsibility to *"not rely on the doctors"* to feed her the necessary information. She tells us, *"you know, you're just signing these things . . . and you don't really read it, the small print saying these statistics and asking you about your medical history. If I had really paid attention, [her son] wouldn't have received the shots* [that resulted in his developmental disability]."

Advocate/caregivers describe how important it is to have other people they can rely upon to help them through difficult times as they search for adequate information about their care receivers' medical situation and as they attempt to find the strength to confront doctors and other medical personnel when they offer options that are not acceptable or feel intuitively wrong or inadequate. A mother talks about how her friends *"empowered"* her, helped her realize that she not only had the right, but the responsibility to *"bother the nurses"* and get complete information about how to use the suction machine. She describes how she, in turn, helped a friend realize that when that person believed her son was not getting adequate medical care, she needed to make a decision to change doctors despite the feeling that *"we don't want to hurt* [the doctor's] *feelings."* Another woman tells of how her mother was available to assist her as she attempted to advocate for her new baby daughter and how her mother, in effect, became an advocate/caregiver for the woman herself.

Careful documentation and record keeping is a strategy believed to construct successful communication in medical encounters by the majority of advocate/caregivers in both focus groups. They discussed how important it is to write out questions, to leave room on the paper to record the answers provided, and then to leave a copy of the paper for the permanent record. One woman, who provides care for an elderly aunt, describes how she documents issues and problems as they occur between appointments. She *"writes down in [her aunt's] very own words about how she feels"* on a daily basis including [her aunt's] food and water intake, blood pressure, sleeping patterns, and how and when [her aunt] takes her pills. She takes the information with her to medical encounters and insists that it be placed in the medical record. She believes that this strategy solves two problems—it allows her aunt to speak about what has occurred without complaining (*"she wouldn't tell them anything even if she could remember!"*) and it helps both of them form and maintain a relationship with the physician.

Another woman and her husband have found that they must *"write down everything that's been happening, all the pills you took, 'cause God forbid if you are missing a pill!"* Because his medication is for pain, he has been *"accused"* of addiction and/or overdosing. Three participants also attend medical encounters with lists of their questions. Several of the advocate/caregivers insist that their questions and answers and documentation regarding the content of the interaction be entered into the record, and report that it thus becomes evidence that *"forces"* the doctor to take their concerns more seriously. In essence, these documenting activities appear to be proactive participation in the social construction of documentary reality.

Most of the advocate/caregivers report that they regularly read the medical records and several of them keep copies of the medical record in their possession. They report having learned that this practice brings a different level of openness and honesty to the discussion of treatment options and the construction of the "reality" (such as the characterization of one advocate/caregiver as an *"overbearing"* or *"schizoid mother"*) by the physician. Additionally, they believe the physician becomes more accountable for how he or she constructs reality in the permanent record. For example, doctors are less likely to document *"outright lies"* if they knows that the advocate/caregiver maintains copies of the record.

One advocate/caregiver reveals her strategy of using audiotapes for documenting medical encounters. She reports that because she and her husband began recording their medical encounters, they no longer experience having misinformation and *"lies"* placed in the permanent record. The other women in the focus group were enthusiastic about the potential helpfulness of audiorecording. They discussed how the taping strategy might *"force the doctor"* to become more engaged in the medical encounter. Such beliefs suggest that written notes and audiorecordings may effectively encourage doctors to listen more actively, *"to more carefully select what they are going to attend to and force the doctor into a framework where he is attending to and selecting the data in this room, this conversation instead of all the others* [that may be going through his or her mind]." Taping the interaction also has the obvious advantage of allowing the advocate/caregiver and her care receiver to recall instructions regarding treatment regimens as well as information provided by the physician in answer to questions.

Autonomy speaks to independence and control over self and the medical situations in which the patient and advocate/caregivers find themselves. It is the power that advocate/caregivers believe they and their care receivers ought to have to make their own reasoned choices. Advocate/caregivers repeatedly expressed concern that the care receiver be the focus of triadic medical encounters and that her or his voice be heard during the interactions in order to ensure her or his autonomy. Addressing this idea one participant describes her efforts to ensure that the doctors *"include"* her aunt in communication in medical encounters, that they direct their comments directly to her aunt and *"take her seriously"* even though she has Alzheimer's disease. Despite the fact that the aunt *"isn't going to remember 2 minutes later what the doctor said,"* this woman has learned to insist that doctors respect her aunt enough to include the elderly woman in the communication moment. She believes this has made it easier for her aunt, who is Christian Scientist and is therefore resistant to medical care, to accept and follow through with treatment plans thus extending and greatly enhancing her quality of life.

A co-researcher shares a story of the concern and discomfort she felt when the oncologists asked her, outside the presence of her husband, to make the decision whether or not to *"put him on a respirator."* She said to them, *"Well, how come you are asking me this, why don't you ask him?"* The recognition of advocate/caregivers that they have the right to not only obtain the medical records of their care receivers, but also contribute to documentation in the medical record speaks to the theme of protecting care receivers' autonomy.

To *"simply tell the doctor,"* as a participant puts it, seems a logical strategy to construct successful communication in medical encounters. Persistence is a characteristic and a behavior that advocate/caregivers consciously strive to develop so that they cannot only *"simply tell the doctor"* but also *"get him* [sic] *to listen."* Such persistence is described in another woman's story about seeing multiple doctors who are *"in a rush and you feel like you are imposing . . . so we just kind of DIG IN our heels and keep talking . . . "* Persistence is a quality and a strategy that requires the advocate/caregiver to be assertive and *"insist"* she be listened to; that medical professionals pay attention to her and her information. It occasionally requires the advocate/caregiver to be willing to, as one woman explains it, *"plant myself on the porch steps in the early morning saying, 'no! LISTEN TO ME! This is different!'"* Yet another tells how she *"has a little fire"* in her now that she didn't used to have. Still another quotes a memorized passage from her journal that portrays persistence in the description of how she *"by-passed assertiveness and went directly to aggression."*

There seems to be doggedness in the quality of persistence these advocate/givers have struggled to develop. This doggedness is demonstrated both in the words and also in the non-verbal behaviors of some co-researchers during one of the focus group conversations. A soft-spoken co-researcher characterizes herself as *"aggressive when I need to be."* She rises from her seat to provide a nonverbal demonstration of how she might grab a doctor's shirtfront to get his or her attention. Others often fantasize about physically aggressive behaviors such as *"wanting to smack them,"* or *"just bash through the door"* and one frequently pounds one clenched fist into the open palm of her other hand for emphasis in this regard.

The implication throughout the focus group conversations is that each of the women have expended much time and effort developing both the willingness and the ability to be persistent and assertive on behalf of their care receivers and that it might be *"taught to young mothers, maybe it ought to be required in college,"* as one suggests, so that advocate/care-givers don't *"have to work so hard to get good at being a good mother."* A participant cites, when she speaks to the development of persistence, the realization that while it requires a tremendous amount of *"emotional energy"* it is necessary to take *"this journey of getting from A to B in the education-empowerment process* [and to learn to get past feeling] *uncomfortable and confront him . . . "* Advocate/caregivers in the research conversations appear to agree with Beckman et al. (1989) who suggest training to enhance patient negotiation and assertiveness skills may result in *". . . creating more realistic treatment plans and goals"* (p. 226).

SUMMARY

Several subthemes coalesce in the focus group conversations to form overarching themes. These themes include ideas that lie on a problems–strengths continuum of understanding such as powerlessness–power–empowerment, doctor expertise–caregiver expertise, and information control–education. Based on co-researcher experiences and the review of extent literature, the power and status that physicians have enable them to control the course of communication in triadic medical encounters. There emerges from these conversations a certain feeling of helplessness regarding the overwhelming sense of powerlessness in which advocate/caregivers begin their journeys; of being in the doctor's world wherein her or his attitudes and character and the system have control over the construction of communication and ultimately over the health of care receivers. The obstacle to be faced by the advocate/care-giver is primarily learning to negotiate a place for her voice in the social hierarchy of the medical encounter/interview and in the decision-making process involving her care receiver.

Also present in the focus group conversations is a sense of advocate/caregivers' proactive resistance to physician control over communication. This resistance is associated with a theme of personal empowerment. Empowerment of the advocate/caregiver enables her to find solutions to the problematic areas of communication in triadic medical encounters and to balance the socially constructed power of the physician. It is expressed by co-researchers primarily in terms of a war metaphor; the advocate/caregivers speak of the *"weapons"* and *"defense"* tactics they find useful to assist them in their *"struggle"* as advocates to communicate effectively on behalf of their care receiver and to *"make it work."* Those weapons and tactics are the strategies they use in their role as watchdog and include walking away, educating self, documenting, protecting autonomy, and persisting. There is also a common journey metaphor that describes the development of persistence.

The problems–strengths continuum is also demonstrated in the dialectical tensions produced by the conflicting, socially constructed identity of the advocate/caregiver as a "good girl." This is clearly a gendered dilemma in which on the one hand she must fulfill her responsibility to seek the expertise of physicians and *"take advantage of their knowledge."* She must be respectful of doctor knowledge and deferential of her or his status. She must take care to appear compliant and be sure that nothing she does or says will *"make him angry," "hurt his feelings," or "tick him off."* This one-down, gendered perception remains, regardless of the gender of the physician, perhaps due to the persisting nature of medicine as a paternalistic social environment.

On the other hand is the advocate/caregiver's identity or role of watchdog wherein she relies on her own expertise to help her protect and defend the health of the care receiver. As one woman declares, *"We have to be listened to!"* The watchdog is persistent, assertive, and insistent, protective of the autonomy of herself and her care receiver, listening to her instincts and intuition, her own expertise, whereas the good girl is compliant and protective of the power and ego of the higher status authority and expertise of the physician.

This theme of power and status includes advocate/caregivers' *"buy in"* to the socially constructed notion of the physician's God complex *("Doctor knows best, honey"), which* is supported by their own communication behaviors stemming from good girl syndrome. The struggle to communicate effectively, in the medical encounter, is intensified as the socially constructed identities of the caregiver (as the good girl and as the watchdog of the advocate/caregivers'–care receivers' world) are in constantly fluctuating juxtaposition with the physicians' socially constructed identity in the doctors' world; a place where the God complex seems to be reality.

A final obstacle is relative to the matter of knowledge. The advocate/caregiver must negotiate her way through a process of coming to understand disease and the medical treatment of that disease. Related here is negotiating a place of value for her own experiential knowledge. Hers is knowledge of the particular; her care receiver, her care receiver's symptoms, beliefs, and lifestyle; and her care receiver's feelings, mental states, and fears. The advocate/caregiver must find the fine line between what is broadly known of a disease and what she knows from her hands-on experience. And she must learn to find and maintain that line by a careful focus on both sides of the line.

The narratives of these advocate/caregivers demonstrate an experiential evolution from feelings of dependence and helplessness to effectiveness; to what O'Hair et al. (2003) label agency. Agency, O'Hair tells us is

> a state or condition where individuals become empowered to the extent that they understand the choices they want to make, advocate for their own rights, take control of their own destiny, and demonstrate the competency necessary for acting in their own best interests. Agency is about having choices and the competencies to act on them. (p. 10)

Advocate/caregivers, acting with authenticity in the interests of their care receivers, come to the medical encounter seeking just such agency for their care receivers and themselves.

The invisible service given to children, parents and other family members by mostly female advocate/caregivers addresses an entire range of debilitating disease from cancer to Alzheimer's to developmental disorders. The women who act as advocate/caregivers for their family members put in a full week of "third shift" work. Their "third shift" work is "invisible," often overlooked, and often unappreciated either personally or socially. Their position as the third party in the triadic medical interview/encounter is past due its full, scholarly recognition. Scholarship, particularly communication scholarship, must very soon develop practical support for both the advocate/caregiver and the medical community so that both sides of the social equation can better prepare to actively improve the health experience of care receivers.

The potential value of this research, then, is much the same process for the health communication scholar as for the advocate/caregiver. One must focus on the knowledge social science has produced and look to studies such as this for a "fleshing out;" for knowledge produced by human science. Experiential knowledge, science of the particular, puts a human face on the scientific knowledge used to make generalizations and can produce a "complete picture" of this significant, rapidly growing location of human interaction. Understanding the experience of the advocate/caregiver will be essential in providing care to the "baby boomers" about to become the primary end consumers of US cancer care.

REFERENCES

Abel, E. K. (1991). *Who cares for the elderly: Public policy and the experiences of adult daughters.* Philadelphia, PA: Temple University Press.

Babers, T. (2003). Voices from the third shift: Advocate/caregiver perceptions of effective communication in medical encounters. Unpublished master's thesis, University of Alaska, Fairbanks.

Ballard-Reisch, D. (1993). Health care providers and consumers: Making decisions together. In B.C. Thornton & G. L. Kreps (Eds.), *Perspectives on health communication* (pp. 51-65). Prospect Heights, IL: Waveland Press.

Beckman, H., Kaplan, S. H., & Frankel, R. (1989). Outcome based research on doctor patient communication: A review. In M. Stewart & D. Roter (Eds.), *Communicating with medical patients* (pp. 223-227). London: Sage.

Beisecker, A. E. (1989). The influence of a companion on the doctor–elderly patient interaction. *Health Communication, 1,* 55-70.

Beisecker, A. E., Brecheisen, M. A., Ashworth, J., & Hayes, J. (1996). Perceptions of the role of cancer patients' companions during medical appointments. *Journal of Psychosocial Oncology, 14*(4), 29-45,

Beisecker, A. E., & Moore, W. P. (1994). Oncologists' perceptions of the effects of cancer patient's companions on physician-patient interaction. *Journal of Psychosocial Oncology, 12*(1), 23-29.

Brown, J., McWherter P., & Leipzig, J. (1995). Using communication resources to impact corporate health care costs. In M. Cross & W. Cummins (Eds.), *Proceedings of the eighth conference on corporate communications: New forces in corporate communication,* (pp. 225-233). Madison, NJ: Fairleigh Dickinson University.

Cegala, D. J., Gade, C., Broz, S. L., & McClure, L. (2004). *Physicians' and patients' perceptions of patients' communication competence in a primary care medical interview.*

Cegala, D. J., Mainelli, T., & Post, D. (2001). The effects of patient communication skills training on compliance. *Archives of Family Medicine 9*, 57-94. Available google.com.

Cegala D.J., Socha McGee, D., & McNeilis, K.S. (1996). Components of patients' and doctors' perceptions of communication competence during a primary care medical interview. *Health Communication, 8*, 1-28.

Charles, C., Gafni, A., & Whelan, T. (1998). Decision-making in the physician-patient encounter: Revisiting the shared decision-making model. *Social Science and Medicine, 49*, 651-661.

duPre, A. (1999). *Communication about health: Current issues and perspectives*. New York: McGraw-Hill.

Ellingson, L. L. (2000). The roles of companions in the geriatric oncology-interdisciplinary health care provider interaction. NCA Doctoral Honors Seminar Conference Paper. Evanston, IL. Available at google.com

Ellis, B., Miller, K. I., & Given, C. W. (1989). Caregivers in home health care situations: Measurement and relations among critical concepts. *Health Communication, 1*(4), 207-226.

Feeser, T. L., & Thompson, T. L. (1988). A test method of increasing patient question asking in physician-patient interactions. *Cosmetic Dermatology, 6*(9), 51-55.

Foster, S. E., & Brizius, J. A. (1991). *Caring too much? American women and the nation's caregiving crisis*. Southport, CT: Southport Institute for Policy Analysis.

Gafni, A., Charles, C., & Whelan, T. (1998). The physician-patient encounter: The physician as a perfect agent for the patient versus the informed treatment decision-making model. *Social Science and Medicine, 47*, 347-354.

Gergen, K. (1994). *Realities and relationships: Soundings in social construction*. Cambridge, MA: Harvard University Press.

Gergen, K. (2001). *Social construction in context*. Thousand Oaks, CA: Sage.

Gerstel, N., and Gallager, S. (1994). Caring for kith and kin: Gender, employment, and the privatization of care. *Social Problems, 41*(4), 519-538.

Greene, M., Majerovitz, K., Adelman, R., & Rizzo, C. (1994). The effects of the presence of a third person in the physician-older patient medical interview. *Journal of the American Geriatric Society, 42*, 413-419.

Greenfield, S., Kaplan, S., & Ware, J. (1985). Expanding patient involvement in care. *Annals of Internal Medicine, 102*, 520-528.

Harré, R., & Gillett, G. (1994). *The discursive mind*. Thousand Oaks, CA: Sage.

Harré, R., & Stearns, P. (1995). *Discursive psychology in practice*. Thousand Oaks, CA: Sage.

Kaplan, S., Greenfield, S., & Ware, J. (1989). Impact of the doctor-patient relationship on the outcomes of chronic disease. In M. Stewart & D. Roter (Eds.), *Communicating with medical patients* (pp. 228-245). London: Sage.

Kreps, G. (1993). Relational communication in health care. In B.C. Thornton & G.L. Kreps (Eds.), *Perspectives on health communication* (pp. 51-65). Prospect Heights, IL: Waveland Press.

Kreps, G., & Thornton, B. (1984). *Health communication: Theory and practice*. Prospect Heights, IL: Waveland Press.

Kvale, S. (1996). *InterViews: An introduction to qualitative research interviewing*. Thousand Oaks, CA: Sage.

McCorkle, R., & Pasacreta, J. (2001). Enhancing caregiver outcomes in palliative care. *Cancer Control, 8*(1) 36-45.

McGee, D., & Cegala, D. (1998). Patient communication skills training for improved communication competence in the primary care medical consultation. *Journal of Applied Communication Research, 26*, 412-430.

Miller, K., & Zook, E. (1997). Care partners of persons with HIV/AIDS: Implications for health communication. *Journal of Applied Communication Research, 25*, 57-74.

O'Hair, D., Villagran, M., Wittenberg, E., Brown, K., Hall, T., Ferguson, M., & Doty, T. (2003). Cancer survivorship and agency model (CSAM): Implications for patient choice, decision-making, and influence. In L. Sparks (Ed.), *Cancer communication and aging. Special Issue of Health Communication, 15*(2).

O'Hair, D., & McNeilis, K. (1993). Advocates for elderly patients: Negotiation of patient and physician roles. In E. B. Ray (Ed.), *Case studies in health communication* (pp. 61-71). Hillsdale, NJ: Erlbaum.

O'Hara, D. (2001). The invisible caregiver: How can doctors care for them too? *American Medical News*. Available at www.amednews.com.

Parrott, R. (1993). Pediatrician-parent conversations: A case of mutual influence. In E. B. Ray (Ed.), *Case studies in health communication* (pp. 49-59). Hillsdale, NJ: Erlbaum.

Polkinghorne, D. E. (1988). *Narrative knowing and the human sciences.* Albany: State University of New York Press.

Quinn, N. (1997). Research on shared task solutions. In C. Strauss & N. Quinn (Eds.), *A cognitive theory of cultural meaning* (pp. 137-188). Cambridge: Cambridge University Press.

Roter, D. (1997). Patient participation in the patient–provider interaction: The effects of patient question asking on the quality of interaction, satisfaction, and compliance. *Health Education Monographs, 5,* 281-310.

Rutman, D. (1996). Caregiving as women's work: Women's experiences of powerfulness and powerlessness as caregivers. *Qualitative Health Research, 6,* 90-106.

Smith, D. E. (1999). *Writing the social: Critique, theory and investigation.* Toronto: University of Toronto Press.

Street, R., & Millay, B. (2001). Analyzing patient participation in medical encounters. *Health Communication, 13,* 61-73.

Tates, K., & Meeuwesen, L. (2001). "Let Mum have her say": Turn-taking in doctor-parent-child communication. *Patient Education and Counseling, 40,* 151-162.

Thompson, T. L. (1984). The invisible helping hand: The role of communication in the health and social service professions. *Communication Quarterly, 32*(2), 148-163.

van Maanen, M. (1990). *Researching lived experience: Human science for an action sensitive pedagogy.* London: SUNY.

von Friederichs-Fitzwater, M. M., & Gilgun, M. (2001). Relational control in physician–patient encounters. *Health Communication, 13,* 75-87.

Watzlawick, P., Bavelas, J., & Jackson, D. (1967). *Pragmatics of human communication.* New York: Norton.

Wolcott, H.F. (1994). *Transforming qualitative data: Description, analysis, and interpretation.* Thousand Oaks, CA: Sage.

12 | Communication and Support Groups For People Living With Cancer

Kevin B. Wright
The University of Oklahoma

Lawrence R. Frey
University of Colorado at Boulder

What's wonderful about [cancer support] groups is that you have others to laugh with and to cry with, others that you can speak to and express everything you feel in a genuine way. You don't have to pull any punches, like you do with your family. You don't have to pretend. And that brings back into our lives that "something" that is lost when we're diagnosed. It brings back that connection with others, that bond, that realization that you are not all alone, that feelings are similar to those of other people. It really gives us back that sense of control, and reconnects us to life.

— Pamela, cancer survivor (as cited in Schimmel, 1999, p. 14)

Support groups for people coping with a variety of illnesses have become a popular source of health information and comfort for more than 25 million Americans (Kessler, Mickelson, & Zhao, 1997), and they are the most common way that individuals in this country attempt to change health behaviors (Davison, Pennebaker, & Dickerson, 2000). Support groups have a long history in the United States, arising from a variety of grassroot efforts in which people bypass professional health care institutions and structures to form communities based on their collective experience of facing similar illnesses and medical conditions (Katz, 1993; Katz & Bender, 1976; Yalom, 1995). These and other grassroots healthcare practices (e.g., residential health care facilities) have added an important, alternative voice to the traditional authorities (e.g., hospitals) that have defined health care (see Adelman & Frey, 1997).

191

Support groups for people with cancer represent a large proportion of these groups. In a recent study of the prevalence of support groups in four major U.S. cities (New York, Chicago, Los Angeles, and Dallas) and on the Internet, Davison et al. (2000) found that cancer groups were the third most common type of health-related support groups in these cities and the most frequent type of support group on the Internet. According to Alexander, Peterson, and Hollingshead (2003), "The results of a quick search on the Internet show over 100 Internet support groups for those living with cancer and their families alone" (pp. 309-310). The National Cancer Institute and the American Cancer Society have lists of numerous support groups throughout the United States for virtually all types of cancer. The prevalence of these support groups is probably due to cancer currently being the second-leading cause of death in the United States (American Cancer Society, 2001a).

Support groups for people with cancer differ in terms of their affiliation, structure, and focus. Some support groups are affiliated with hospitals, cancer centers, and other health care facilities; other support groups, such as those found on the Internet, operate independent of any health care organization. Cancer support groups are also distinguished by whether they are facilitated by health professionals (typically, a counselor or an oncology nurse) or are self-led (often with informal or no leadership) by people with cancer. In addition, such groups differ in the type of support they offer members, with some groups focusing primarily on providing information about cancer (e.g., educating people about the nature of the disease, helping them to cope with lifestyle changes, and suggesting treatment options), some groups primarily providing peer-based emotional support, and some offering both informational and emotional support.

Social scientists from several disciplines, including communication, have conducted numerous studies of support groups for people with cancer, focusing on a number of issues (e.g., participation in these groups, participants' personal characteristics, comparison of support groups to traditional support networks, types of supportive messages exchanged in such groups, and the effects of participation on various outcomes). However, the precise nature and role of communication within cancer support groups is unclear, and there have been few attempts to synthesize findings from studies of cancer support groups or to identify themes in the literature that may help scholars, practitioners, and even participants to understand more fully the role that communication plays in such groups.

The purpose of this chapter is to examine the current literature on social support groups from a communication perspective. Specifically, we focus on the communicative reasons people with cancer join support groups, characteristics of cancer support group members, cancer support group communication processes, and outcomes associated with participating in these groups. We use this framework to summarize what we currently know about support group communication for those living with cancer and to suggest directions for future research.

COMMUNICATIVE REASONS PEOPLE WITH CANCER JOIN SUPPORT GROUPS

Although many people who have been diagnosed with cancer may never feel the need to join a cancer support group, many other individuals experience difficulties with the social implications of having cancer and in communicating with others about this disease. In particular, some individuals with cancer appear to be drawn to support groups because of problems they experience with traditional support providers (e.g., family members and close friends) in their existing social network who do not always behave in supportive ways when dealing with the issue of cancer.

Inadequate support is not just a social problem for people facing illness; it has been linked to negative health outcomes, such as suppressed immune systems, prolonged recovery time, disease vulnerability, and increased stress (Cohen & Wills, 1985; DiMatteo & Hays, 1981). Conversely, satisfaction with one's support network has been found to be associated with positive health outcomes, including reduced stress and better adjustment to living with a disease (Lepore, Allen, & Evans, 1993; Wills, 1985; Wortman, 1984). Such effects are important because successful adjustment to cancer has been associated with longer survival times (Jones & Reznikoff, 1989), improved psychological well-being and sense of control (Fritz, Williams, & Amylon, 1988; Sullivan & Reardon, 1985), and improved ability to cope with the experience of pain (Spiegel & Bloom, 1983).

Researchers have, thus, argued that effective communication with members of one's support network is critical for psychological adjustment to cancer, although the precise ways in which communication and adjustment to cancer are linked are unclear (Gotcher, 1995; Walsh-Burke, 1992). However, we do know that communication problems within traditional networks for people with cancer may occur at both the macro, societal level, due to the stigma of the disease and the resulting social isolation that stigma creates, and at the micro, interpersonal level, because of the inability to communicate effectively about the disease.

The Stigma of Cancer and Sense of Social Isolation

Cancer, like many other diseases and medical conditions (although less than some other diseases, such as HIV), has been found to carry a social stigma in the United States, as it does in many other cultures (see Goffman, 1963; Mathieson, Logan-Smith, Phillips, MacPhee, & Attia, 1996; Sullivan & Reardon, 1985), that negatively affects the provision of social support (MacDonald & Anderson, 1984). Perhaps because of the stigma associated with cancer, the social implications of being diagnosed with it can lead people to struggle with their identity. This identity crisis is exacerbated because cancer may limit people's ability to perform various taken-for-granted roles they engage in on a daily basis (e.g., work and family roles), and the strain of changes in these roles contributes to feelings of being socially and emotionally isolated (Bloom & Spiegel, 1984).

The feeling of being socially stigmatized by an illness and, consequently, embarrassed by having it, can often lead people to a sense of alienation and isolation from individuals in their current social network. Spiegel, Bloom, and Yalom (1981) contended that individuals within the social network of a person with cancer "often in subtle but unmistakable ways, distance themselves from the dying" (p. 528) due to societal-induced fears about disease and death. Spiegel (1992) found that discussion of cancer often arouses relational partners' fears, which may lead to avoidance of the person with cancer or a lack of discussion of cancer-related topics when interacting with him or her. Such responses can contribute to the person with cancer feeling alienated and isolated, feelings that can create even greater psychological stress, which, in turn, can exacerbate the person's physical health problems (Cohen & Wills, 1985; DiMatteo & Hays, 1981). Indeed, social isolation has also been empirically linked to mortality among those with cancer, although there are some discrepancies among studies. Reynolds and Kaplan (1990), for example, in a longitudinal study of cancer patients, found that socially isolated women had a significantly elevated risk of dying from cancer and that men with few social connections had significantly poorer survival rates.

The creation of social connections within cancer support groups and the positive effects of those connections on participants' health suggest that such groups provide participants with "social capital." Originally used by Hanifan (1916) to describe "those tangible substances [that] count for most in the daily lives of people" (p. 130), and later by Putnam (2000) to refer to "connections among individuals—social networks and the norms of reciprocity and trustworthiness that arise from them" (p. 19), primarily for the purpose of contributing to civic life, this research on the social network effects of cancer support groups adds to the growing body of scholarship that suggests that people with more social capital enjoy better mental and physical health (see Baker, 2000).

In addition to the more general sense of isolation due to the social stigma of cancer, people with cancer may feel socially isolated due to embarrassing aspects of cancer symptoms and treatment. For instance, Weber, Roberts, and McDougall (2000) argued that "the diagnosis and treatment for prostate cancer may cause incontinence and sexual dysfunction, [about which] men often feel embarrassment and shame" (p. 251). As another example, Bloom (1982) contended that mastectomy as a treatment for breast cancer often undermines a woman's sense of her attractiveness, leading to both embarrassment and mutual withdrawal from relationships with significant others. A woman who has had a mastectomy may be hesitant to engage in intimate interaction with her spouse; in turn, he "perceives her withdrawal as rejection and responds by further withdrawal" (p. 1330). This mutual withdrawal can lead a woman with breast cancer to feel isolated and disconnected from a vitally important potential source of social support.

The difficulties of caring for a person with cancer can also damage relationships within an individual's primary support network due to factors such as stress and burnout (Chesler & Barbarin, 1984; Helgeson & Gottlieb, 2000), which may foster a greater sense of isolation for the individual with cancer. Scholars have suggested that simply expressing their needs can be problematic for people facing illness because this may lead to a secondary stigma of feeling inadequate, non-active, and/or weak (Chesler & Barbarin, 1984; DiMatteo & Hays, 1981). Samarel and Fawcett (1992) reported that the diagnosis of cancer often leads to difficulty maintaining the previous quality of people's interpersonal relationships, creating dissatisfaction with traditional sources of support.

Such isolation and alienation from traditional sources of support may help to make peer support groups attractive for people with cancer. According to Davison et al. (2000), "Alienation from one's usually supportive network may be precisely the kind of social anxiety that in turn increases the value of the mutual support context" (p. 213). These researchers found that the amount of support health-related support group participants sought was highly correlated with their feelings of embarrassment due to the social stigma assigned to their disease or condition.

Difficulties Communicating About Cancer

Cancer can be a difficult topic to discuss because it may make people think about their mortality, lead to the expression of strong, often uncontrollable, emotional feelings (e.g., crying), and create general discomfort because people may not have the skills to communicate about sensitive topics such as illness. Because of these and other difficulties, members of the support network of a person with cancer may not encourage him or her to express negative emotions about the illness, either because those members believe that it is unhealthy or because it makes them feel uncomfortable. They may lead network members to minimize the concerns of the person with cancer, avoid interacting with him or her, and/or steer conversational topics away from emotional talk about the disease or from discussion of cancer altogether (Dakof & Taylor, 1990; Heinrich, Schag, & Ganz, 1984; Helgeson, Cohen, Schultz, & Yasko, 2000; Sullivan & Reardon, 1986; Wortman & Dunkel-Schetter, 1979). It is not surprising, therefore, that people with cancer report inadequate support or unhelpful supportive behaviors from their traditional networks (see, e.g., Dakof & Taylor, 1990; Martin, Davis, Baron, Suls, & Blanchard, 1994).

Even when traditional support network members are receptive, people with cancer often find it difficult to discuss cancer with them, even when they wish to do so, because of their desire not to burden them with problems caused by the disease (DiMatteo & Hays, 1981; Gotcher & Edwards, 1990). They may feel that bringing up the subject of cancer during conversations may be crossing interpersonal boundaries of closeness and intimacy in the relationship (Chesler & Barbarin, 1984).

The desire to provide support to a person with cancer also brings up the issue of reciprocity. People who are ill and receive support from others often feel uncomfortable when they do not have the ability to reciprocate (Chesler & Barbarin, 1984; La Gaipa, 1990). This discomfort is based on a sense of inequity that may lead a person with cancer to feel over-benefited if he or she cannot help his or her friends in a similar manner. According to Arntson and Droge (1987), "Accepting help without being able to reciprocate can foster feelings of dependence, resentment at the imbalance in the relationships, and implies that one is socially incompetent because he or she has nothing of worth to offer other people" (p. 168).

One might suspect, given the collapse of traditional support networks that often occurs, that people with cancer might talk about their illness with medical personnel, such as those in a hospital, but research shows that they often do not feel comfortable doing so (Ford, Fallowfield, & Lewis, 1996). Siminoff and Fetting (1991), in fact, found that the emotions of people living with cancer are often the least discussed topic in a medical setting. This may be an additional reason why people with cancer often participate in support groups (see Alexander et al., 2003).

CHARACTERISTICS OF CANCER SUPPORT GROUP PARTICIPANTS

At present, there have been no large-scale surveys conducted of cancer support group membership. Factors associated with cancer support groups—such as the typical group norm of preserving the anonymity of members, the affiliation of many of these groups with hospitals and medical centers that protect the privacy of members, and the transient nature of membership within some groups—present numerous challenges to studying the characteristics of cancer support group members (Helgeson & Gottlieb, 2000). In addition, most studies of cancer support groups have relied on convenience samples, making it difficult to generalize sample characteristics to larger populations of cancer support group members. Moreover, given that the majority of studies of cancer support groups have been cross-sectional rather than longitudinal, there is little research on individuals who stop participating in cancer support groups. With these caveats acknowledged, studies of support group membership, in general, and some relatively small-scale surveys of cancer support groups give some insight into the types of people who participate in these groups with regard to race, ethnicity, social status, age, and gender.

According to Kessler et al. (1997), a survey of self-help group membership in the United States revealed that Whites were three times more likely to participate in self-help groups than were African Americans. This figure may well apply to support groups for people with cancer, as the studies reviewed for this chapter were comprised mostly of Whites. The low incidence of studies about cancer support group participants representing other ethnic/racial groups is disturbing, considering that there are high rates of many types of cancer among African Americans, Native Americans, and Latinos/Latinas (Miller et al., 1996). Moreover, in terms of social status, most individuals who participate in support groups, including those for cancer, appear to be middle class, with at least a high school diploma and with the majority of individuals having at least some college education or a college degree (Deans, Bennett-Emslie, Weir, Smith, & Kaye, 1988; Kessler et al., 1997).

As far as the age of cancer support group participants is concerned, Kessler et al. (1997) found, in a nationwide study of self-help groups, that the average age of participants was 43.1 years. However, for cancer support groups, participants are likely to be much older given the greater incidence of cancer among the elderly population (Deans et al., 1988). The risks of developing specific types of cancer, such as breast and prostate cancer, have been found to increase dramatically as people age (National Cancer Institute, 2002; Weber et al., 2000). Moreover, people may be more likely to seek support in cancer support groups as they age, as Funch and Marshall (1983) found that older individuals with cancer perceived themselves having less social support from family and friends than did younger individuals.

Finally, with regard to gender, existing studies of cancer support groups indicate that women are much more likely than men to be members (Anderson, 1994; Cella & Yellen, 1993; Taylor, Falke, Shoptaw, & Lichtman, 1986). Moreover, women not only are more likely than men to participate in cancer support groups but they also are more likely to rely on traditional support networks to cope with cancer (Fife, Kennedy, & Robinson, 1994). However, given that the majority of studies has focused on breast cancer groups, and, therefore, relatively little is known about the characteristics of men who belong to cancer support groups, the proportion of men who participate may be underestimated. This lack of information about the participation by men should be of concern, given, for instance, that prostate cancer has the second highest mortality rate in the United States (American Cancer Society, 2001a), and because men may experience more problems communicating about prostate cancer among members of their traditional support network than do women about breast cancer (Weber et al., 2000). Perhaps, however, men's participation depends, in part, on what communication processes characterize the support group, as research shows that men who do participate in cancer support groups typically prefer an informational or educational focus, whereas women prefer groups that emphasize personal experience and emotional support (Klemm, Hurst, Dearholt, & Trone, 1999; Sullivan, 1997, 2003; Taylor et al., 1986). We now turn to a discussion of communication processes in such groups.

CANCER SUPPORT GROUP COMMUNICATION PROCESSES

A substantive portion of the existing literature on support groups, including groups for people with cancer, has focused on the processes characterizing these groups (see Arntson & Droge, 1987; Cline, 1999; Sullivan, 2003). Studies emphasize the central role of communication in support group processes, particularly in terms of the topics discussed, the exchange of social support messages, and the role that narratives play in the support process.

Topics Discussed in Cancer Support Groups

Group norms within support groups encourage discussion of topics that are discouraged in other social contexts, especially discussion of health-related issues. Arntson and Droge (1987) noted that "members have the freedom to bring up topics that may be no longer welcome in other contexts and the time to talk about them" (p. 155), and Spiegel et al. (1981) pointed out that "members are not only permitted but encouraged to voice all of their morbid concerns, which become a common bond rather than a cause for isolation" (p. 528). In fact, cancer support groups may be beneficial precisely because they offer participants opportunities to communicate about their illness. Given that members of a person with cancer's traditional network often avoid talking about cancer, as previously explained, support groups may serve as one of the few places where people can discuss cancer-related topics. Sullivan (2003) found that cancer support group members often "vented about doctors, treatments, side effects such as, hair loss, weight gain, and relationships" (p. 90), topics they felt were difficult to discuss in their more traditional social networks. Cella and Yellen (1993) found that the most common themes of discussion in cancer support groups included the emotional impact of illness, the meaning of illness, family difficulty, problems of intimacy, a sense of isolation/stigma, role changes, cancer-specific concerns, and negotiating the health care system. Discussion of these types of topics led Weber et al. (2000) to conclude that support "group dynamics provide members the opportunity to interact with each other to counter the avoidance that may be present between patient and well-meaning family members who often have misinformation and fears" (p. 252).

Social Support Messages Exchanged in Cancer Support Groups

The primary purpose of cancer support groups, as the title of the group suggests, is to offer participants opportunities to gain social support. Alexander et al. (2003) identified four types of social support that are exchanged in support groups: (a) *informational* support, which "provides recipients with information to help deal with stressful situations"; (b) *emotional support*, which "deals with individuals' feelings, primarily in terms of relieving negative emotions and sometimes supplementing them with positive emotions"; (c) *esteem support*, which "is used to make others feel good about themselves by demonstrating respect through compliments, validation of opinions and beliefs, alleviation of guilt felt by others, and offers of encouragement"; and (d) *tangible assistance*, which "provides recipients with direct help by offering to lend a helping hand in the form of, for instance, money, babysitting, or meals" (pp. 313-314).

Alexander et al. (2003) conducted a comparative case analysis of four Internet support groups—cancer, attention-deficit disorder (ADD), depression, and alcoholism (Alcoholics Anonymous; [AA]) support groups—with regard to the type of social support provided in these groups. Using participant-observation and self-reports, Alexander et al. analyzed Internet messages produced during a 3-week period of time, as well as responses to questionnaires from some of the Internet support group participants. The examination of these messages showed that although all four Internet support groups focused on health issues, the groups functioned quite differently and served different purposes for their members. For instance, the distribution of informational support, emotional support, esteem support, and tangible assistance differed in these groups, with informational support being exchanged the most in the cancer group (72% of the group's discourse) compared with the ADD (57%, the largest proportion), AA (43%, the largest proportion), and depression (27%, the second largest proportion) support groups. In contrast, emotional support accounted for only 16% of the support exchanged in the cancer group compared to 18% in the AA, 27% in the ADD, and 48% in the depression groups, and esteem support accounted for only 9% in the cancer group compared with 15% in the ADD, 24% in the depression, and 37% in the AA groups. Finally, tangible assistance accounted for 3% or less in all of the groups. In terms of satisfaction, the members of the cancer group were more satisfied with their group ($M = 5.93$, on a seven-point scale) than were members of the AA ($M = 5.33$) and ADD ($M = 3.88$) groups, but less satisfied than members of the depression group ($M = 6.47$). Members of the cancer support group were especially satisfied with the amount and quality of the information they received and "some members even stated that they used the group as a source of information because they mistrusted doctors and other members of the medical community" (Alexander et al., p. 326). The researchers hypothesized that as support groups grow larger in size (with the cancer group being the largest of the four support groups studied), communication tends to focus more on information exchange than on emotional support.

There also appear to be gender differences in the types of supportive messages that are shared within cancer support groups and perceptions of their usefulness. Sullivan (1997, 2003) found that women in online breast cancer groups were more likely to exchange emotionally supportive messages (encouragement, in particular), whereas men were more likely to exchange information. Klemm, Reppert, and Visich (1998) also found that men with prostate cancer were more likely to discuss social activism in an online cancer forum than were women with breast cancer. These gender differences are in line with findings from studies of face-to-face cancer support groups, where, in general, men perceive informational support to be more useful than emotional support, whereas women prefer emotional support over informational support, although there appears to be a great deal of variability in terms of individual male and female preferences (see, e.g., Harrison, Maguire, & Pitceathly, 1995).

Narratives in Cancer Support Groups

Cancer support groups, like other types of support groups, encourage participation among members through group norms of "telling one's story" to the group on a voluntary basis (Arntson & Droge, 1987; Cline, 1999; Yalom, 1995). This process usually begins with a member providing a brief history of his or her experience with cancer and then discussing current issues and feelings with which he or she is dealing (Helgeson & Gottlieb, 2000). Rappaport (1993) contended that members of self-help groups use narratives like this as a means of forming a social identity. As we previously discussed, people with cancer and other life-threatening diseases and conditions often experience feelings of isolation, and support groups provide an environment where these individuals feel they share a common identity with the other members. Cancer support group members learn to identify with other members' experiences and feelings about cancer through the sharing of narratives, and this appears to both validate their own experiences and feelings and to lessen their sense of isolation (Mok & Martinson, 2000; Wright & Bell, 2003). According to Davison et al. (2000), "The stories told and heard in this context carry the weight of shared experience, the emotional potency of common suffering, and an avenue for social learning" (p. 206).

In addition to identifying with other members' experiences and feelings, newer members of support groups often find experienced members' stories particularly credible (Wright, 1997). Moreover, the experiences of other health-related support group members is often perceived as more credible than information obtained from other people, even healthcare professionals, especially information about the psychosocial aspects of their disease, due to the fact that other support groups members are actually living with the disease on a daily basis. However, the tendency to privilege information obtained from fellow support group members over professional advice has been criticized; as Rosenberg (1984) argued, "The self-help movement appears to be anti-intellectual, holding the belief that 'having been there' and working through the problem is the superior, and perhaps, only basis for emotional understanding" (p. 183).

Communication researchers have suggested that narratives play an important role in changing the worldview of support group members when it comes to dealing with health-related issues (Antze, 1976; Arntson & Droge, 1987; Cline, 1999; Wright, 1997). Mok's (2001) study of cancer self-help groups in China reported that the communication process that "cancer group members experienced is an important cognitive process that helped to shape their perception of reality of self, the world, and the self-in-the-world" (p. 127). According to Davidson et al. (2000), "Each individual account contributes to a larger collective narrative that paints a portrait of identity by diagnosis" (p. 210). By promoting such collective understandings, the storytelling process within support groups helps to establish a sense of community among members (Adelman & Frey, 1997; Cawyer & Smith-Dupré, 1995; Cline, 1999).

Arntson and Droge (1987) pointed to some specific functions served by the sharing of narratives within support groups that may benefit both the narrator and those who listen to his or her story. For example, because narratives typically place events within a sequence, they "organize the relevant symbols in one's environment, making it possible to gain meaning from the past, give meaning to the present, and reduce uncertainty about the future" (p. 161). Such meaning may help those with cancer to perceive health-related events as less unpredictable, which may strengthen their sense of control over the disease. Moreover, listening to stories told in support groups is a way to receive advice nondidactically, and individuals are free to follow or disregard it (Arntson & Droge, 1987). Advice is rarely given directly within support groups but it is often embedded in a narrator's story (Wright, 2000a). For example, a narrator might disclose through a story that a certain type of medication was helpful in alleviating nausea during chemotherapy, without actually telling others that they should take the medication themselves. In addition, support group participants may identify not only with the information shared in a narrator's story but also with the emotions that the stories convey, serving to validate those feelings and to increase one's sense of similarity to the others members (Wright, 1997).

Some of the messages exchanged within cancer support groups appear to be useful in terms of changing members' perceptions of the disease. As previously mentioned, society tends to attach a negative stigma to cancer, and many individuals equate cancer with death, despite the fact that there are many forms of cancer, and that the prognosis for the different types of cancer vary widely. The common societal perception of the hopelessness of recovery from cancer may lead some individuals to view themselves as victims of the disease, which may result in passive coping strategies (Kreps, 1993) or a type of self-fulfilling prophecy, in which they do not aggressively seek treatment for the disease or adhere to lifestyle changes that may improve their chances for survival. Support group members, however, learn to develop less negative perceptions of cancer. According to Spiegel et al. (1981), within cancer support groups, "compassionate experience with dying persons seems to detoxify rather than exaggerate the fear of dying and thus underscores the positive aspects of living" (p. 528). Mok (2001) found that through talk, cancer support group members learned that "cancer is not equivalent to death, having cancer is not shameful, cancer is curable, and cancer is simply one kind of illness to be treated" (p. 127). As such, cancer support groups appear to result in a number of important outcomes, a topic to which we now turn.

OUTCOMES FOR CANCER SUPPORT GROUP PARTICIPANTS

The relationships between participation in cancer support groups and relevant outcomes are, in general, complicated because social support is provided in a variety of ways and its effects are mediated by a number of variables (see Schwarzer & Leppin, 1991). However, a number of studies provide insight into possible relationships between participation in cancer support groups and various outcomes; these include dealing with the stigma of cancer; expansion of people's social support network; being helped by helping; active coping, empowerment, and activism; and some additional health benefits.

Dealing with the Stigma of Cancer

Cancer support groups often take a proactive role in helping to minimize the social stigma of the illness through the interactions in which group members engage. Societal misconceptions about illness are often challenged during group discussion, and members, consequently, often feel less marginalized as a result. Arntson and Droge (1987) asserted that "self-help groups attack the social origins of the stigma by giving members an opportunity to renegotiate their ascribed roles through helping other people" (p. 167).

Other researchers, however, have argued that support groups could potentially increase members' perceived stigma and isolation if interactions in those groups lead members to feel even more different from individuals within their traditional social network or to perceive those individuals as being unable or unwilling to help at all (Helgeson & Gottlieb, 2000). The degree to which the benefits of support group membership offset new problems that members may experience with traditional network members after joining a support group remains unclear. Researchers, therefore, should conduct more controlled studies using pretest/

posttest measures to see what new problems may occur from participating in support groups and whether the benefits accrued outweigh any new problems incurred.

Expansion of People's Social Support Network

Support groups create opportunities for people with cancer to expand their social networks to include others living with cancer (Mok, 2001; Mok & Martinson, 2000; Sharf, 1997; Weber et al., 2000; Wright, 2002). Because it is unlikely that people know several individuals within their current social networks who have the same type of cancer as they do, cancer support groups provide an important place for people to meet similar others with whom they can exchange informational, emotional, esteem, and tangible support. Although some people attend support groups that include people with multiple types of cancer, studies suggest that people prefer support groups that focus on the type of cancer they have, as this allows for a more specialized understanding of their particular problems and solutions (see, e.g., Samarel & Fawcett, 1992).

One reason for the increased expansion of social networks is due to the many online cancer support groups that now exist. Support groups on the Internet allow people with cancer and other medical conditions to transcend geographical and temporal constraints to greatly expand their social networks (Davison et al., 2000; Klemm et al., 1999; Klemm et al., 1998; Street & Rimal, 1997). In a recent study of an online cancer community, Wright (2002) found that participants perceived the greatest advantage of online cancer support groups to be their ability to put people in touch with others who had similar types of cancer and specialized knowledge of symptoms and treatments. Sharf (1997), in a study of a breast cancer listserv, found that participation in the listserv increased the likelihood of people connecting with others with very similar health circumstances and their ability to draw on the expertise of those who had used certain medications and procedures, and the lifestyle changes needed to use them successfully.

The expansion of one's social network through support groups is thought to increase opportunities for social comparison, in which individuals make assessments about their own health and coping mechanisms by comparing them to others in the group (Davison et al., 2000; Helgeson & Gottlieb, 2000). According to Helgeson and Gottlieb, *lateral comparisons,* comparisons to similar others, may normalize people's experiences and reduce uncertainty and stress for those dealing with health concerns. However, when individuals compare themselves to others within support groups, their self-assessment could be either positive or negative. For example, if a person feels that he or she is coping less effectively than others in the support group, this may create *upward comparisons,* which could produce feelings of frustration or could serve as a source of inspiration to the person to cope more effectively by emulating the successful behaviors of those other members. Conversely, *downward comparisons* to others in a support group, such as when an individual feels that he or she is coping better than other members, can lead to positive self-assessments and/or to negative feelings about the group if interaction with the other members is perceived as being unhelpful. Helgeson and Gottlieb (2000) pointed out that individuals with low self-esteem, in comparison with those with high self-esteem, may make more negative downward comparisons in a support group. In short, the expansion of one's network through support groups could lead to positive or negative outcomes depending on the individual and his or her perception of others within the group.

Being Helped by Helping

One-on-one counseling typically creates an atmosphere where people living with cancer are relatively passive recipients of help from an expert; in contrast, support groups provide participants with opportunities to proactively help others (Mok, 2001). The norm of helping others is usually part of a support group's ideology that is reinforced during group interaction (Antze, 1976; Frank & Frank, 1991; Wright, 1997).

Cancer support groups, like other support groups, typically consist of individuals who vary in terms of the amount of time they have been members of the group, and members who have participated for longer periods of time are in a better position to proactively help others. They can be especially influential in providing new members with opportunities to learn vicariously about cancer; helping them to understand how to cope with physical, psychological, and social issues associated with the disease; offering them emotional support; and sharing information with them about treatment options (Wright, 2002).

Although newer members certainly receive a great deal of support from more experienced members, support groups are not a one-way street in terms of helping behaviors; the act of helping others appears to have psychological benefits as well. Social support groups, thus, encourage members who have been with the group for a longer period of time to share their experiences with newer members through the idea that helping others is important to one's own recovery. Helping others has been found to increase helpers' sense of self-worth and value and, simultaneously, to reduce their feelings of powerlessness (Spiegel et al., 1981; Yalom, 1995). According to Spiegel et al. (1981), "Patients who feel helpless and demoralized learn that they can be enormously useful to others" (p. 528). Moreover, Rosenberg (1984) said that "members feel that by improving their own competence in handling the situation they are also improving the competence of other group members and perhaps the social conditions of the group as a whole" (p. 175). Mok and Martinson (2000), in a study of cancer self-help groups in China, reported that members felt valued and found meaning in life through helping others in the group and, by doing so, that they saw themselves as help-givers and not just as people who received benefits from the group.

Benefiting by helping others has been termed "the helper principle" in the support group literature (Riessman, 1965). According to Cline (1999), the helper principle "encompasses a complex process of cognitive reframing during which rookie helpers become veterans" (p. 524). New support group members go through a socialization process in which they learn that helping others is an important part of the process of coping with the disease. Cline (1999) contended that "as members make the transition from helpee to helper, retelling their stories validates their experiences and reminds them, as well as other members, of their progress" (p. 524). This transformation from helpee to helper also appears to help support group members gain a sense of personal control when discussing their illness (Arntson & Droge, 1987; Cline, 1999).

Active Coping, Empowerment, and Activism

A crisis such as cancer can evoke a number of coping responses as individuals attempt to manage the disease; some people withdraw from social contact to cope privately, whereas others prefer to interact with people as a coping mechanism (Mattlin, Wethington, & Kessler, 1990).

The strategies that people use to cope with illness range from active to passive (Billings & Moos, 1981): *active strategies* are problem-focused, directed at remedying a threatening or harmful situation, whereas *passive strategies* are emotion-focused coping, taking the form of venting emotions in response to the negative situation. In addition, people often choose *avoidance-focused* coping strategies, in which they physically or mentally disengage from the threatening situation (Kohn, 1996). In general, active coping strategies have been linked to positive adaptation to problems when people perceive that the problem is not insurmountable, whereas passive coping strategies may be more effective when the problem is perceived to be beyond one's control. The evidence for adaptation to a problem situation is mixed for individuals who chose avoidance-focused strategies, depending on the person and his or her unique situation (Endler & Parker, 1990; Kohn, 1996).

Support groups that include caregivers of people with cancer or are designed specifically for them may encourage them to take a more active role in learning about symptoms, treatments, and productive ways of supporting those with the disease for whom they are caring. Chesney and Chesler (1993), for instance, found that participation in support groups for parents of children with cancer was highly correlated with parents' increased activism (e.g., working with others to raise awareness about cancer issues in the communities), use of active coping strategies, and help-seeking. In addition, the study found that support group participation was negatively correlated with parents' subsequent use of passive coping strategies, especially a tendency to cope solely by themselves with their child's illness.

Additional Health Outcomes of Cancer Support Groups

There are some more specific health outcomes that have been found as a result of participation in cancer support groups. For instance, in a longitudinal study of 86 women with metastatic breast cancer, Spiegel et al. (1981) randomly assigned women (and, thereby, eliminated the self-selection bias that is common in many other studies of cancer support groups) to participate in a support group or in a control group that received no treatment over a 1-year period of time. They found at the end of that time period that the support group women reported less tension, less depression, less fatigue and more vigor, less confusion, fewer maladjusted coping responses, and fewer phobias over time than the women in the control group. In addition, support group members reported that the group helped them to focus on and clarify numerous problems they faced as a result of being diagnosed with cancer. For example, the group helped the members to (a) manage information about cancer and treatment options, (b) deal with their anxieties toward illness and death, (c) reduce their sense of isolation, and (d) become more actively involved in making decisions about their health when communicating with their oncologists.

Cain, Kohorn, Quinlan, Latimer, and Schwartz (1985) investigated the psychosocial benefits of using a thematic counseling model with 80 females with cancer randomly assigned to one-on-one counseling sessions that employed the model, a cancer support group that employed the model, or a control one-on-one counseling condition that did not include the thematic counseling model. The model consisted of eight themes, including the nature and causes of cancer; the impact of treatment; relaxation techniques; diet and exercise; relating to caregivers, family, and friends; and goal-setting. The researchers found no significant differences in outcomes between the one-on-one counseling sessions and the support group; however, women in these two conditions, in comparison to those assigned to the standard counseling condition, were significantly less anxious about having cancer, more knowledgeable about their illness and treatment, and had more positive attitudes toward their health care providers. Cain et al. concluded that the thematic counseling model helped women to learn more about their illness and treatment, better express their feelings, communicate more effectively with members of their social network and with healthcare providers, and find ways to relax, diet, and exercise more efficiently.

Helgeson et al. (2000) argued that research on the benefits of social support groups for people with cancer have been inconclusive largely because few studies have examined individual differences in intervention responses. These researchers examined a variety of individual difference among 312 women with breast cancer, including education level, income, stage of disease, age, social support, negative interactions with network members, and personal resources (such as self-esteem and uncertainty about illness). Participants were randomly assigned to one of three support interventions: peer discussion only, education only, or a group that combined education and peer discussion. Health quality of life (including mental and physical health dimensions) was measured prior to and again 2 weeks after the intervention.

These authors found that although education groups produced more positive effects than peer-discussion groups for the entire sample, a subgroup of women within the sample who lacked emotional support from or who reported more negative interactions with their relational partners benefited more from the peer-discussion group than from the education group. The researchers concluded that women who were satisfied with their support networks prior to the intervention tended not to benefit from the peer-discussion group, whereas women who had deficits in their support networks tended to benefit from it. Moreover, in some cases, the peer-discussion group may have altered the perceptions of women who, prior to the intervention, had positive feelings toward their support network, leading them to question the quality of support they had been receiving from their social network and, thereby, form more negative perceptions of that network. In short, the researchers concluded that the effects of support groups are moderated by individuals' differing needs for support, which depends on the quality of their pre-existing support networks, and that, specifically, people with deficits in those social networks are more likely to benefit from cancer support groups. The researchers also suggested, however, that the inclusion of people with strong support networks within cancer support groups may help those who have weak support networks to increase their ability to manage their illness and stress more effectively.

IMPLICATIONS AND DIRECTIONS FOR FUTURE RESEARCH ON COMMUNICATION IN CANCER SUPPORT GROUPS

The research reviewed here reveals much about the role of communication. In the following, we discuss some of the implications of the findings from the extant literature and identify theoretical and empirical gaps in that literature to which future research on cancer support groups should be devoted.

With regard to the communicative reasons people with cancer join support groups, one important issue to consider when deciding whether a person will benefit from participating in a cancer support group is the strength of his or her traditional support network of family and friends. Specifically, those with weak traditional support networks appear to benefit the most. In fact, as Helgeson et al. (2000) found, those with strong traditional networks don't necessarily benefit from participating in cancer support groups and may even demonstrate negative effects on their traditional support networks. However, it may be the case that even though individuals may have a strong traditional support network, they often (a) feel uncomfortable communicating about the disease with these individuals, (b) feel embarrassed or stigmatized because of having cancer, or (c) may simply believe that traditional support network members lack the specialized knowledge or perspective that only other individuals who have cancer. Future studies of cancer support groups need to assess more fully what communicative reasons are predictive of cancer support group membership and benefits to determine when support groups may and may not be an effective means for helping people to cope with cancer.

With regard to the characteristics of cancer support group participants, there exists a significant gap in the current literature that needs attention. More studies are needed about the characteristics of cancer support group participants, especially longitudinal studies that examine the characteristics of individuals who stay and those who quit participating. In addition, there is a lack of information in existing studies about the participation of minorities, men, and people from lower socioeconomic backgrounds in cancer support groups. What research does exists suggest that these groups of people do not participate much in cancer support groups. However, it may also be the case that there are possible cultural barriers that inhibit their participation in these groups. If that is the case, research needs to discover ways in which cancer support groups can be made more responsive to the needs of members of these groups.

It is possible that some racial/ethnic groups or individuals with lower socioeconomic status may lack information about the possible benefits of cancer support groups, or they may simply be unaware of the availability of such groups in their community. Because many cancer support groups are affiliated with hospitals and medical centers, it is possible that people who lack basic health insurance may not have access to these groups, or they may be unaware that most groups do not charge a fee for participation.

Research also needs to explore the psychological characteristics that may lead to or prevent people from participating in cancer support groups. Psychological barriers might include, for instance, an individual's health locus of control, in that people who have an external health locus of control might perceive talking about cancer to be unhelpful given that they believe the disease is beyond their control (see Sullivan & Reardon, 1985). In terms of communicative barriers, men often do not feel comfortable talking about their feelings in public (Weber et al., 2000), and it is possible that other personal communication characteristics variables, such as perceived communication competence (see Query & Wright, in press), group communication apprehension (see Wright, 2000b), or willingness to communicate about health, may influence a person's decision to participate in these types of groups. In addition, cultural conceptions of health and, in particular, communicating about health may make these groups more or less attractive to certain individuals.

With regard to support group communication processes, although there have been many studies of support group processes, in general, only a small proportion of these studies have examined specific communication variables or cancer-specific support groups (Sullivan, 2003). As Alexander et al. (2003) demonstrated, there appears to be substantial variability between different types of support groups in terms of the types of messages exchanged among members, the purpose and utility of those messages, and the subsequent satisfaction of group members. People with cancer face a much different set of issues than people in substance abuse support groups or support groups dealing with other health-related topics.

There is a need for researchers to identify the unique issues that exist within cancer support groups that may facilitate or inhibit supportive exchanges between members. Thus, it is important that communication scholars develop a clearer understanding of the interaction processes that occur within cancer support groups. Theories of intrapersonal, interpersonal, group, organizational, and health communication may be particularly helpful in contributing to an understanding of the interaction that takes place within these groups.

Finally, with regard to outcomes, the literature identified a number of outcomes that result from participation in cancer support groups. These outcomes are, in part, presumably the result of the communication processes that characterized these groups; however, we still know little about the relationship between communication and such outcomes. More research, thus, needs to examine the relationships between particular processes occurring within cancer support groups and specific health outcomes for participants. Much of the extant research has treated group participation (or not participating) as the salient independent variable and has ignored the interaction processes—the messages exchanged—within these groups. Rather than simply randomly assigning research participants to a cancer support group or a control group, experimental designs should examine the degree to which participation in or satisfaction with particular group processes (such as the sharing of personal narratives) is related to individual and group outcomes. Moreover, it would be helpful for scholars to identify potential communication problems that occur within cancer support groups that may lead to negative outcomes, as this information would be useful for developing interventions that could potentially increase the efficacy of these groups or participants' satisfaction with them. By including these processes into the design of research studies, a better understanding can be gained of how communication plays a role in how people with cancer use these groups to effectively cope with living with this disease.

CONCLUSION

Although support groups are certainly not a panacea for what ails people living with cancer, they have proven their worth in helping many people to live with cancer. It is no wonder, then, that the National Board of the American Cancer Society (2001b) adopted in November 1992 the following policy statement: "As many well-controlled studies indicate that appropriately designed and supervised support groups improve the quality of life of cancer patients, the American Cancer Society encourages them as a valuable and cost-effective component of comprehensive psychological services in cancer care" (p. 3). At the core of cancer support groups are a set of communication practices that encourage participants to talk openly about the disease, exchange information about how to manage it, and, most important of all, to acquire the social support needed to sustain living with the disease, where, in the words of songwriter Peter Gabriel, "words support like bone."

REFERENCES

Adelman, M. B., & Frey, L. R. (1997). *The fragile community: Living together with AIDS*. Mahwah, NJ: Erlbaum.

Alexander, S. C., Peterson, J. L., & Hollingshead, A. B. (2003). Help is at your keyboard: Support groups on the Internet. In L. R. Frey (Ed.), *Group communication in context: Studies of bona fide groups* (2nd ed., pp. 309-334). Mahwah, NJ: Erlbaum.

American Cancer Society. (2001a). Cancer statistics. Accessed November 1, 2002. Available at http://www.cancer.org/cancerinfo/.

American Cancer Society. (2001b). *Cancer support groups: A guide for facilitators*. Washington, DC: Author.

Anderson, B. L. (1994). Surviving cancer. *Cancer, 74*, 1484-1495.

Antze, P. (1976). The role of ideologies in peer psychotherapy organizations: Some theoretical considerations and three case studies. *Journal of Applied Behavioral Science, 12*, 323-346.

Arntson, P., & Droge, D. (1987). Social support in self-help groups: The role of communication in enabling perceptions of control. In T. L. Albrecht, M. B. Adelman, & Associates (Eds.), *Communicating social support* (pp. 148-171). Newbury Park, CA: Sage.

Baker, W. (2000). *Achieving success through social capital: Tapping the hidden resources in your personal and business networks*. San Francisco, CA: Jossey-Bass.

Billings, A. G., & Moos, R. H. (1981). The role of coping responses and social resources in attenuating the impact of stressful life events. *Journal of Behavioral Medicine, 4*, 139-157.

Bloom, J. R. (1982). Social support, accommodation to stress and adjustment to breast cancer. *Social Science Medicine, 16*, 1329-1338.

Bloom, J. R., & Spiegel, D. (1984). The relationship of two dimensions of social support to the psychological well-being and social functioning of women with advanced breast cancer. *Social Science Medicine, 19*, 831-837.

Cain, E. N., Kohorn, E. I., Quinlan, D. M., Latimer, K., & Schwartz, P. E. (1985). Psychosocial benefits of a cancer support group. *Cancer, 57*, 183-189.

Cawyer, C. S., & Smith-Dupré, A. (1995). Communicating social support: Identifying supportive episodes in an HIV/AIDS support group. *Communication Quarterly, 43*, 243-258.

Cella, D. F., & Yellen, S. B. (1993). Cancer support groups: The state of the art. *Cancer Practice, 1*, 56-61.

Chesler, M. A., & Barbarin, O. A. (1984). Difficulties of providing help in a crisis: Relationships between parents of children with cancer and their friends. *Journal of Social Issues, 40*, 113-134.

Chesney, B. K., & Chesler, M. A. (1993). Activism through self-help group membership: Reported life changes of parents with children with cancer. *Small Group Research, 24*, 258-273.

Cline, R. J. (1999). Communication within social support groups. In L. R. Frey (Ed.), D. S. Gouran & M. S. Poole (Assoc. Eds.), *The handbook of group communication theory and research* (pp. 516-538). Thousand Oaks, CA: Sage.

Cohen, S., & Wills, T. A. (1985). Stress, social support, and the buffering hypothesis. *Psychological Bulletin, 98*, 310-357.

Dakof, G. A., & Taylor, S. E. (1990). Victim's perceptions of social support: What is helpful from whom? *Journal of Personality and Social Psychology, 58*, 80-89.

Davison, K. P., Pennebaker, J. W.., & Dickerson, S. S. (2000). Who talks? The social psychology of illness support groups. *American Psychologist, 55*, 205-217.

Deans, G., Bennett-Emslie, G. B., Weir, J., Smith, D. C., & Kaye, S. B. (1988). Cancer support groups—who joins and why? *British Journal of Cancer, 58*, 670-674.

DiMatteo, M., & Hays, R. (1981). Social support and serious illness. In B. Gottlieb (Ed.), *Social networks and social support* (pp. 117-148). Beverly Hills, CA: Sage.

Endler, N. S., & Parker, J. A. (1990). *Coping inventory for stressful situations: Manual.* Toronto, Canada: Multi-Health Systems.

Fife, B. L., Kennedy, V. N., & Robinson, L. (1994). Gender and adjustment to cancer: Clinical implications. *Journal of Psychosocial Oncology, 12*, 1-21.

Ford, S., Fallowfield, L., & Lewis, S. (1996). Doctor-patient interactions in oncology. *Social Science and Medicine, 42*, 1511-1519.

Frank, J. D., & Frank, J. B. (1991). *Persuasion and healing.* Baltimore, MD: Johns Hopkins University Press.

Fritz, G. K., Williams, J. R., & Amylon, M. (1988). After treatment ends: Psychosocial sequelae in pediatric cancer survivors. *American Journal of Orthopsychiatry, 54,* 552-561.

Funch, D. P., & Marshall, J. (1983). The role of stress, social support, and age in survival from breast cancer. *Journal of Psychosomatic Research, 27,* 77-83.

Goffman, E. (1963). *Stigma: Notes on the management of spoiled identity.* Englewood Cliffs, NJ: Prentice-Hall.

Gotcher, J. M. (1995). Well-adjusted and maladjusted cancer patients: An examination of communication variables. *Health Communication, 7,* 21-33.

Gotcher, J. M., & Edwards, R. (1990). Coping strategies of cancer patients: Actual communication and imagined interactions. *Health Communication, 2,* 255-266.

Hanifan, L. J. (1916). The rural school community center. *Annals of the American Academy of Political and Social Science, 67,* 130-138.

Harrison, J., Maguire, P., & Pitceathly, C. (1995). Confiding in crisis: Gender differences in patterns of confiding among cancer patients. *Social Science Medicine, 41,* 1255-1260.

Heinrich, R. L., Schag, C. C., & Ganz, P. A. (1984). Living with cancer: The cancer inventory of problem situations. *Journal of Clinical Psychology, 40,* 972-980.

Helgeson, V. S., Cohen, S., Schultz, R., & Yasko, J. (2000). Group support interventions for women with breast cancer: Who benefits from what? *Health Psychology, 19,* 107-114.

Helgeson, V. S., & Gottlieb, B. H. (2000). Support groups. In S. Cohen, L. G. Underwood, & B. H. Gottlieb (Eds.), *Social support measurement and intervention* (pp. 221-245). New York: Oxford University Press.

Jones, D. N., & Reznikoff, M. (1989). Psychosocial adjustment to a mastectomy. *Journal of Nervous and Mental Disease, 177,* 624-631.

Katz, A. H. (1993). *Self-help in America: A social movement perspective.* New York: Twayne.

Katz, A. H., & Bender, E. I. (1976). Self-help groups in Western society: History and prospects. *Journal of Applied Behavioral Science, 12,* 265-282.

Kessler, R. C., Mickelson, K. D., & Zhao, S. (1997). Patterns and correlates of self-help group membership in the United States. *Social Policy, 27,* 27-46.

Klemm, P., Hurst, M., Dearholt, S. L., & Trone, S. R. (1999). Cyber solace: Gender differences on Internet support groups. *Computers in Nursing, 17,* 65-72.

Klemm, P., Reppert, K., & Visich, L. A. (1998). A nontraditional cancer support group: The Internet. *Computers in Nursing, 16,* 31-36.

Kohn, P. M. (1996). On coping adaptively with daily hassles. In M. Zeidner & N. S. Endler (Eds.), *Handbook of coping* (pp. 181-201). New York: Wiley.

Kreps, G. L. (1993). Refusing to be a victim: Rhetorical strategies for confronting cancer. In B. C. Thornton & G. L. Kreps (Eds.), *Perspectives on health communication* (pp. 42-47). Prospect Heights, IL: Waveland Press.

La Gaipa, J. J. (1990). The negative effects of informal support systems. In S. Duck & R. C. Silver (Eds.), *Personal relationships and social support* (pp. 122-139). Newbury Park, CA: Sage.

Lepore, S. J., Allen, K. A. M., & Evans, G. W. (1993). Social support lowers cardiovascular reactivity to an acute stressor. *Psychosomatic Medicine, 55,* 518-524.

MacDonald, L. D., & Anderson, H. R. (1984). Stigma in patients with rectal cancer: A community study. *Journal of Epidemiology and Community Health, 38,* 284-290.

Martin, R., Davis, G. M., Baron, R. S., Suls, J., & Blanchard, E. B. (1994). Specificity in social support: Perceptions of helpful and unhelpful provider behaviors among irritable bowel syndrome, headache, and cancer patients. *Health Psychology, 13,* 432-439.

Mathieson, C. M., Logan-Smith, L. L., Phillips, J., MacPhee, M., & Attia, M. L. (1996). Caring for head and neck oncology patients: Does social support lead to better quality of life? *Canadian Family Physician, 42,* 1712-1720.

Mattlin, J., Wethington, E., & Kessler, R. C. (1990). Situational determinants of coping and coping effectiveness. *Journal of Health and Social Behavior, 31,* 103-122.

Miller B. A., Kolonel, L. N., Bernstein L., Young, Jr. J. L., Swanson G. M., West D., Key C. R., Liff, J. M., Glover C. S., Alexander G. A.\ et al. (Eds.). (1996). *Racial/ethnic patterns of cancer in the United States 1988-1992.* Bethesda, MD: National Cancer Institute.

Mok, B. H. (2001). Cancer self-help groups in China: A study of individual change, perceived benefit, and community impact. *Small Group Research, 32,* 115-132.

Mok, E., & Martinson, I. (2000). Empowerment of Chinese patients with cancer through self-help groups in Hong Kong. *Cancer Nursing, 23,* 206-213.

National Cancer Institute (2002). Lifetime probability of breast cancer in American women. Available at Retrieved http://cis.nci.nih.gov/fact/5_6.htm. Accessed December 4, 2002.

Putnam, R. D. (2000). *Bowling alone: The collapse and revival of American community.* New York: Simon & Schuster.

Query, J. L., Jr., & Wright, K. B. (2003). Assessing communication competence in an on-line study: Towards informing subsequent interventions among older adults with cancer, their lay caregivers, and peers. *Health Communication, 15,* 205-219.

Rappaport, J. (1993). Narrative studies, personal stories, and identity transformation in the mutual help context. *Journal of Applied Behavioral Science, 29,* 239-256.

Reynolds, P., & Kaplan, G. A. (1990). Social connections and risk for cancer: Prospective evidence from the Alameda County study. *Behavioral Medicine, 16,* 101-110.

Riessman, F. (1965). The "helper" therapy principle. *Social Work, 10,* 27-32.

Rosenberg, P. P. (1984). Support groups: A special therapeutic entity. *Small Group Behavior, 15,* 173-186.

Samarel, N., & Fawcett, J. (1992). Enhancing adaptation to breast cancer: The addition of coaching to support groups. *Oncology Nursing Forum, 19,* 591-596.

Schimmel, S. R. (1999). *Cancer talk: Voices of hope and endurance from "The Group Room," the world's largest cancer support group.* New York: Broadway Books.

Schwarzer, R., & Leppin, A. (1991). Social support and health: A theoretical and empirical overview. *Journal of Social and Personal Relationships, 8,* 99-127.

Sharf, B. F. (1997). Communicating breast cancer on-line: Support and empowerment on the Internet. *Women & Health, 26,* 65-84.

Siminoff, L. A., & Fetting, J. H. (1991). Factors affecting treatment decisions for a life-threatening illness: The case of medical treatment of breast cancer. *Social Science and Medicine, 32,* 813-818.

Spiegel, D. (1992). Effects of psychosocial support on patients with metastatic breast cancer. *Journal of Psychosocial Oncology, 10,* 113-121.

Spiegel, D., & Bloom, J. R. (1983). Pain in metastatic breast cancer. *Cancer, 52,* 149-153.

Spiegel, D., Bloom, J. R., & Yalom, I. (1981). Group support for patients with metastatic cancer: A randomized prospective outcome study. *Archives of General Psychiatry, 38,* 527-533.

Street, R. L., Jr., & Rimal, R. N. (1997). Health promotion and interactive technology. In R. L. Street, Jr., W. R. Gold, & T. Manning (Eds.), *Health promotion and interactive technology: Theoretical applications and future directions* (pp. 1-18). Mahwah, NJ: Erlbaum.

Sullivan, C. F. (1997, April). *Cancer support groups in cyberspace: Are there gender differences in message functions?* Paper presented at the meeting of the Central States Communication Association, St. Louis, MO.

Sullivan, C. F. (2003). Gendered cybersupport: A thematic analysis of two on-line cancer support groups. *Journal of Health Psychology, 8,* 83-103.

Sullivan, C. F., & Reardon, K. K. (1985). Social support satisfaction and health locus of control: Discriminators of breast cancer patients' style of coping. In M. L. McLaughlin (Ed.), *Communication yearbook* (Vol. 9, pp. 707-722). Beverly Hills, CA: Sage.

Taylor, S. E., Falke, R. L., Shoptaw, S. J., & Lichtman, R. R. (1986). Social support, support groups, and the cancer patient. *Journal of Consulting and Clinical Psychology, 54,* 608-615.

Walsh-Burke, K. (1992). Family communication and coping with cancer. Impact of the We Can Weekend. *Journal of Psychosocial Oncology, 10,* 63-81.

Weber, B. A., Roberts, B. L., & McDougall, G. J. (2000). Exploring the efficacy of support groups of men with prostate cancer. *Geriatric Nursing, 41,* 250-253.

Wills, T. A. (1985). Supportive functions of interpersonal relationships. In S. Cohen & S. L. Syme (Eds.), *Social support and health* (pp. 61-82). Orlando, FL: Academic Press.

Wortman, C. (1984). Social support and the cancer patient: Conceptual and methodological issues. *Cancer, 53,* 2339-2362.

Wortman, C., & Dunkel-Schetter, C. (1979). Interpersonal relationships and cancer. *Journal of Social Issues, 35,* 120-155.

Wright, K. B. (1997). Shared ideology in Alcoholic Anonymous: A grounded theory approach. *Journal of Health Communication, 2,* 83-99.

Wright, K. B. (2000a). The communication of social support within an on-line community for older adults: A qualitative analysis of the SeniorNet community. *Qualitative Research Reports in Communication, 1,* 33-43.

Wright, K. B. (2000b). Social support satisfaction, on-line communication apprehension, and perceived life stress within computer-mediated support groups. *Communication Research Reports, 17,* 139-147.

Wright, K. B. (2002). Social support within an on-line cancer community: An assessment of emotional support, perceptions of advantages and disadvantages, and motives for using the community from a communication perspective. *Journal of Applied Communication Research, 30,* 195-209.

Wright, K. B., & Bell, S. B. (2003). Health-related support groups on the Internet: Linking empirical findings to social support and computer-mediated communication theory. *Journal of Health Psychology, 8,* 37-52.

Yalom, I. (1995). *The theory and practice of group psychotherapy.* New York: Basic Books.

13 | Spiritual Care

Kenneth M. Brown
Washburn University

Alexis D. Bakos
National Institute of Nursing Research,
National Institutes of Health

Health communication is described and defined by Kreps (2001) as a "rich, exciting, and relevant research area that investigates and elucidates the many ways that human and mediated communication dramatically influence the outcomes of health care and health promotion efforts" (p. 232) Kreps goes on to declare "health communication must move toward a sophisticated trans-disciplinary agenda that will examine the role of communication in health care at multiple communication levels and in a broad range of communication contexts" (p. 237).

The study of health communication is recognizing that it is wider than the traditional parameters of public health campaigns and patient–provider interaction. A multitude of health communication processes take place before, after, and around the medical consultation between patient and provider (usually meaning the physician). More frequently, *provider* is viewed as all professional providers (e.g., nurses, pharmacists, nutritionists, clergy, etc.) as well as family and friends. Health communication can be instrumental in bringing attention to a holistic approach to health care that encompasses spiritual care. This chapter focuses on the function of spiritual care as a component to holistic cancer care.

THE ROLE OF SPIRITUAL CARE

In the past, the concept of spirituality received minimal attention by health professionals both in clinical practice and in research. Roberts, Brown, Elkins, and Larson (1997) state religion has been largely disregarded in the professional literature. Researchers who are currently studying spirituality, however, are finding it to be a powerful resource for coping with health-related problems. Health communication must address spirituality in the health care setting. Specifically, we must learn what impact spirituality has on health status and recovery issues, as well as what effects spirituality has on the processing of messages in the health care realm.

Hermann (2000) defined *spirituality* as a multifaceted, fundamental part of each person that drives a search for meaning and purpose in life. This search is often expressed through religion and involves relationship with self, others, and a transcendent being. Thomas and Retsas (1999) pointed out that some writers equate spirituality with ideas such as faith, hope, trust, and the central life force of a person's wholeness. Therefore, when confronting the crisis of cancer, the person seeks reasons for the crisis to give meaning to its intrusion into their life. Additionally, Hermann (2000) pointed out nurses have traditionally equated spirituality with religion. It is likely that the average person makes the same equation of meaning and therefore, the literature distinctions of definition would be without meaning or significance.

Hermann represents much of the literature that distinguishes spirituality as broader than religion and religion as one vehicle for the expression of spirituality. Fryback and Reinert (1999), in describing spirituality as a bridge between hopelessness and meaningfulness in life, found that subjects identified a spiritual domain of health. The domain consists of three main concepts: belief in a higher power (church attendance/religion, spiritual beliefs, transcendence); recognition of mortality (appreciation of life, appreciation of nature, live in the moment), and self-actualization (self-love/acceptance, finding meaning/purpose in life and disease). The spiritual domain is a point where the patient recognizes a more profound realm beyond the physical aspect of illness. Thus, the illness is not necessarily the most important realm of existence, but a place where meaning, purpose, and hope are primary. Additionally, hope is not restricted to the possibility of healing from the disease. Rather, it is a place of "ease" within the disease of an uncertain physical outcome. Hope, therefore, pertains to death and beyond in addition to the present and illness.

Emanuel and Emanuel (1999) stated that the health care profession has long recognized the importance and urgency of spiritual issues. It is the reason for the existence of pastoral care departments in hospitals and clergy as essential participants in hospice care. However, issues of spirituality in practice have been secondary to medical concerns and medical providers have not been equipped or trained to deal with spirituality. Kristeller, Zumbrun, and Schilling (1999) found that physicians and nurses identify themselves as responsible for addressing spiritual issues but give it low priority in favor of more pressing medical concerns. Oncologists and nurses each identified themselves as the individual with primary responsibility to address spiritual issues.

Each identified themselves as primarily responsible for spiritual issues, even more than they viewed it as the responsibility of a chaplain. Despite this, they gave spiritual concerns very low priority in comparison to competing demands. Spiritual issues in cancer patients are likely underaddressed due to time constraints, lack of confidence in effectiveness, and role uncertainty.

Some of the literature that does exist makes some distinction in the meaning of the words *spirituality*, *faith*, and *religion*. For the purpose of this chapter, however, these terms used synonymously and interchangeably unless otherwise specified. In addition, the focus of this chapter is on spirituality within the context of cancer diagnoses, the resulting prognoses, and communication.

DIAGNOSIS AND SPIRITUAL NEED

The diagnosis of cancer is a devastating experience. A cancer finding can range in severity from a reasonably sure prognosis of survival to the diagnosis of pancreatic cancer, which is usually a grim, traumatic, death sentence. It is a disease that permits less than 1% of its sufferers to achieve a 5-year survival. The more common prognosis for pancreatic cancer is a painful life expectancy of 3 to 6 months (Holland et al., 1986).

Cole and Pergament (1999) highlighted that people facing traumatic events find religion and spirituality to be helpful in the coping process. Additionally, among people with cancer, strong religious beliefs have been associated with decreased levels of pain, anxiety, hostility, and social isolation.

A common experience of cancer patients, however, is unmet spiritual needs. In their study, Moadel et al. (1999) reported a range of 25% to 51% of spiritual needs going unmet. These unmet needs consisted of overcoming fear; finding hope, peace of mind, and meaning in life; and identifying spiritual resources.

High spiritual needs were identified as particularly significant for Hispanics, followed by African Americans. Although not as salient for Whites, these researchers found a strong association between quality of life and existential well-being. These findings give guidance in understanding the need of culturally tailored support factors for individual patients.

The patient is not the only person who endures this trial. Counseling professionals have, for three decades, suggested that a cancer diagnosis should be regarded as an illness that affects the entire family (Veach & Nicholas, 1998). The model for treatment must include the family members as well as the patient, and must consider the likely disease duration and outcome.

Spiritual and religious issues and questions frequently become dominant concerns in cases of cancer. Spirituality has often been neglected as part of the cancer treatment and support regimen. Perhaps this is due to the difficulty of qualifying examining the religious components of life being difficult to quantify and examine. However, the most dominant strategy employed by long-term cancer survivors is a spiritual one (Creagan, 1997). As spiritual and religious beliefs continue to emerge as potent factors in multiple medical diagnoses, including cancer, it is important that health care and health communication scholars and researchers investigate and attempt to understand and explain this growing phenomenon.

In light of the trauma presented to a cancer patient and his or her family, this chapter examines the issues faced by the patient and his or her family, the spiritual components at work in the lives of patient and the family, and some suggestions regarding future research in this particular area.

Cancer patients have frequently been plagued by a lack of adequate communication regarding their diagnosis and prognosis. This lack of information heightens the stress factors that accompany a cancer diagnosis. The perceived life-threatening nature of the disease, coupled with inadequate information, hinders the possibility of effective communication with cancer patients (Glimelius, Birgegard, Hoffman, Kvale, & Sjoden, 1995). The most stunning factor the pancreatic cancer patient faces is the almost certain likelihood of death in a relatively brief amount of time. The high probability of death is a stressful burden accompanied by fear, denial, shock, and a sense that the situation is unreal. Additionally, the news of cancer can produce indecision and lead to a feeling of isolation (McCollum, 1978), as well as an intensified feeling of loneliness (Rokach, 2000).

The crisis of possible impending death is not far from the patient's mind as he or she processes the news of cancer and all it encompasses. Roberts, Brown, Elkins, and Larson (1997), recounting a study of women diagnosed with breast cancer, discovered that fewer than half the subjects expected the physician to either cure or contain the disease. The bleak forecast for some forms of cancer likely dims survival hopes of its victims to an even greater degree. Coming to terms with death is essential to a survival strategy. That is, the recognition of whether it is the certainty of death (i.e., from this disease at an estimated point in time), or as only a possible outcome of the cancer diagnosis. In either case, this prepares the way for a spiritual identification of life's meaning and purpose and "making the most" of the time remaining.

EMOTIONS

The emotions experienced by the cancer patient are difficult to identify. There is no definitive correlation between the emotions anticipated and the ones actually expressed (Hunt & Meerabeau, 1993). Hunt and Meerabeau pointed out the possibility that the emotions experienced are created through the various interactions in which the patient engages. Additionally, there is no definitive formula to calculate what amount or type of emotions should be expressed. In fact, consideration must be given to the idea that unexpressed grief can be just as helpful as expressed grief. The appropriateness of emotional expression or its lack should be individualized according to the patient, context, timing, and any number of variables at work for the patient and family and friends.

Depression is a significant factor in the emotional aspect of pancreatic cancer (Peterson, Popkin, & Hall, 1983). Holland et al., (1986) reported that an analysis of differences between groups shows a significantly greater disturbance in pancreatic cancer patients on the individual dimensions of depression, fatigue, tension, anxiety, and confusion bewilderment. In addition, the same difference is reflected in global mood disturbance. There are likely two reasons for this occurrence. First, the pancreas can produce a peptide that affects the area of the brain that controls mood. This could explain the high number of pancreatic cancer patients who present with depression prior to the cancer diagnosis. Second, the dismal prognosis of pancreatic cancer could at least partly account for the depressive state.

The serious nature of a pancreatic cancer prognosis and its accompanying incidences of depression emphasize a need for counseling. Roberts et al. (1997) detailed a study of women diagnosed with cancer expressing their greatest need as "straight talk" regarding their illness and outcomes. The conclusions drawn from the study demonstrate the patients' need to be sufficiently informed to feel a sense of control in their situations and thus be able to manage their fear and be equipped to make decisions.

COPING CHALLENGES

Schaefer (1985) noted that living with a life-threatening disease presents many coping challenges. This crisis may necessitate a variety of coping skills and different types of coping skills required by the progression of the disease. Schaefer (1985) proceeded to delineate a short-term group treatment model with five components.

1. Validation of one's own wellness: Sharing experiences, concerns, coping strategies with others to develop a baseline for one's own self-assessment.
2. Patient education: Understanding the medical aspects of one's own disease.
3. Prevention: Coping skills to prevent maladaptive coping patterns.
4. Mutual aid: Supporting and inspiring each other to combat feeling of being in this alone.
5. Ego-oriented goal-directed counseling: Identifying goals and means of attainment.

Jevne (1987) explained that as part of a broad range of interventions, counseling to achieve a "stillpoint" can be an effective coping mechanism to strengthen oneself in dealing with the impact of a disease. Stillpoint is defined as achieving an inner place where patients are confident their internal and external environments have some predictability and reasonable expectations can be anticipated. A stillpoint can provide patients a sense of assurance in dealing with things that are beyond their control.

The diagnosis of cancer and the terminal forecast of some cancers, such as pancreatic cancer, underscores the need to focus on (QOL) issues for the patient. The need to address this issue has spawned several QOL measures. These show, however, that QOL assessments are not necessarily uniform among terminally ill individuals (Greenwald, 1987). The symptoms and dysfunctions reported can be very diverse. QOL outcomes are determined to be equally important to treatment regimens designed to prolong life. This becomes increasingly important with the marginal success of attempts to prolong life in pancreatic cancer patients. In studying the perceptions of patients in reference to QOL issues, Fitzsimmons, George, Payne, and Johnson (1999) identified two central areas of anxiety. Patients are concerned with the threat posed by the disease. Threat was perceived to focus on timing, symptoms, and circumstances. Additionally, patients acknowledged maintaining control in the face of threat was significant to their QOL. Five coping strategies emerged from these areas of concern:

1. Defending/avoidances: Problem is ignored as long as possible.
2. Blaming: Problem is blamed on external event.
3. Rationalizing: Problem seen as "normal part of the illness."
4. Turning to others: Patient turns to family and/or health professionals to explain symptoms and provide support in tackling symptom.
5. Taking a direct action: Patient takes affirmative action against symptom.

These strategies demonstrate patients taking a holistic approach to QOL and dealing with both positive and negative aspects of their illness in this process (Fitzsimmons et al., 1999).

These strategies and coping mechanisms assist patients in the coping challenges of cancer as they relate to the spiritual realm. A place of spiritual peace becomes an aid to managing patient environments and assessing and making QOL decisions.

PAIN

A further component of QOL is the issue of pain. Newshan (1998) reported that love and relatedness play a role in experiencing pain. Being alone was perceived to make pain worse, whereas being with a spouse or participating in family activities helped with pain. In addition, one's spiritual perspective can influence the meaning ascribed to pain. Spiritual health is viewed as identifying pain as a challenge through which the sufferer is strengthened. Newshan (1998) described spiritual health and pain in terms of hope. Hope is expressed in two ways: curative hope, which is the hope for cure; and palliative hope, which is the hope for relief from pain and a peaceful death.

Therefore, a component of hope is seeking realistic information about one's condition and expressing hope for a positive outcome. In contrast, indicators of spiritual distress include suppressing feelings and failing to wonder or ask questions. O'Leary (2002) pointed out that attitudes about pain may be influenced by beliefs that may offer a rationale for pain. Otis-Green, Sherman, Perez, and Baird (2002) stressed that physical pain is very common with the cancer experience and 75% of patients with advanced or end-stage disease experience pain, and close to 33% of these individuals experience severe or excruciating pain. Thus, it is essential for the medical team to have full knowledge of how the patient's beliefs and perceptions may be contributing to pain issues. A thorough spiritual assessment, accompanied by ongoing spiritual care implemented at the time of diagnosis, could minimize much of the pain and suffering that patients experience while living and dying with cancer.

ALL IN THE FAMILY

As stated previously, the patient is not the only individual affected when cancer is diagnosed. The patient's family members are also stricken, even though they do not personally possess the cancer cells. A pancreatic cancer diagnosis initiates a death crisis for the patient and the family. However, the death crisis continues with the family well beyond diagnosis, trauma, and the death of the patient. During the terminal illness phase, family members will reflect on the upcoming situation of life without the patient. Following death, the struggle continues as adjustment is made to life without the patient (McCollum, 1978).

During the terminal illness phase, family members experience several responsibilities. First, they assume responsibilities for the care of the ill family member (Northouse & Northouse, 1987). These tasks are notably more difficult as they must be performed while family members deal with their own emotional turmoil regarding the circumstance. Second, the psychological reactions of family members are important to the treatment process. It is important for the entire health care team to attend to the needs of the family in order to reinforce useful psychological reactions (McCollum, 1978).

Communication plays an important role in easing the family's stress level. It is possible that communication can become limited during this stressful time as a means of avoiding personal pain (Northouse & Northouse, 1987). The family perseveres through the adjustment process of life without the patient (McCollum, 1978). The findings of research regarding communication are mixed. There is a positive correlation between adjustment and open communication, but some families are able to cope more effectively via silence (Northouse & Northouse, 1987).

In order for a care delivery model for a terminally ill patient to be effective, it must result from the cooperative effort and design of the care providers, patient, and family members. It is not adequate for care to be designed exclusively by the care providers without consideration of the needs and concerns of the patient and family. Research cites focus group results that attest to this and suggests it as a model for all facilities that treat the terminally ill (Anonymous, 1998). The ideas that emerged from these focus groups are as follows:

1. It is important to pay attention to a loved one's last days because it is an opportunity to grow and heal in the spiritual and emotional realms. These opportunities are often missed because professional care givers focus on physical symptoms and therefore are not cognizant of, nor sensitive to, other signs.
2. Survivors complain that the loved one's final days were made difficult because health care professionals ignored living wills and advance directives and insisted on using technology to keep the patient alive. Additionally, this often prevented loved ones from being with the dying family member.
3. Physicians are not well trained in caring for the dying.
4. It is not easy to make the transition from curing to caring. Caring can offer the patient a great deal when curing cannot be reasonably achieved (Anonymous, 1998).

INCREASING INTEREST IN SPIRITUAL CARE

Cancer care and treatment have enjoyed several years of emphasis in research and in the public arena. One area that has been largely neglected, however, is the spiritual dimension of cancer diagnosis, treatment, and end-of-life concerns. As stated previously, this neglect could be a result of the difficulty in quantifying and replicating the study of spiritual matters (Creagan, 1997). In recent years, however, religion has been making a comeback in the world of cancer and cancer treatment. Increasingly religion and spirituality are being viewed as important in issues of QOL and patient relations. This return to an interest in religion has been sparked by a growing general interest in spirituality and alternative medicines. Additionally, it is a recognition that this is something patients desire and consider important. In particular, many cancer patients rely on religion after the cancer diagnosis (Ziegler, 1998). In particular, faith in God is a principle means of acquiring strength for the trial of dealing with cancer and a sense of inner peace regardless of the pending outcome of the disease.

Spirituality infiltrates all aspects of what it means to be human. It is very difficult to separate spirituality from other psychological, social, and physical aspects of life. Therefore, every problem has at least a spiritual component (Carroll, 2001). Spiritual care is both important and difficult. It is important because the spiritual realm permeates every compartment of life. It is difficult because it can be complicated to isolate the spiritual component amidst more overt needs such as pain and nausea (Carroll, 2001).

The spiritual dimension of the illness situation focuses on two issues. The issues are the perception of relationship to, and dependence on, a Supreme Higher Being, and second, a relationship to a member of the clergy, family members, and/or individuals who are members of the same "faith body."

Spiritual well-being can be described as the affirmation of life in relationship to a higher being or God, self, community, and environment that nurtures the development of wholeness (Fernsler, Klemm, & Miller, 1999). Being religious is reported by cancer patients as helpful when facing questions about the quality and meaning of life. Eighty-five percent of patients surveyed reported believing in God; 75% reported praying (Norum, Risberg, & Solberg, 2000). It can be concluded that spiritual factors do have an impact on QOL and possibly on survival. Creagan (1997) pointed out that patients are shown to have a statistically significant benefit from praying and being prayed for by others.

PRAYER

Many cancer patients view prayer is as important ingredient in spiritual well-being issues of their disease. The prayer experience involves discussion of the result of prayer. Prayer is held as personally beneficial. Taylor and Outlaw (2002) reported respondent expectations to be "answered" prayers, which frequently entailed literal outcomes. Only a few informants hoped that their prayers would bring a cure or prolonged life, most expected other outcomes. These included God's ultimate best, comfort, peace, hope, less anxiety and fear, forgiveness and salvation, or nothing. Typically, patients prayed for "God's will," although not knowing specifically what that would be. Prayer is frequently an instrument for coping with cancer. Prayer is typically viewed as a religious practice, a form of communication between individuals and a divine being. It is both speaking and listening (Taylor, Outlaw, Bernardo, & Roy, 1999).

Additionally, the predominant strategy of long-term cancer survivors is spiritual. Fernsler et al. (1999) reported that researchers who have studied spirituality find it to be a powerful resource for coping with health-related problems. These studies also demonstrate an integral relationship between spiritual well-being and the demands of the illness.

RELIANCE ON FAITH

National longitudinal research data were used to examine why and how men and women seek religious comfort during illness. Results show that seeking religious consolation is most likely among those who already have some form of religious affiliation. Cancer was associated with higher religious seeking particularly among women. The findings also suggest that seeking religious consolation intensifies among religious people during traumatic experiences (Ferraro & Kelley-Moore, 2000). Roberts et al. (1997) reported a study of women with recent cancer diagnoses. The study revealed that 76% stated religion had an important place in their lives and 93% indicated their religious commitment helped sustain their hopes.

Patient reliance on religious faith is not only becoming a popular topic in the general press, it is increasingly becoming a topic of scientific research. Religious affiliation and reliance on God to influence decisions are having a crucial impact in understanding attitudes toward life-sustaining treatments and end-of-life issues and determinations. For health care to be effective and individualized, health care professionals must pay attention to the belief systems and personality characteristics of their patients (Ejaz, 2000). It is suggested that measures of spirituality and illness-related demands may be used as screening tools to identify individuals in need of interventions (Fernsler et al., 1999).

Faith, religion, and spirituality play a vital role in managing the battle with loneliness that accompanies a cancer diagnosis. Rokach (2000) examined the manner in which those with terminal illness cope with loneliness. Religion and faith appear to confirm that individuals need to feel connected to and worship a divine entity, God, or Supreme Being. Feeling connected to God and to other worshippers with whom the patient affiliates appears to provide strength, inner peace, and a sense of community and belonging.

THE ROLE OF THE CLERGY

Another aspect of the interplay between spirituality and terminal illness is the relationship the patient and family members have to a member of the clergy (Rokach, 2000). The clergy person can be a hospital chaplain, but is most often the pastor/minister/priest/rabbi of the patient and/or family. Additionally, the pastor is the person with whom the patient and family prefer to have this relationship. The general level of satisfaction with the clergy is very high. It is directly correlated with, and increases with, the willingness of the minister to engage in spiritual activities. The pastor praying with and for the patient and family is very highly regarded. However, it is also possible for the experience with clergy to be displeasing. The most frequently mentioned cause for this is lack of communication, understanding, interest, and/or concern (Spilka, Spangler, & Nelson, 1983). Spilka et al. also pointed out that clergy training has been poor in this area in the past but current training is improving. Additionally, continuing education opportunities are needed and can be offered through workshops. Training and continuing education are becoming more readily available in these areas. A perusal of seminary catalogs demonstrates more offerings of this nature today than when this author was a seminary student in the mid-1970s. Additionally, continuing education opportunities are offered more frequently through hospitals, educational institutions, and church/denomination sponsored entities.

CULTURE AND ADVANCE DIRECTIVES

The role of culture is important in the correlation between spirituality and cancer Taylor (2001) found non-whites are less likely to know about and have an advance directive. The advance directive is an instrument created by and for patients to give prior instructions on their desires regarding wishes to receive, or not to receive, resuscitation and/or heroic medical efforts. Most minorities are less likely to agree to the discontinuation of life support. Additionally, several minority groups believe in not fully disclosing bad news to the patient and in the importance of family (vs. patient) decision making.

Hispanic and African-American cancer patients are more likely to use religious or spiritual healing practices and coping strategies to manage their cancer, and experience more positive outcomes from their religiosity (e.g., coping, hope, quality of life; Taylor, 2001). In addition, Moadel et al. (1999) found the lack of a significant partner, and chronological proximity to the time of diagnosis, to be important issues of need.

LESSONS FROM HIV/AIDS

The correlation between spiritual concerns and terminal illness is a topic of interest for the entire population of terminally ill clients. Valuable lessons can be learned for understanding spiritual dynamics by drawing on items learned through spiritual counseling with HIV/AIDS clients. Three issues have been found to be particularly relevant. First, the fear of death is a natural manifestation of the prospect of death from an illness, especially in the latter stages of the illness. Often, this fear results in doubts about the patient's relationship with others and with God. In the death confrontation, however, clients find comfort in spirituality. Second, clients find a need to express themselves regarding hope and the changing stages of hope as the terminal illness progresses. Spirituality frequently becomes a resource for dealing with an otherwise hopeless situation. Hope is a companion to the terminally ill patient but it must be properly understood. It is not a pretend hope that all will turn out okay and the disease will go away. Instead, it is the path of obtaining a means to living a positive life, and not focused on finding a cure. Third, terminal illness involves examining the meaning of life. Terminally ill patients find life meaning by facing the inevitability of their own death. Turning to the spiritual dimension may be an attempt to find some meaning and an effective coping strategy (Holt, Houg, & Romano, 1999).

The work of O'Connor, Meakes, McCarroll-Butler, Gadowsky, and O'Neill (1997) uncovered a unique focus of terminally ill patients that was different than that proposed in the literature. The principle concern identified in the literature is "meaning of life." O'Connor et al., however, found the primary theme and concern to be making the most of life now, and markedly little concern for what may lie beyond death.

The increasing emphasis on spiritual care, and the need to be informed on the multiple ramifications of its delivery, highlight the great need for work in this area. The phrase "spiritual care" indicates that the spiritual is part of, and inseparable from, the whole. Thus, spiritual care is an integral part of overall care and cannot be ignored or minimized (Carroll, 2001). As a result, it is necessary for all who are involved with cancer patients to be willing to address these needs and to be as prepared as possible for these occasions. Spiritual issues lie at the center of the crisis of terminal illness. When spiritual care is ignored, it seriously limits the understanding of, and response to, the patient's illness (Kearney & Mount, 2000). In addition, Carroll (2001) underscored that on occasion "just being there" and attending to the patient's physical needs was all the patient wanted and was in fact a means of providing spiritual care.

PROBLEMATIC INTEGRATION THEORY

Recent research into the role of religion and spirituality in the lives of terminally ill patients and their families reveals this is a topic of significance that must be further explored and cannot be ignored. Research that is theory-based can be useful in further understanding the role of faith in the terminal illness condition and employing that knowledge to further improve matters of meaning and QOL for the patient.

A potential theory to help facilitate research into the connection between religion and health may be the Problematic Integration Theory. Problematic Integration Theory is a general perspective on uncertainty and communication. Uncertainty is a central figure of illness and exacerbates stress and threats to health (Babrow, Hines, & Kasch, 2000). Uncertainty is possibly the primary issue religion and spirituality address. Coming to terms with the terminal illness circumstance involves coming to a place where uncertainty can be managed. Managing uncertainty does not necessarily mean reducing uncertainty. Managing uncertainty can mean reducing, maintaining, or increasing uncertainty. Also, managing uncertainty may not be a "one-shot" operation but rather an ongoing process. Serial management of uncertainty may be needed as the disease progresses (Babrow et al., 2000).

Problematic Integration Theory posits that people form probabalistic orientations to the world (i.e. what is it? What are its characteristics?). In addition, people form evaluative orientations (i.e., Is it good or bad?). Therefore, Problematic Integration Theory assumes people assess and evaluate probabilities. Thus, expectations and evaluations are interdependent and the relationship between them is complex, dynamic, and constantly changing. In, this regard, Problematic Integration Theory goes beyond Uncertainty Reduction Theory (linear, mechanistic prediction) by focusing on the complexity of the dynamic relationship between probabilistic assessment and evaluation (Babrow et al., 2000). Problematic Integration Theory works from a perspective that every situation has an optimal level of uncertainty (a comfort zone) that is sometimes high and sometimes lower and we try to achieve and maintain that level. Thus, as applied to health care and health communication, Problematic Integration Theory is used to attempt to understand and apply to efforts to cope with the challenging uncertainties of end-of-life issues. Problematic Integration Theory recognizes uncertainty is individualistic and contextually sensitive and constructed and focuses on both individual- level and social integration problems (Babrow et al., 2000).

One of the difficulties encountered in the study of religion and faith as a communication factor for terminally ill patients is having a measure of the level of religious faith existent in each patient. Although attention to associations between religious involvement and health outcomes for cancer patients has been growing, research has been hampered by a lack of suitable measures of religiosity. One recently developed measure that shows promise in this area is the Santa Clara Strength of Religious Faith Questionnaire. To date, this measurement instrument has demonstrated high test–retest reliability and internal consistency (Sherman et al., 2001). This presents as one representative religiosity scale that has potential for providing a means of assessing each individual's level of religiosity/faith/spirituality in order to determine the role religiosity plays in issues such as message processing in particular health care and health communication circumstances and situations.

LOOKING AHEAD

Matters of religion, spirituality, and faith are being identified as crucial elements in the care and treatment of cancer patients and their families. Health communication scholars can assist in understanding the impact and effect this produces in the lives of terminally ill patients and families as well as other health care situations. The issues of spirituality are no longer as silent and ignored as they once were. The emergence of spirituality as a component of health care and health communication cries out to communication scholars to bring our unique perspective to spirituality's impact on communication and interpretation in these settings.

The secular and medical "worlds" both identify the necessity and power of the spiritual realm, faith, and hope in health care. However, it is too common for important issues to achieve merely a "fad" status in the secular world and soon disappear from the scene. The medical world is inundated with the unrelenting pressures of time and cost that all too easily manifest themselves in pushing aside things that are nonclinical.

Health communication professionals can provide a service for the greater good of the community by being a force for the increased recognition and importance of the place of communication in health care settings. The great and growing societal importance of health care and health communication provides an opportunity and responsibility to develop theory that pertains holistically to this realm. Spiritual care is a vital and dynamic part of this equation. Health communication in general and spiritual care in particular are ripe for development in research.

REFERENCES

Anonymous. (1998a). Best care for the dying: Listen to their needs. *RN, 61*(9), 24L.

Anonymous. (1998b, November 2–9). Study will look at religion's effect on breast cancer patients. *Women's Health Weekly*, p. 4.

Babrow, A. S., Hines, S. C., & Kasch, C. R. (2000). Managing uncertainty in illness exploration: An application of Problematic Integration Theory. In B. B. Whaley (Ed.), *Explaining illness: Research, theory, and strategies* (pp. 41-67). Mahwah, NJ: Erlbaum.

Carroll, B. (2001). A phenomenological exploration of the nature of spirituality and spiritual care. *Mortality, 6*(1), 81-98.

Cole, B., & Pergament, K. (1999). Re-creating your life: A spiritual/psychotherapeutic intervention for people diagnosed with cancer. *Psycho-Oncology, 8,* 395-407.

Creagan, E. T. (1997). Attitude and disposition: Do they make a difference in cancer survival? *Mayo Clinic Proceedings, 72*(2), 160-164.

Ejaz, F.K. (2000). The influence of religious and personal values on nursing home residents' attitudes toward life-sustaining treatments. *Social Work in Health Care, 32*(2), 23-39.

Emanuel, E. J., & Emanuel, L. L. (1999). The promise of a good death. *The Lancet, 351,* 21-29.

Fernsler, J. I., Klemm, P., & Miller, M. A. (1999). Spiritual well-being and demands of illness in people with colorectal cancer. *Cancer Nursing, 22*(2), 134-140.

Ferraro, K. F., & Kelley-Moore, J. A. (2000). Religious consolation among men and women: Do health problems spur seeking? *Journal for the Scientific Study of Religion, 39*(2), 220-234.

Fitzsimmons, D., George, S., Payne, S., & Johnson, C. D. (1999). Differences in perception of quality of life issues between health professionals and patients with pancreatic cancer. *Psycho-Oncology, 8,* 135-143.

Fryback, P. B., & Reinert, B. R. (1999). Spirituality and people with potentially fatal diagnoses. *Nursing Forum, 34*(1), 13-22.

Glimelius, B., Birgegard, G., Hoffman, K., Kvale, G., & Sjoden, P. (1995). Information to and communication with cancer patients: Improvements and psychosocial correlates in a comprehensive care program for patients and their relatives. *Patient Education and Counseling, 25,* 171-182.

Greenwald, H. P. (1987). The specificity of quality-of-life measures among the seriously ill. *Medical Care, 25*(7), 642-651.

Hermann, C. (2000). A guide to spiritual needs of elderly cancer patients. *Geriatric Nursing, 21*(6), 324-325.

Holland, J. C., Korzun, A. H., Tross, S., Silberfarb, P., Perry, M., Comis, R., & Oster, M. (1986). Comparative psychological disturbance in patients with pancreatic and gastric cancer. *American Journal of Psychiatry, 143*(8), 982-986.

Holt, J. L., Houg, B. L., & Romano, J. L. (1999). Spiritual wellness for clients with HIV/AIDS: Review of counseling issues. *Journal of Counseling & Development, 77*(2), 160-170.

Hunt, M., & Meerabeau, L. (1993). Purging the emotions: The lack of emotional expression in subfertility and in the care of the dying. *International Journal of Nursing Studies, 30*(2), 115-123.

Jevne, R. F. (1987). Creating stillpoints: Beyond a rational approach to counseling cancer patients. *Journal of Psychosocial Oncology, 5*(3), 1-15.

Kearney, M., & Mount, B. (2000). Spiritual care of the dying patient. In H.M. Chochinov & W. Breitbart (Eds.), *Handbook of psychiatry in palliative medicine* (pp. 352-370). New York: Oxford University Press.

Kristeller, J. L., Zumbrun, C. S., & Schilling, R. F. (1999). "I would if I could": How oncologists and oncology nurses address spiritual distress in cancer patients. *Psycho-Oncology, 8*(5) 451-458.

Kreps, G. L. (2001). The evolution and advancement of health communication inquiry. In W.B. Gudykurst (Ed.), *Communication yearbook* (pp. 231-253). Thousand Oaks, CA: Sage.

McCollum P. S. (1978). Adjustment to cancer: A psychosocial and rehabilitative perspective. *Rehabilitation Counseling Bulletin, 21*(3), 216-223.

Moadel, A., Morgan, C., Fatone, A., Grennan, J., Carter, J., LaRuffa, G., Skummy, A., & Dutcher, J. (1999). Seeking meaning and hope: Self-reported spiritual and existential needs among an ethnically-diverse cancer patient population. *Psycho-Oncology, 8,* 378-385.

Newshan, G. (1998). Transcending the physical: Spiritual aspects of pain in patients with HIV and/or cancer. *Journal of Advanced Nursing, 28*(6), 1236-1241.

Northouse, P.G., & Northouse, L.L. (1987). Communication and cancer: Issues confronting patients, health professionals, and family members. *Journal of Psychosocial Oncology, 5*(3), 17-46.

Norum, J., Risberg, T., & Solberg, E. (2000). Faith among patients with advanced cancer: A pilot study on patients offered "no more than" palliation. *Support Care Cancer, 8,* 110-114.

O'Connor, T. S. J., Meakes, E., McCarroll-Butler, P., Gadowsky, S., & O'Neill, K. (1997). Making the most and making sense: Ethnographic research on spirituality in palliative care. *The Journal of Pastoral Care, 51*(1), 101-112.

O'Leary, U. (2002). Psychosocial influences on pain perceptions in cancer. *Nursing Times, 96*(43), 36-38.

Otis-Green, S., Sherman, R., Perez, M., & Baird, P. (2002). An integrated psychosocial-spiritual model for cancer pain management. *Cancer Practice, 10*(1), 58-65.

Peterson, L. G., Popkin, M. K., & Hall, R. C. (1983). Psychiatric presentations of cancer and sequelae of treatment. *Psychiatric Medicine, 1*(1), 79-92.

Roberts, J. A., Brown, D., Elkins, T., & Larson, D. B. (1997). Factors influencing views of patients with gynecological cancer about end-of-life decisions. *American Journal of Obstetrics and Gynecology, 176*(1), 166-172.

Rokach, A. (2000). Terminal illness and coping with loneliness. *Journal of Psychology, 134*(3), 283-297.

Schaefer, S. M. (1985). An ego-oriented, goal-directed, short-term treatment model of groupwork with cancer patients and their families. *Social Work With Groups, 8*(2), 154-157.

Schilling, R. F. (1999). "I would if I could": How oncologists and oncology nurses address spiritual distress in cancer patients. *Psycho-Oncology, 8,* 451-458.

Sherman, A. C., Simonton, S., Adams, D. C., Latif, U., Plante, T. G., Burns, S. K., & Poling, T. (2001). Measuring religious faith in cancer patients: Reliability and construct validity of the Santa Clara Strength of Religious Faith Questionnaire. *Psycho-Oncology, 10,* 436-443.

Spilka, B., Spangler, J. D., & Nelson, C. B. (1983). Spiritual support in life threatening illness. *Journal of Religion & Health, 22*(2), 98-104.

Taylor, E.J. (2001). Spirituality, culture, and cancer care. *Seminars in Oncology Nursing, 17*(3), 197-205.

Taylor, E. J., & Outlaw, F. H. (2002). Use of prayer among persons with cancer. *Holistic Nursing Practice, 16*(3), 46-60.

Taylor, E. J., Outlaw, F. H., Bernardo, T. R., & Roy, A. (1999). Spiritual conflicts associated with praying about cancer. *Psycho-Oncology, 8,* 386-394.

Thomas, J., & Retsas, A. (1999). Transacting self-preservation: A grounded theory of the spiritual dimensions of people with terminal cancer. *International Journal of Nursing Studies, 36,* 191-201.

Veach, T. A., & Nicholas, D. R. (1998). Understanding families of adults with cancer: Combining the clinical course of cancer and stages of family development. *Journal of Counseling & Development, 76*(2), 144-156.

Ziegler, J. (1998). Spirituality returns to the fold in medical practice. *Journal of the National Cancer Institute, 90*(17), 1255-1258.

IV

SPECIAL PATIENT POPULATIONS

14 | Cancer Care and the Aging Patient

Complexities of Age-Related Communication Barriers

Lisa Sparks
Chapman University

For the aging patient, the new cultural world of cancer is frequently burdened with a new technical- and medical-oriented language along with a new set of unknown relationships. The focus of this chapter is to highlight the significant potential contributions to our understanding of cancer communication that can be made by integrating scholarship from the communication and aging area. We must begin to pay attention to the subtle complexities of age-related communication barriers, how older adults use strategies of selection and optimization with compensation to deal with such barriers, and how such unique cognitive message processing and information seeking may impact communication with the aging patient diagnosed with cancer. In order to provide the best care for aging patients, we must first understand such complexities that many older adults face and how these barriers can get in the way of older adult preferences for and ability to process messages, which could potentially influence health outcomes.

Recent estimates indicate that nearly 9 million Americans have a history of cancer (http://dccps.nci.nih.gov/ocs/). Cancer was second only to heart disease as the leading cause of death in the United States for those aged 65 and over (NCHS, 2000). Older adults account for 61% of all new cancer cases and 70% of all cancer deaths, and it is estimated that those

Sparks

aged 65 and over have 11 times the cancer risk of those under the age of 65 years (Lewis et al., 2003). Moreover, the number is expected to increase as the U.S. population ages, even with increased improvements in early detection and treatment of cancer (Edwards et al., 2002; Yancik, 1997). Cancer survivors aged 65 and older are already estimated to be 16% and rising (http://srab.cancer.gov/prevalence/index.html). Increasingly, older adults are diagnosed with cancer more than any other segment of the population (see Hewitt, Rowland, & Yancik, 2003; Sparks, 2003). However, older adults diagnosed with cancer are the population group over and above any other, which are at increased risk for poor communication with health professionals (Adelman & Greene, 2000; Greene & Adelman, 2001, 2002). At this time more than any other, it is crucial that we begin to understand how to communicate with aging cancer patients across the continuum of cancer care from diagnosis to survivorship. Thus, the study of communication practices during cancer care for the aging patient is critical for improving geriatric care as well as for considering the lives of those affected by the disease. Consequently, the unique aspects of cancer care for the aging patient will become increasingly important.

Research involving the communication of cancer care for the aging patient includes such topics as social identity (Harwood & Sparks, 2003), successful adaptation across the life span (Nussbaum, Baringer, & Kundrat, 2003), narratives (Anderson & Geist-Martin, 2003), palliative care (Ragan, Wittenberg, & Hall, 2003), social support (Robinson & Turner, 2003), communicative competence online (Query & Wright, 2003), decision-making processes (O'Hair et al., 2003), and communicating about cancer risk (Rowan, Sparks, Pecchioni, & Villagran, 2003). Furthermore, Kreps (2003) stated that the study and application of health communication has the greatest potential to help reduce cancer risks, incidence, morbidity, and mortality, while enhancing quality of life across the continuum of cancer care (prevention, detection, diagnosis, treatment, survivorship, and end-of-life care).

In order to implement more sound communicative practices during cancer care, it is crucial that we first begin to understand that just as not all cancer diagnoses are alike, not all patients are alike. Individuals of similar chronological age often undergo very different life experiences. These different experiences can influence communication in relationships. One life- experience that can differ between individuals of the same chronological age is the presence or absence of a cancer diagnosis. Health care providers of various specialties beyond oncology are often the first to discover the cancer and have to cope with communicating the bad news to the fearful and angry patient (Ong et al., 1998).

The impact of such a diagnosis, and subsequent interactions related to the diagnosis, can be remarkably overwhelming for older adults as well as for those caring for the older adult patient. Although many older adults have known others who have been diagnosed with cancer, more often than not these individuals have little to no experience with the cancer culture and any norms associated with this unknown world (Sparks, 2003). The communication surrounding each diagnosis for older adult patients must begin to be tailored to account for such complexities.

Recognizing the complexities of effective cancer care communication with the aging patient must no longer be ignored. Cancer communication messages must be designed and delivered to match the communication skills, needs, and predispositions of specific audiences such as the older adult population. To influence entrenched health behaviors, messages need to be relevant and compelling, with health information that provides direction and rationale for making the best health-related decisions and adopting health-preserving behaviors (Maibach, Kreps, & Bonaguro, 1996).

Cancer poses a series of significant health threats that demand effective health communication (Kreps & Chapelsky Massimilla, 2002). Effective health communication can encourage cancer prevention, inform cancer detection and diagnosis, guide cancer treatment, support successful cancer survivorship, and promote the best end-of-life care. Implications of this analysis are drawn for directing informed cancer communication research and practice. This chapter sheds light on the powerful potential to strategically use health communication to reduce cancer risks, incidence, morbidity, and mortality, while enhancing quality of life across the continuum of cancer care germane to the aging patient (prevention, detection, diagnosis, treatment, survivorship, and end-of-life care; Byock, 2000; Hiatt & Rimer, 1999). This chapter reviews the unique physical, cognitive, language, and interactive relationship characteristics of caring for the aging patient as well as the family members connected to the patient in the complex, confusing, and overwhelming cancer cancer-related health environment. It should be evident that age-related physiological changes, cognitive changes, and life experiences of older individuals tend to complicate the ways health care providers and family members care for the aging patient who has been diagnosed with cancer. From a perspective grounded in life life span developmental communication, the notion of understanding conversational barriers that are unique to caring for the aging patient is first put forth followed by an explanation of the selection and optimization with compensation model that aids older adults in adjusting to their communicative, psychological, affective, and behavioral environment. Once such conversational barriers are addressed and better understood in terms of older adult adaptation to such deficits across the life span, researchers, practitioners, and family members involved in caring for aging patients will have more clearly defined ways of constructing messages that aging patients will likely comprehend and process, which may contribute to better health outcomes. Cancer messages must be designed specifically for the older adult population. Insight into the unique difficulties of all related communication barriers that get in the way of older adult cognitive message processing and information-seeking strategies is pertinent and long over due. This chapter attempts to answer that call so that more effective and relevant health campaigns can ultimately be launched to reach this specific, albeit complex and interesting aging population. Persuasion and health communication scholars alike must focus on designing messages and interventions focused on encouraging younger and aging patients to be active participants in health communication environments, particularly when it comes to cancer care for the aging patient.

COMPLEXITIES OF AGE AGE-RELATED COMMUNICATION BARRIERS

Throughout this chapter it is suggested that a significant relationship exists between communication messages and the satisfaction that people obtain from such messages, whether such exchanges stem from interpersonal, small-group, organizational, public, or mass-oriented contexts. The next reasonable argument then would be that an individual's ability to create and maintain satisfaction with interactions and message exchanges ultimately affects the individual's health. Epidemiological researchers Berkman and Syme (1979) suggested that individuals without close interpersonal interactions and relationships are two times as likely to die than those with strong interpersonal ties. Thus, further understanding of how older adults' communicative interactions play out in the construction and processing of such messages across the communication continuum (e.g., interpersonal, small-group, organizational, public, mass) is another element that may contribute greatly to increased health outcomes for aging patients.

The importance of understanding the complexities underlying communicating with the aging patient diagnosed with cancer works in another important way. Communication not only plays a crucial role in assessing the mental and physical health of patients, but, additionally, after they are diagnosed with an illness such as cancer, their communicative relationships seem to influence how they will get well (Nussbaum, Pecchioni, Robinson, & Thompson, 2000). Due to the complexities of the health care provider–older adult patient relationship, barriers that older adults and their partners and caregivers face in conversation and some implications of such barriers must be better understood, as well as the connection to the ways in which older adults adapt to deficits acquired across the life span. As Cohen (1994) stated, the nature and management of cancer for older adults not only depends on biological processes, but on psychological and social processes as well.

BARRIER 1: AGING CHARACTERISTICS

Before diving into communication and relational barriers, one must understand Busse's (1969) discussion of primary and secondary characteristics of aging. Gerontological theorist, Busse first recognized that many of the declining characteristics associated with aging were not a function of growing old, but most often were tied to other elements of one's life. The primary characteristics of aging include developmental changes that result solely from the process of aging (i.e., wrinkles), whereas secondary characteristics are changes that occur due to events that take place during the life span (e.g., poor diet). Eisdorfer and Cohen's (1980) research suggests that much of the cognitive decline associated with aging is not the result of the aging process, but is due to high blood pressure, which can occur at any age. Thus, it is important to first understand that communication barriers in cancer care for the aging patient can be caused by both primary and secondary characteristics of aging (Nussbaum et al., 2000).

BARRIER 2: AGING AND PRESBYOPIA

Presbyopia is a thickening of the crystalline lenses of the eye, along with a decrease in elasticity of the lenses of the eye (Corso, 1971; Kline & Scialfa, 1996; McFarland, 1968), and begins around the age of 40. At this point, many individuals begin to hold printed material farther away from their eyes than they did before. At age 50, most individuals have trouble seeing small objects and details, with an increased need for glasses when reading (Botwinick, 1978). By the age of 70, less than 30% have retained 20/20 eyesight and most do not have normal vision even with correction (Botwinick, 1978). Thus, older adults increasingly have to adjust to problems related to seeing objects both near and far. Certain losses due to aging also begin to affect everyday activities (Kline & Scialfa, 1996). Such increased difficulties include spatial acuity, depth perception, motion perception, and being able to see in shadowed areas.

BARRIER 3: AGING AND PRESBYCUSIS

Not surprisingly, the aging process also impacts the ability to process aural information. *Presbycusis* is the term used to describe the hearing loss associated with aging. Characteristics of presbycusis include a decrease in the ability to distinguish between consonants and among adjacent frequencies as well as a reduced sensitivity to higher frequency sounds (Botwinick, 1977, 1978; Corso, 1971; Willeford, 1971). Hearing problems increase considerably after the age of 45, although older adult deafness is rare with only 15% of individuals over the age of 75 considered to be deaf (Darbyshire, 1984; Verbrugge, 1984). Still, 20% of older adults over the age of 75 or older suffer from mild hearing loss. Often, the declining ability to hear, combined with a decline in confidence about hearing, results in more requests for repetition of information from the interactant or an avoidance of conversations (Nussbaum et al., 2000). Elderly individuals experiencing hearing loss will try to overcompensate via a number of strategies, including an attempt to fill in the semantic and syntactic gaps whenever possible (Villaume, Brown, & Darling, 1994). Of course, as with any conversational snafu, inappropriate fillers can create uncomfortable conversations. When conversations do not follow conventional norms, the wrong words bring about unintended difficulties. Even the slightest impairments in both sight and hearing are often worse when combined, than a more significant impairment in either sight or hearing. Such sensory difficulties contribute to decreases in confidence with one's conversational abilities, which in turn may contribute to problems in other areas, such as message processing or particular information-seeking strategies for older adults.

Hearing problems have been linked to difficulties in the production of speech sounds for older adults (Hutchinson & Beasley, 1981). Message exchange and understanding is likely to be impacted by such declines acquired across one's life span. Another problem in the message exchange is the increase in time it takes for older adults to encode and decode messages (Nussbaum et al., 2000). The increase in such coding processes is attributed to physiological changes in the brain and a decrease in the information-processing efficiency of the central nervous system (Birren, Woods, & Williams, 1980; MacKay & Abrams, 1996; Smith, Thompson, & Michalewski, 1980; Takeda & Matsuzawa, 1985). Although encoding and decoding process problems are likely to be minor, delays during conversation are often awkward and seem to be longer than usual, which can be attributed to negative personality characteristics of the older adult.

BARRIER 4: AGING AND MESSAGES

Word retrieval, name recall, and planning what to say during a conversation can also present problems along with delays in processing (Cohen, 1994; MacKay & Abrams, 1996), all of which can impact the typical conversational flow. Such difficulties lead interactants to begin to question the older speaker's competence. Thus, memory difficulties are just some of the problems associated with message transmission and exchange.

Information seeking with aging patients, however, does have added barriers. Although a number of cancer interventions and campaigns are currently launched, it is unknown the extent to which older adults pay attention to, or even seek out this information. In fact,

Pecchioni and Sparks' (2004) data tell us that the only source of health information that older adults use consistently is their doctor. After doctors, the most important information sources were (in order) as follows: family members, nurses, friends, the Internet, other medical personnel, and other patients. Yet, the source of information with which patients were most satisfied was their friends and family. The source of information with which they were least satisfied was listed as their doctor. These data indicate a serious discrepancy between information sought, and information persons are satisfied with (see also Sparks, Pecchioni, & Mittapalli, 2003, 2004). For aging patients in particular, it is important to understand the extent by which satisfaction with information is correlated with message effectiveness. If this is indeed the case, then it is reasonable to assume that older adults will be most persuaded by information provided by friends and family. This is a critical issue for health practitioners because friend and family information may lack up-to to-date research, clarity, or even accuracy. Thus, it is imperative that we examine the complexities of age-related communication barriers by understanding how aging patients process cognitive, affective, and behavioral information in unique ways, how older adults are persuaded to seek out information, and thus be active participants in their health care.

BARRIER 5: AGING AND COGNITIVE FUNCTION

A simplistic relationship between aging and decline in cognitive ability does not exist, however, some dimensions of intelligence slightly decrease as we age, particularly for those over the age of 70 (see, e.g., Jarvik & Bank, 1983; Schaie, 1983, 1996). Moreover, research indicates that some of the cognitive decline related to aging can be overcompensated for with mental and physical activity (see, e.g., Botwinick, 1977; Schaie, 1996). Recent research in cognitive aging indicates that for normal cognitive aging, older adults will maintain the relative strengths and weaknesses acquired and practiced earlier in their lives (Anstey, Hofer, & Luszcz, 2003). In other words, these new and contrasting findings suggest that even the very old are able to retain their unique patterns of cognitive strengths and weaknesses. Prior research suggests that explanations for cognitive deficits across the life span are primarily due to genetic factors, neurochemical factors, and central nervous system efficiency and integrity (Anstey, Lord, & Williams, 1997; Anstey & Smith, 1999; Li, 2002; Li & Lindenberger, 1999). Another theme in the cognitive aging literature that is worth noting is the importance of distinguishing between chronological age as an index of time and the physiological and contextual processes that may be a better indicator of adult development that is more informative for explaining cognitive change (Birren & Cunningham, 1985; Wohlwill, 1970). Individuals of the same chronological age are not automatically in the same physical or mental state of mind (Rubin & Rubin, 1986). Contextual age is "a transactional view of aging that incorporates physiological, psychological, social, and communication influences on life-position" (Rubin & Rubin, 1986, p. 30). It is the state affected by physical health, interpersonal interactions, mobility, life satisfaction, social activity, and economic security (Rubin & Rubin, 1986). Despite differences in chronological age, contextual age allows individuals to identify with one another in ways that are sometimes invisible (Kundrat & Nussbaum, 2003).

Evidence related to drastic declines in cognition processes for older adults does not strongly support a negative relationship and has been overstated. However, significant declines in cognitive ability have been found to occur in older adults about 5 years before death (Kleemeier, 1962). The decline is likely to be related to distance from death more than being related to age (Berg, 1996). Cohen's (1979) research suggests that when older adults are able to understand a spoken message in the same manner as a younger adult, they are often not able to use the information. Older adults frequently have a more difficult time than younger adults in making inferences from information obtained from an interaction, which leads conversants to believe that the older adult is not getting the point of the conversation.

Everyday problem solving can also be a problem for older adults simply because the strategies employed differ from those used by younger adults (Willis, 1996). Nussbaum et al. (2000) state that such differences are shown on declarative (i.e., searching for the information) and procedural (i.e., using prior experiential knowledge) levels. On the declarative level, older adults can sift through vast amounts of information and pull out the relevant pieces of information necessary for choosing the best option available. Younger adults tend to act more like novices by searching for extensive information. If successful decision making is established by the amount of information gathered, then older adults show a poorer performance than their younger counterparts. On the procedural level of problem solving, older adults rely on well-established procedural strategies for obtaining solutions to the problem. Poor problem solving may emerge when old skills are applied to newer problems (Nussbaum et al., 2000).

Schaie's (1975) research has suggested that the intellectual abilities and skills of reasonably healthy older adults have not diminished but have instead become obsolete. Older adults simply need retraining to adjust to contemporary society. Some dimensions of intelligence decrease with age and are typically divided into two categories—crystallized and fluid. As Nussbaum et al. (2000) described, crystallized intelligence includes verbal skills, comprehension skills, and vocabulary typically acquired via education and personal experience and remain relatively stable until the age of 70 (Botwinick, 1977). Fluid intelligence is typically unrelated to experience or education, but rather refers to mainly nonverbal skills such as abstract reasoning, response time, and mathematics. Fluid intelligence tends to decline after the age of 35 and is usually due to a decreased functioning of the central nervous system (Horn & Donaldson, 1980). One way to greatly slow down the decreases in fluid intelligence is through interaction with others (Nussbaum et al., 2000). Research into the influence of fluid intelligence on conversation is untouched and desperately needed.

BARRIER 6: AGING AND MEMORY

Similar to the research on aging and cognitive abilities, research studying the influence of aging on memory indicates memory to be a multidimensional construct (Nussbaum et al., 2000). In short, the relationship between age and memory is incredibly complex. Three types of memory tend to dominate the aging and memory literature—sensory, short-term, and long-term term—and all are differentially impacted by the aging process. *Sensory memory* is defined as one's ability to remember an image or memory of stimuli within a fraction of a second after exposure (see e.g., Baltes, Reese, & Lipsitt, 1980). The authors further state that sensory memory does not appear to diminish with age if sensory limitations fail to get in the way of the reception of stimuli. *Short-term memory* is defined as the ability to remember an image or memory of stimuli within seconds or minutes after exposure and tends to slowly decline with age (see e.g., Baltes et al., 1980). Decline in short-term memory processes varies with each individual owing to aspects such as cognitive style (Monge, 1969), complexity of material (Botwinick & Storandt, 1974), amount of emotional threat in terms of stress the older adult receives, rapid pace of presentation, amount or complexity of organizing needed to encode vast amounts of information (Arenberg & Robertson-Tchabo, 1977; Craik & Rabinowitz, 1985), fear of failure (Okun, 1976), and recognizable recall material (Chase & Simon, 1973; Hanley-Dunn & McIntosh, 1984). Conversational difficulties tend to arise for older adults because of problems with simultaneously processing and storing information (Smith, 1996). In terms of short-term memory recall of information, younger adults have an advantage over older adults. Although such declines in short-term memory associated with aging make conversations slightly more difficult for older adults, research indicates that such difficulties can be reduced and increases in affect can be achieved simply by conversing in a relaxed and nonevaluative style (Nussbaum, Robinson, & Grew, 1983, 1985). *Long-term memory* is comprised of specific experiences or episodic memory, knowledge or semantic memory, and procedural memory (Smith, 1996). Declines in age-related long-term memory tend to be more drastic in some components than those for short-term memory (Craik, 1977). Such dramatic declines are primarily the result of encoding or organizational difficulties, or the procedural component of memory (see e.g., Arenberg & Robertson-Tchabo, 1977; Craik & Rabinowitz, 1985; Smith, 1996). A number of other factors contribute to declines in long-term memory. It takes more time for older adults to retrieve information from memory (Craik, 1977). Other factors impacting long-term recall include recognition of the material being recalled (see, e.g., Chase & Simon, 1973; Hanley-Dunn & McIntosh, 1984), as well as one's learning style (Monge, 1969), salience of information, number of items to remember, type of task and task structure (Botwinick, 1973), and motivation level (Elias & Elias, 1977). However, older adults have been found to have better narrative recall and tend to remember stories in more accurate detail than their younger counterparts. Furthermore, older adults have a more complex and developed scripted knowledge of daily activities and tend to be more efficient at identifying problems and finding reasonable solutions (Blanchard-Fields & Abeles, 1996). Older adults and younger adults have different problem-solving strategies and social-knowledge scripts because they do not share the same schema (Nussbaum et al., 2000). Understanding such differences is the first step toward reducing misunderstandings and miscommunication of health messages.

BARRIER 7: AGING AND RELATIONSHIPS

Nussbaum, Baringer, and Kundrat (2003) state that an understanding of successful adaptation and effective management of cancer by older adults cannot be accomplished without the study of the interpersonal communication of older adults. First, the nature and management of cancer for older adults not only depends on biological processes, but psychological and social processes as well (Cohen, 1994). The Socioemotional Selectivity Theory advanced by Carstensen (1992) proposes that older adults reduce their overall social interactions while maintaining those relationships that provide the most emotional support. This can enlighten our understanding of where a diagnosis of cancer will be most disruptive in an older adult's relational world. Understanding how family and friend relationships function in old age can help us to predict and explain the process of an older individual's successful adaptation to living with cancer (Nussbaum et al., 2003).

Cancer information is often highly emotionally charged, due to the serious, often life-threatening, nature of many forms of cancer. Receiving a diagnosis of cancer can be a major shock to most people. It is important that cancer communications programs are strategically designed to address the important psychological and socioemotional issues surrounding different individuals' experiences with cancer (Kreps, 2003). Care must be taken to coordinate content and relational aspects of communication to both inform people about cancer and cancer treatment, without confusing or upsetting them (Buckman, 1996; Gillotti, Thompson, & McNeilis, 2002).

SELECTIVE OPTIMIZATION WITH COMPENSATION MODEL

Underlying the notion that older adult cancer patients adapt to their illness through communication is a meta-model of adaptation developed by Baltes and Baltes (1990). Baltes and Baltes view aging as a lifelong adaptive process by suggesting that as we grow older, adaptation to the losses associated with aging can be best explained by examining the relationships among the processes of selective optimization based on compensation. Based on social exchange theory, it is believed that people make determinations about the behaviors they will enact based on the goals they have selected, the resources and opportunities available to them, and their perceptions of their ability to enact behaviors that will help them attain those goals. Although individuals may not be able to perform a particular task as well as they once did, through the selective optimization with compensation (SOC) process, older adults are able to maintain satisfying, successful, efficacious, and arguably healthier lives.

The SOC model can be explained succinctly by defining three terms. *Selection* is viewed as adaptation through limiting the number of goals the individual may pursue. *Optimization* is a positioning of skills and resources within a limited goal or life domain to remain effective. *Compensation* is used to describe the individual's response to a loss in behavioral capacity. Because our skills often exceed requirements of the task, a slight loss in a skill or ability as a consequence of aging may not present much of a problem because the losses tend to occur in those skill or ability areas that are not typically used.

DESIGNING HEALTH MESSAGES FOR OLDER ADULTS

Health communication scholars must focus on designing messages and interventions that encourage older adults to be active participants in health communication contexts, especially in the cancer communication context, which is often frightening and unknown territory. We need to focus on message strategies that will prove effective with the unique complexities and barriers facing the elderly population. That said, such a goal must be pursued by focusing on an understanding of older adult cognitive processes followed by particular message framing that will more likely reach this unique population. Prior research by Mitchell (2000) and Mitchell, Brown, Morris Villagran, and and Villagran (2001) indicates that when exposed to messages that are negatively framed, persons are more likely to enact health protective behaviors. But, is this still the case for older adults?

Seeking out cancer cancer-related health information is a risky endeavor. That is, knowledge gained from such information-seeking strategies will not cure cancer, but rather it can aid in finding out if one is at risk for cancer. Health communication and persuasion scholars, as well as health practitioners have utilized Prospect Theory by using the framing postulate as a way to understand the communication involved in risky decisions (see, e.g., Kahneman & Tversky, 1979). The theory suggests that individuals will act differentially to information presented as gains or losses. The framing postulate further hypothesizes that individuals avoid risks when considering gains but prefer risks when considering losses. Older adult patients may differentially face decisions about cancer treatments relative to their unique characteristics and life circumstances (e.g., chemotherapy regimens, etc.) in considering gains and losses germane to the aging population.

Negatively framed messages are referred to in terms of losses, whereas positively framed messages are typically referred to in terms of gains. The message-framing postulate of Prospect Theory has been utilized in the health domain fairly extensively, particularly given that the outcome of disease detection is an uncertain and often risky behavior (see, e.g., Banks, Zimmerman, Ishak, & Harter, 1995; Meyerowitz & Chaiken, 1987; Rothman, Salovey, Antone, Keough, & Martin, 1993). For instance, Meyerowitz and Chaiken's research suggests that female participants were more convinced to conduct breast self-examinations after being exposed to negatively framed messages, than positively framed messages. Negatively framed messages have also been found to be more effective in persuading persons in terms of detection behaviors such as seeking health information or discovering a lump or mole (see Rothman et al., 1993). One way in which health messages differ is whether they recommend preventing a health risk or a hazard (e.g., wearing seatbelts) or recommend detecting a health risk or a hazard (e.g., breast self self-examinations). Information seeking is often considered a detection behavior (see e.g., Mitchell, 2000). Detecting a health problem is viewed as more risky because in the process of gathering health information about particular symptoms, individuals may find out they have a serious health problem, such as cancer. Presumably, not knowing about a disease is less risky than knowing that one has a disease. Prevention is less risky because one is taking measures to ensure not becoming sick or hurt. That said, negatively framed messages are more likely to smooth the progress of detection behaviors, largely because risky options are preferred when individuals are considering losses (Rothman et al., 1993). In fact, research has indicated that individuals who are exposed to negatively framed messages are more likely to change their behavioral intentions toward health detection behaviors.

In such a discussion of message framing, it is interesting to point out that positively and negatively framed information are equal numerically speaking—but it is the tone of the information that leads individuals to perceive it differently. And, therefore, individuals will cognitively process messages differentially based on framing, particularly older adults. Researchers have long recognized the magnitude of examining cognitive processing as mediating the link between messages and subsequent behavior. For instance, Mitchell (2000) and Mitchell et al. (2001) examined the role of cognitive processing in understanding the emotion by message message-quality interaction. By experimentally varying emotion, involvement, and message quality, the researchers investigated the impact that emotion and message quality jointly have on cognitive processes in terms of thought valence, counterarguing, and message recall. Results indicated that overall message quality is the best predictor of attitude change, and that cognitive processing is a key mediator of that relationship. Furthermore, Lapinski and Levine

(2000) found similar results with this finding across cultural groups. Both studies also showed a strong linear correlation between counterarguments and attitude change such that, as participants' ability to counterargue increases, their attitude change decreases. This line of research suggests that communication scholars need to begin addressing the unique ways by which older adults process and receive messages, as well as the ways the older adult population begin to adapt to such difficult health diagnoses such as cancer in different ways than their younger counterparts.

CONCLUSION

This chapter reviewed the unique physical, cognitive, language, and interactive relationship characteristics likely to be involved when caring for the aging patient as well as the family members connected to the patient in the complex, confusing, and overwhelming cancer-related health environment. Age-related physiological, cognitive, and life changes and experiences often complicate the ways care is provided for an older adult diagnosed with cancer. By better understanding such conversational barriers, researchers, practitioners, and family members involved in caring for aging patients will be able to deliver relevant and compelling messages that aging patients can better understand and process, and better health outcomes will be achieved. Designing and delivering cancer communication messages to match the specific communication skills, needs, and predispositions of the older adult population is a crucial component of health care delivery. This chapter provided concrete suggestions for a focus on message design and framing for health interventions tailored to the older adult population. Such systematic, communication research-based campaigns can assist older adults in becoming active participants in health communication environments. By focusing on such complexities of particular age-related communication barriers that may hinder or help in caring for the aging patient, researchers, family members, and health practitioners can provide much better cancer care.

Furthermore, the SOC model (Baltes & Baltes, 1990) is important as it explains how adaptation occurs in a general sense and provides a framework for understanding the middle range theories employed above to generate specific hypotheses. SOC also provides a rationale for what constitutes an optimal match in terms of a good or desirable message. From the social exchange perspective, which underlies the SOC model, a good message is one where the rewards of listening to and absorbing the message exceed the costs—relative to the available message alternatives. Thus, the SOC model and designing of relevant and compelling messages for aging patients can aid in pushing through the age-related barriers older adults face to achieve increased health outcomes. By gaining this knowledge, researchers and health care providers can give better care to aging patients and aging patients as well as partners and family members can more easily acquire health information that will help them to help themselves in more productive and efficient ways.

Health communication scholars must do a better job of translating relevant communication theories and literature into the lives of aging patients, caregivers, and health care provider teams. Communication theories from interpersonal relationship development to persuasion and mass-mediated processes provide sound building blocks for those interested in using reliable research-based empirical evidence to aid in explaining the critical features of a successful older adult who has received the news of a cancer diagnosis. Thus, further understanding of how older adults' communicative interactions play out in the construction and processing of such messages across the communication continuum (e.g., interpersonal, small-group, organizational, public, mass) is an essential step that is greatly needed to increase health outcomes for aging patients. Recognizing the complexities of effective cancer care communication with the aging patient must no longer be ignored. Cancer communication messages must be designed and delivered to match the communication skills, needs, and predispositions of such specific audiences. To influence entrenched health behaviors, messages (from interpersonal to mediated) need to be relevant and compelling, with health information that provides direction and rationale for making the best health-related decisions and adopting health-preserving behaviors. Effective health communication can encourage cancer prevention, inform cancer detection and diagnosis, guide cancer treatment, support successful cancer survivorship, and promote the best end-of-life care in unique ways.

The goal of this chapter was to highlight the powerful potential to strategically construct health communication messages to reduce cancer risks, incidence, morbidity, and mortality, while enhancing quality of life across the continuum of cancer care germane to the aging patient (prevention, detection, diagnosis, treatment, survivorship, and end-of-life care). It is argued that, by first understanding such unique age-related communication barriers, researchers, practitioners, and family members can then begin to construct interpersonal and mediated messages in a systematic, understandable way. Such tailored, research-based messages will have a greater likelihood of reaching and impacting the aging patient diagnosed with cancer. Health communication scholars have a plethora of theoretical, methodological, and pragmatic communication-based approaches to greatly contribute to the complex yet unique communicative contexts of cancer care for the aging patient. There is no better way to inform the health care and research community than to engage in care and to get involved in interdisciplinary research teams by translating such research efforts into practice.

REFERENCES

Adelman R., & Greene, M. (2000). Communication between older patients and their physicians. *Clinics in Geriatric Medicine, 16*(1), 1-24.

Adelman, M. B., Parks, M. R., & Albrecht, T. L. (1987). Beyond close relationships: Support in weak ties. In T. L. Albrecht & M. B. Adelman (Eds.), *Communicating social support* (pp. 126-147). Newbury Park, CA: Sage.

Albrecht, T., Burleson, B., & Goldsmith, D. (1994). Supportive communication. In M. Knapp & G. Miller (Eds.), *Handbook of interpersonal communication* (pp. 419-459). Thousand Oaks, CA: Sage.

Anderson, J., & Geist-Martin, P. (2003). Narratives and healing: Exploring one family's stories of cancer survivorship. *Health Communication, 15*(2), 133-144.

Anstey, K. J., Hofer, S. M., & Luszcz, M. A. (2003). Cross-sectional and longitudinal patterns of differentiation in late-life cognitive and sensory function: The effects of age, ability, attrition, and occasion of measurement. *Journal of Experimental Psychology: General, 32*(3), 470-487.

Anstey, K. J., Lord, S. R., & Williams, P. (1997). Strength in the lower limbs, visual contrast sensitivity, and simple reaction time predict cognition in older women. *Psychology and Aging, 12,* 137-144.

Anstey, K. J., & Smith, G. A. (1999). Interrelationships among biological markers of aging, health, activity, acculturation, and cognitive performance in older adults. *Psychology and Aging, 14,* 615-618.

Anstey, K. J., Stankov, L., & Lord, S. R. (1993). Primary aging, secondary aging, and intelligence. *Psychology and Aging, 8,* 562-570.

Arenberg, D., & Robertson-Tchabo, E. (1977). Learning and aging. In J. Birren & K. Schaie (Eds.), *Handbook of the psychology of aging* (pp. 721-749). New York: Van Nostrand Reinhold.

Baltes, P. B., & Baltes, M. M. (1990). Psychological perspectives on successful aging: The model of selective optimization with compensation. In P. B. Baltes & M. M. Baltes (Eds.), *Successful aging: Perspectives from the behavioral sciences*. New York: Cambridge University Press.

Baltes, P. B., Reese, H., & Lipsitt, L. (1980). Life-span developmental psychology. In M. Rosenzweig & L. Porter (Eds.), *Annual review of psychology* (pp. 65-110). Palo Alto, CA: Annual Reviews.

Banks, A. T., Zimmerman, H. J., Ishak, K. G., & Harter, J. G. (1995). Diclofenac-associated hepatotoxicity: Analysis of 180 cases reported to the Food and Drug Administration as adverse reactions. *Hepatology, 22*(3), 820-827.

Berg, S. (1996). Aging, behavior, and terminal decline. In J. E. Birren & K. W. Schaie (Eds.), *Handbook of the psychology of aging* (4th ed., pp. 323-337). San Diego, CA: Academic Press.

Berkman, L., & Syme, S. (1979). Social networks, host resistance, and mortality. *American Journal of Epidemiology, 109,*186-204.

Birren, J. E., Woods, A., & Williams, M. (1980). Behavioral slowing with age: Causes, organization, and consequences. In L. Poon (Ed.), *Aging in the 1980s* (pp. 293-308). Washington, DC: American Psychological Association.

Birren, J. E., & Cunningham, W. (1985). Research on the psychology of aging: Principles, concepts, and theory. In J. E. Birren & W. Schaie (Eds.), *Handbook of the psychology of aging* (2nd ed., pp. 3-34). New York: Van Nostrand Reinhold.

Blanchard-Fields, F., & Abeles, R. (1996). Social cognition and aging. In J. E. Birren & K. W. Schaie (Eds.), *Handbook of the psychology of aging* (4th ed., pp. 150-161). San Diego, CA: Academic Press.

Booth-Butterfield, M. (2003). Embedded health behaviors from adolescence to adulthood: The impact of tobacco. *Health Communication, 15*(2), 171-185.

Botwinick, J. (1973). *Aging and behavior.* New York: Springer.

Botwinick, J. (1977). Intellectual abilities. In J. Birren & K. Schaie (Eds.), *Handbook of the psychology of aging* (pp. 580-605). New York: Van Nostrand Reinhold.

Botwinick, J. (1978). *Aging and behavior* (2nd ed.). New York: Springer.

Botwinick, J., & Storandt, M. (1974). *Memory related functions and age.* Springfield, IL: Thomas.

Buckman, R. (1996). Talking to patients about cancer. *British Medical Journal, 31,* 699-700.

Busse, E. (1969). Theories of aging: In E. Busse & E. Pfeiffer (Eds.), *Behavior and adaptation in later life* (pp. 11-32). Boston: Little, Brown.

Byock, I. (2000). Completing the continuum of cancer care: Integrating life-prolongation and palliation. *CA: A Cancer Journal for Clinicians, 50,* 123-132.

Carstensen, L. L. (1992). Social and emotional patterns in adulthood: Support for socioemotional selectivity theory. *Psychology and Aging, 7,* 331-338.

Chase, W., & Simon, H. (1973). The mind's eye in chess. In W. G. Chase (Ed.), *Visual information processing* (pp. 215-281). New York: Academic Press.

Cohen, G. (1979). Language comprehension in old age. *Cognitive Psychology, 11,* 423-429.

Cohen, G. (1994). Age-related problems in the use of proper names in communication. In M. L. Hummert, J. M. Wiemann, & J. F. Nussbaum (Eds.), *Interpersonal communication in older adulthood: Interdisciplinary theory and research* (pp. 40-57). Thousand Oaks, CA: Sage.

Corso, J. (1971). Sensory processes and age effects in normal adults. *Journal of Gerontology, 26,* 90-105.

Craik, F. (1977). Age differences in human memory. In J. Birren & K. W. Schaie (Eds.), *Handbook of the psychology of aging* (pp. 384-420). New York: Van Nostrand Reinhold.

Craik, F., & Rabinowitz, J. (1985). The effects of presentation rate and encoding task on age-related memory deficits. *Journal of Gerontology, 40,* 309-315.

Darbyshire, J. (1984). The hearing loss epidemic: A challenge to gerontology. *Research on Aging, 6,* 384-394.

Edwards, B. K., Howe, H. L., Ries, L. A. G., Thun, M. J., Rosenberg, H. M., Yancik, R., Wingo, P. A., Jemal, A., & Feigal, E. G. (2002). Annual report to the nation on the status of cancer, 1973-1999, featuring implications of age and aging on the US cancer burden. *Cancer, 94*(10), 2766-2792.

Eisdorfer, C., & Cohen, D. (1980). The issue of biological and psychological deficits. In E. Borgatta & N. McCluskey (Eds.), *Aging and society: Current research and policy perspectives* (pp. 49-70). Beverly Hills, CA: Sage.

Elias, M. F., & Elias, P. K. (1977). Motivation and activity. In J. Birren & K. W. Schaie (Eds.), *Handbook of the psychology of aging* (pp. 357-383). New York: Van Nostrand Reinhold.

Festinger, L. (1954). A theory of social comparison processes. *Human Relations, 7*(1), 152-163.

Gillotti, C., Thompson, T., & McNeilis, K. (2002). Communicative competence in the delivery of bad news. *Social Science and Medicine, 54,* 1011-1023.

Greene, M. G., & Adelman, R. D. (2001). Building the physician–older patient relationship. In M. L. Hummert & J. F. Nussbaum (Eds.), *Aging, communication, and health: Linking research and practice for successful aging* (pp. 101-120). Mahwah, NJ: Erlbaum.

Greene, M., & Adelman, R. (2002, January). Physician–older adult patient communication about cancer. In G. L. Kreps (Chair), *Consumer–Provider Communication Symposium*, Bethesda, MD.

Hanley-Dunn, P., & McIntosh, J. (1984). Meaningfulness and recall of names by young and old adults. *Journal of Gerontology, 39,* 583-585.

Harwood, J., & Sparks, L. (2003). Social identity and health: An intergroup communication approach to cancer. *Health Communication, 15*(2), 145-170.

Hewitt, M., Rowland, J., & Yancik, R. (2003). Cancer survivors in the United States: Age, health, and disability. *The Journals of Gerontology, Series A, 58*(1), 82-92.

Hiatt, R. A., & Rimer, B. K. (1999). A new strategy for cancer control research. *Cancer Epidemiology, Biomarkers, & Prevention, 8,* 957-964.

Horn, J. L., & Donaldson, G. (1980). Cognitive development in adulthood. In O. G. Brim, Jr. & J. Kagen (Eds.), *Constancy and change in human development* (pp. 445-529). Cambridge, MA: Harvard University Press.

Hutchinson, J., & Beasley, D. (1981). Speech and language functioning among the aging. In H. Oyer & E. Oyer (Eds.), *Aging and communication* (pp. 155-174). Baltimore, MD: University Park Press.

Jarvik, L., & Bank, L. (1983). Aging twins: Longitudinal psychometric data. In K. Schaie (Ed.), *Longitudinal studies of adult psychological development* (pp. 40-63). New York: Guilford.

Kahneman, D., & Tversky, A. (1979). "Prospect theory": An analysis of decision under risk. *Econometrica, 47,* 263-291.

Kleemeier, R. (1962). Intellectual changes in the senium. *Proceedings of the Social Statistics Section of the American Statistics Association, 1,* 290-295.

Kline, D. W., & Scialfa, C. T. (1996). Visual and auditory aging. In J. E. Birren & K. W. Schaie (Eds.), *Handbook of the psychology of aging* (4th ed., pp. 181-203). San Diego, CA: Academic Press.

Kreps, G. L. (1988). Relational communication in health care. *Southern Speech Communication Journal, 53,* 344-359.

Kreps, G. L. (2003). Impact of communication on cancer risk, incidence, morbidity, and quality of life [Special Issue]. *Health Communication, 15*(2), 163-170.

Kreps, G. L., & Chapelsky Massimilla, D. (2002). Cancer communications research and health outcomes: Review and challenge. *Communication Studies, 54*(4), 318-336.

Kreps, G. L., & Viswanath, K. (2001). Communication interventions and cancer control: A review of the National Cancer Institute's health communication intervention research initiative. *Family and Community Health, 24*(3), ix-xiv.

Kundrat, A., & Nussbaum, J. F. (2003). The impact of invisible illness on identity and contextual age across the life span. *Health Communication, 15*(3), 331-347.

Lapinski, M. K., & Levine, T. R. (2000). Culture and manipulation theory: The effects of self-construal and locus of benefit on information manipulation. *Communication Studies, 51*(1), 55-73.

Lewis, J., Ng, K., Hung, K. E., Bilker, W. B., Berlin, J. A., Brensinger, C., & Rustgi, A. K. (2003). Detection of proximal adenomatous polyps with screening sigmoidoscopy: A systematic review and meta-analysis of screening colonoscopy. *Archives of Internal Medicine, 163*(4), 413-421.

Li, S.-C. (2002). Connecting the many levels and facets of cognitive aging. *Trends in Cognitive Neuroscience, 11,* 38-43.

Li, S.-C., & Lindenberger, U. (1999). Cross-level unification: A computational exploration of the link between deterioration of neurotransmitter systems and differentiation of cognitive abilities in old age. In L.-G. Nilsson & H. Markowitsch (Eds.), *Cognitive neuroscience and memory* (pp. 103-146). Toronto, Ontario, Canada: Hogrefe & Huber.

MacKay, D. G., & Abrams, L. (1996). Language, memory, and aging: Distributed deficits and the structure of new-versus-old connections. In J. E. Birren & K. W. Schaie (Eds.), *Handbook of the psychology of aging* (4th ed., pp. 251-265). San Diego, CA: Academic Press.

Maibach, E. W., Kreps, G. L., & Bonaguro, E. W. (1996). Developing strategic communication campaigns for HIV/AIDS prevention. In S. Ratzan (Ed.), *AIDS: Effective communication for the 90s* (pp. 15-35). Washington, DC: Taylor & Francis.

McFarland, R. (1968). The sensory and perceptual processes in aging. In K. Schaie (Ed.), *Theory and methods in research on aging* (pp. 9-52). Morgantown: West Virginia University Press.

Meyerowitz, B. E., & Chaiken, S. (1987). The effect of message framing on breast self-examination attitudes, intentions, and behaviors. *Journal of Personality and Social Psychology, 52*(3), 500-511.

Mitchell, M. M. (2000) Motivated, but not able? The effects of positive and negative mood on persuasive message processing. *Communication Monographs, 67,* 215-225.

Mitchell, M. M., Brown, K. M., Morris Villagran, M. & Villagran, P. D. (2001). The effects of anger, sadness and happiness on persuasive message processing: A test of the negative state relief model. *Communication Monographs, 68,* 347-359.

Monge, R. (1969). Learning in adult years set or rigidity. *Human Development, 12,* 131-140.

National Center for Health Statistics. (2000). *Health, United States, 2000.* Hyattsville, MD: U.S. Department of Health and Human Services.

Nussbaum, J. F., Baringer, D., & Kundrat, A. (2003). Health, communication, and aging: Cancer and the older adult [Special Issue]. *Health Communication, 15*(2), 185-194.

Nussbaum, J. F., Pecchioni, L., Robinson, J. D., & Thompson, T. (2000). *Communication and aging* (2nd ed.). Mahwah, NJ: Erlbaum.

Nussbaum, J. F., Robinson, J. D., & Grew, D. (1983, May). *Nursing staff-resident communication within the long-term health care facility.* Paper presented at the International Communication Association, Dallas, TX.

Nussbaum, J. F., Robinson, J. D., & Grew, D. (1985). Communicative behavior of the long-term health care employee: Implications for the elderly resident. *Communication Research Reports, 2,* 16-22.

O'Hair, H. D., Villagran, M. M., Wittenberg, E., Brown, K., Ferguson, M., Hall, H. T., & Doty, T., (2003). Cancer survivorship and agency model (CSAM): Implications for patient choice, decision-making, and influence [Special Issue]. *Health Communication, 15*(2), 195-202.

Okun, M. (1976). Adult age and cautiousness in decision. *Human Development, 19,* 220-233.

Ong, L., Visser, M., Kruyver, I., Bensing, J. M., Brink-Muinen, A., Stouthard, J., Lammes, F., & de Haes, J. (1998). The Roter Interaction Analysis System (RIAS) in oncological consultations: Psychometric properties. *Psycho-oncology, 7,* 387-401.

Pecchioni, L., Ota, H., & Sparks, L. (2004). Cultural issues in communication and aging. In J. F. Nussbaum & J. Coupland (Eds.), *Handbook of communication and aging research* (pp. 167-207). Mahwah, NJ: Erlbaum.

Pecchioni, L., & Sparks, L. (2002). *Health information sources of individuals with cancer and their family members.* Paper presented to the Health Communication Division of the Eastern Communication Association, New York.

Query, J., & Wright, K. (2003). Assessing communication competence in an online study: Towards informing subsequent interventions among older adults with cancer, their lay caregivers and peers [Special Issue]. *Health Communication, 15*(2), 203-218.

Ragan, S., Wittenberg, E., & Hall, H. T. (2003). The communication of palliative care for the elderly cancer patient {Special Issue]. *Health Communication, 15*(2), 219-228.

Robinson, J. D., & Turner, J. (2003). Interpersonal and hyperpersonal social support: Cancer and the elderly adult [Special Issue]. *Health Communication, 15*(2), 229-238.

Rothman, A. J., Salovey, P., Antone, C., Keough, K., & Martin, C. D. (1993). The influence of message framing on intentions to perform health behaviors. *Journal of Experimental Social Psychology, 29*(5), 408.

Rowan, K., Sparks, L., Pecchioni, L., & Villagran, M. (2003). The CAUSE model: A research supported aid for physicians communicating about cancer risk. *Health Communication, 15*(2), 239-252.

Rubin, A. M., & Rubin, R. B. (1986). Contextual age as a life-position index. *International Journal of Aging and Human Development, 23*, 27-45.

Schaie, K. (1975). Age changes in adult intelligence. In D. Woodruff & J. Birren (Eds.), *Aging* (pp. 111-124). New York: Van Nostrand.

Schaie, K. (1983). The Seattle longitudinal study: A 21 year exploration of psychometric intelligence in adulthood. In K. Schaie (Ed.), *Longitudinal studies of adult psychological development* (pp. 64-135). New York: Guilford.

Schaie, K. (1996). Intellectual development in adulthood. In J. E. Birren & K. W. Schaie (Eds.), *Handbook of the psychology of aging* (4th ed., pp. 266-286). San Diego, CA: Academic Press.

Smith, B. (1996). Memory. In J. E. Birren & K. W. Schaie (Eds.), *Handbook of the psychology of aging* (4th ed., pp. 236-250). San Diego, CA: Academic Press.

Smith, B., Thompson, L., & Michalewski, H. (1980). Average evoked potential research in adult aging: Status and prospects. In L. Poon (Ed.), *Aging in the 1980s* (pp. 135-151). Washington, DC: American Psychological Association.

Sparks, L. (Ed.). (2003). Cancer communication and aging [Special Issue]. *Health Communication, 15*(2), 123-258.

Sparks, L. (2003). An introduction to cancer communication and aging: Theoretical and research insights. *Health Communication, 15*(2), 123-132.

Sparks, L., Pecchioni, L., & Mittapalli, K. (2003). *Health information sources of individuals diagnosed with lung cancer.* Paper presented to the Health Communication Division of the Eastern Communication Association, Washington, DC.

Sparks, L., Pecchioni, L., & Mittapalli, K. (2004). *Health information sources of family caregivers of individuals diagnosed with lung cancer.* Paper submitted to the Health Communication Division of the Eastern Communication Association, Hartford, CT.

Takeda, S., & Matsuzawa, T. (1985). Age-related brain atrophy: A study with computer tomography. *Journal of Gerontology, 40*, 159-163.

Turner, J. W., Grube, J., & Meyers, J. (2001). Developing an optimal match within online communities: An exploration of CMC support communities & traditional support. *Journal of Communication, 51*(2), 231-251.

Verbrugge, L. (1984). A health profile of older women with comparisons to older men. *Research on Aging, 6*, 291-322.

Villaume, W. A., Brown, M. H., & Darling, R. (1994). Presbycusis, communication, and older adults. In M. L. Hummert, J. M. Wiemann, & J. F. Nussbaum (Eds.), *Interpersonal communication in older adulthood: Interdisciplinary theory and research* (pp. 83-106). Thousand Oaks, CA: Sage.

Walther, J. B., & Boyd, S. (2002). Attraction to computer-mediated social support. In C.A. Lin & D. Atkin (Eds.), *Communication technology and society: Audience adoption and uses of the new media.* Cresskill, NJ: Hampton Press.

Wellman, B., & Gulia, M. (1999). Net surfers don't ride alone: Virtual communities as communities. In M. A. Smith & P. Kollock (Eds.), *Communities in cyberspace* (pp. 167-194). London: Routledge.

Willeford, J. A. (1971). The geriatric patient. In D. Rose (Ed.), *Audiological assessment* (pp. 281-319). Englewood Cliffs, NJ: Prentice-Hall.

Willis, S. L. (1996). Everyday problem solving. In J. E. Birren & K. W. Schaie (Eds.), *Handbook of the psychology of aging* (4th ed., pp. 287-307). San Diego, CA: Academic Press.

Wohlwill, J. F. (1970). The age variable in psychological research. *Psychological Review, 77,* 49-64.

15 | Consumer-Provider Communication Research With Special Populations

Amelie G. Ramirez
Baylor College of Medicine

The bond between consumer and provider is one of the strongest that exists in health care. Cancer treatment and prevention is incomplete without this component, and every effort should be made to ensure consumer–provider research is representative of all consumers and providers in the United States. If doctors and nurses involved in cancer care are to help patients and their families achieve an optimal level of quality of life and psychological adjustment, they must be able to carry out key communication tasks successfully (Maguire, 2000).

As the population of the United States becomes increasingly diverse, understanding consumer–provider communication among distinct consumer groups becomes of paramount importance. The National Cancer Institute's Special Populations Networks initiative has identified people of African-American, Appalachian, Asian and Pacific Islander, Hispanic/Latino, and Native American descent or origin as special populations (National Cancer Institute, 2004). Adding to the complexity, diverse subgroups exist within these broad classifications. Appalachians are defined as individuals and their descendants who originated in parts of 12 states surrounding the Appalachian Mountain chain (Dillard, 1983). Approximately 7.3% of the residents of the Appalachian region are of African-American descent (Williams, 1985). Asian and Pacific Islander Americans encompass more than 30 distinct cultural and linguistic groups (Tanjasiri et al., 1995). Hispanic/Latinos are defined as people of Mexican, Puerto Rican, Cuban, or other Spanish/Hispanic/Latino descent (US Census Bureau, 2004). The Native American population is comprised of 560 federally recognized tribes, each with its own unique political, social, cultural, and spiritual aspects (Burhansstipanov & Dresser, 1993). Each of the special populations and their subgroups have unique cancer care and prevention needs that can be met, at least in part, through more effective consumer–provider communication.

Special populations suffer from a disproportionate cancer burden, often experiencing higher morbidity and mortality rates than the general population (American Cancer Society, 1997; Ramirez et al., 2000a; Ries et al., 2000; Wadman, 1999). Special populations also suffer unequally from specific cancers, such as prostate and breast cancers among African-Americans, lung cancer among Appalachians, stomach and liver cancers among Asian Americans, and cervical cancer among Hispanic/Latinos (American Cancer Society, 1997; Ramirez et al., 2000a; Ries et al., 2000; Wadman, 1999). This burden of cancer illustrates a clear need for consumer–provider communication research to improve cancer prevention and detection among these groups.

Access to quality health care is a central issue among these populations, and cultural competence is a key component in increasing access to care and improving consumer–provider communication. Cultural competence requires the provision of services, education, and training in the language and cultural context that is most appropriate for the individuals for whom the services are intended, including the provision of bilingual services, if necessary (Brach & Fraser, 2000). Within cancer care, cultural competence is a way of increasing access to quality care for all patients by overcoming linguistic barriers and addressing the patient's cultural background, beliefs, and values in the way that cancer treatment and prevention is delivered. Cultural competence is also important to cancer prevention, research, and training.

Health professionals have a responsibility to promote cultural competence and ensure access to quality cancer care to all health care consumers. In the special populations, the diminution of cultural and linguistic barriers can serve to improve communication between consumers and providers. To this end, consumer–provider communication research is required to understand the cancer treatment and prevention communication needs of special populations, identify and overcome the barriers to consumer–provider communication, and direct effective interventions to improve consumer–provider communication for special populations.

A significant number of consumer–provider communications studies have been conducted; however, research specific to special populations is lacking. Although sparse, the majority of consumer–provider communication research in special populations has primarily included African-Americans and Hispanic/Latinos, presumably because these are the largest minority groups and account for nearly 25% of the U.S. population.

BARRIERS TO EFFECTIVE SPECIAL POPULATION CONSUMER–PROVIDER COMMUNICATION

Ethnic/Racial Barriers

The association between patients and physicians of the same ethnicity is referred to as racial concordance (Cooper-Patrick et al., 1999; Saha et al., 1999). This is somewhat misleading because Hispanic/Latinos belong to several races; however, they are often classified as one group or race for the purpose of research. Interestingly, minority patients have been found to be five times as likely as Whites to report that their regular physician is of an ethnic/racial minority (Gray & Stoddard, 1997). Whites are more likely to have a racially concordant physician, due to a greater number of White than non-White physicians, and nonconcordant physicians for Blacks and Hispanic/Latinos are primarily White and Asian (Saha et al., 1999).

Patients from special populations seem to prefer physicians of the same ethnicity/race (Cooper-Patrick et al., 1999; Saha et al., 1999). African-American and Hispanic/Latino patients have been found to be more likely than White patients to see African-American and Hispanic/Latino physicians, respectively (Cooper-Patrick et al., 1999; Gray & Stoddard, 1997). Hispanic/Latino patients are more likely than African-American patients to have a provider of the same race/ethnic group (Gray & Stoddard, 1997).

Racial concordance has been found to be positively associated with patient satisfaction (Cooper-Patrick et al., 1999). African-Americans and Hispanic/Latinos are more satisfied with the care they receive from racially concordant physicians than from physicians of other races (Saha et al., 1999). African-Americans receiving care from Black physicians are more likely to report preventive and necessary medical care and to perceive being treated with respect than other African-Americans (Saha et al., 1999). Factors associated with Hispanic/Latino patient satisfaction are reassurance and support offered by the physician and staff, and the perceived quality of examinations (Morales et al., 2000). Hispanic/Latinos are more satisfied with their health care when the physician and office staff provide a more culturally and linguistically Hispanic setting (Saha et al., 1999).

Few publications exist with regard to consumer–provider communication and Appalachian, Asian/Pacific Islander, or Native American patients. Interestingly, studies that have attempted to include Asians and Native Americans have later excluded these populations because of an inability to recruit a representative sample (Saha et al., 1999). Additionally, there is some ambiguity as to whether the ethnic/racial barrier stands alone or reflects the cultural and linguistic barriers that underlie race.

Cultural Barriers

A prevalent barrier to cultural competence in communication among providers is lack of knowledge of cultural values and practices of patients. Understanding these practices will better equip health professionals to communicate with their special population patients with regard to treatment decisions. For example, African-Americans and Appalachians who migrated from the south share similar cultural values related to the importance of kinship networks, Bible-oriented religious beliefs, and preferences for informal social services (Helton, 1995). Appalachians are more amicable to open-ended questions when obtaining health information and eliciting opinions and beliefs about health care practices (Purnell, 1999). Family is an important element in Appalachian life, and both immediate and extended family members are likely to be consulted about important health decisions (Purnell, 1999). For cancer education and treatment to be effective, support must begin with the family, and providers should consider the entire family, rather than the individual, as the basic treatment unit (Purnell, 1999).

In Appalachian culture, folk medicine is viewed as a natural process rather than an "alternative" to mainstream health care (Helton, 1996). Appalachian mountain people are more likely to try folk remedies that have been passed down from generation to generation before they seek a health professional (Helton, 1995, 1996). Also, the high cost of medical care and the relative isolation of mountain people often render modern health technology inaccessible (Helton, 1996). Furthermore, there is an initial distrust of strangers rooted in the history of outsiders who took over the land for timbering and coal mining (Helton, 1995). Physicians new to the area would, therefore, be wise to gain the trust of patients slowly.

Asian cultures also have strong cultural influences, such as the widely held belief that any procedure that cuts flesh disrupts harmony (McLaughlin & Braun, 1998). Because surgery is a common treatment option for many cancer patients, providers should understand the cultural root of the decision to refuse surgery. Also common is filial piety, or the obligation to take care of family members (McLaughlin & Braun, 1998). Children must ensure that parents are well cared for in old age, and family members feel great shame if they cannot adequately meet this responsibility (McLaughlin & Braun, 1998). This is important to consider when discussing the options of home health care, hospice, or nursing home placement for cancer patients. Owing to filial piety, a traditional Asian family may wait until a situation is extremely difficult before seeking assistance and placement, or refuse help altogether (McLaughlin & Braun, 1998). Yet another cultural element for health providers to consider is the often stoic and reserved nature of Asian Americans. Asians are less inclined to question decisions made by health care professionals and more likely to endure hardship and pain, and keep their wishes silent if they believe their true desires would inconvenience or disturb others (Saldov et al., 1997). Clearly, such behavior has a direct impact on consumer–provider communication.

Many Hispanic/Latinos believe that suffering is part of life, a burden to endure to enter heaven (Juarez et al., 1998a). Enduring pain is also seen as a reflection of personal strength and pride, and as part of the *machismo* mentality for Hispanic/Latino men (Juarez et al., 1998a; Savitz, 2001). Hispanic/Latinos hold strong cultural beliefs about cancer, including the common belief that "cancer is a punishment from God" (Shankar & Figueroa-Valles, 1999). Many Mexican Americans and Puerto Ricans believe cancer is not curable and perceive a greater risk of the disease than Cubans and Central Americans (Ramirez et al., 2000b). Because of lifestyle, tradition, and culture, cancer misconceptions among Hispanic/Latinos seem to perpetuate through generations (Savitz, 2001). Health professionals should seek current information about Hispanic/Latinos in order to tailor consumer–provider communications (Ramirez et al., 2000a). To improve compliance with cancer care in Hispanic/Latinos, providers should try to incorporate the patient's folk practices and beliefs into the plan of care, involve family in the patient's care, and ensure that instructions for medications are available in Spanish (Juarez et al., 1998b).

When working with Native American patients, it is important for health care providers to keep an open mind about folk medicine and prevalent cancer beliefs. Historically, Native Americans were widely considered to be immune to cancer, to have some natural protection from it, or both (Burhansstipanov, 1998). Additionally, providers should be aware of common cultural perceptions of cancer that can delay prevention and timely treatment. These beliefs include the following: cancer is a (a) "a white man's disease," (b) punishment for one's actions, (c) a natural part of one's path and lessons to learn, (d) a curse from someone or result of a personal violation of tribal mores, and (e) a contagious disease (Burhansstipanov, 1998). Providers should also consider the important role of spirituality; most Native Americans participate in traditional and spiritual healing as a supplement to their biomedical care (Burhansstipanov, 1998).

Quality of life (QOL) is an essential issue for health professionals working with cancer patients. QOL is defined as "an individual's perception of their position in life in the context of the culture and value systems in which they live and in relation to their goals, expectations, standards, and concerns" (World Health Organization, 1993). Culture, as a component of QOL, remains a neglected area of research (Juarez et al., 1998b). For example, the perceptions of QOL of Hispanic/Latino patients with cancer are embedded in culturally based values of family life, acceptance of God's will, and religious beliefs (Juarez et al., 1998b).

Among cancer patients, pain can have a significant impact on QOL. Because the disease may be more advanced at diagnosis and mortality rates are higher among minorities and those with low socioeconomic status, greater proportions of these population groups are likely to be suffering from pain (Ramer et al., 1999). Expressions of pain on the part of the patient may be well understood by those within the same culture but not by those outside the culture (Ramer et al., 1999). This may help explain why minorities seek racially concordant physicians.

Significant differences among African-Americans, Hispanic/Latinos, Asians and Pacific Islanders, and Whites have been found with regard to consumer–provider communication about pain (Juarez et al., 1998a). Asians report the most amount of pain, followed by Hispanic/Latinos, African-Americans, and Whites (Ramer et al., 1999). Asians are also the least likely to have been told that treatment of pain is very important, followed by Hispanic/Latinos, African-Americans, and Whites (Ramer et al., 1999). Health providers are often accustomed to giving the same doses of pain medication and may fail to consider differences in pain perception among people of different ethnicities and cultures. This in turn may lead to inadequate pain management for cancer patients within special populations, indicating a continued need for cultural considerations in health provider education. To increase understanding of how culture and ethnicity influence pain perception, pain research should include cancer patients from special populations. Also, more research with special population consumers and providers is needed to identify ways to improve communication about cancer pain and pain management.

Linguistic Barriers

Language barriers, which are frequently encountered in communication with Hispanic/Latino and Asian patients, negatively impact access to quality cancer care. For example, in a qualitative study on pain, the most common reason cited for noncompliance with pharmacological treatment was an inability to understand instructions (Juarez et al., 1998a). A Hispanic/Latino breast cancer survivors study also reported the language barrier as a significant deterrent to seeking care, because inability to adequately communicate leads to fear and despair.

Language is an extremely important aspect of culture. Even for bilingual Hispanic/Latino patients, communication in Spanish adds a strong feeling of trust (Savitz, 2001). Also, because effective communication includes nonverbal means, such as voice tone or eye contact, Spanish-speaking patients in cross-language encounters may not develop the same level of rapport with their physician as other patients and may hesitate to disclose personal concerns or feelings (Buck, 1984). This may also apply to many Asian American patients who have not mastered the English language.

In a patient-centered encounter, the physician seeks to understand the patient's symptoms and facilitate the patient's expression of thoughts, feelings, and expectations (Henbest &

Stewart, 1989). Spanish-speaking patients report significantly fewer symptoms than English-speaking patients, yet physicians exhibit more patient-centredness toward English-speaking Hispanic/Latinos and are more likely to ignore comments from Spanish-speaking patients (Rivadeneyra et al., 2000). No difference in patient-centredness between the English-speaking Hispanic/Latinos and other English-speaking patients has been found, suggesting that language rather than dissimilar ethnic backgrounds precipitates differential participatory interactions (Rivadeneyra et al., 2000).

Health professionals who work in areas where a language barrier exists can encounter distressing, insensitive, and sometimes dangerous situations. For example, although an interpreter may be able to convey a cancer diagnosis to a non-English-speaking patient, when the provider cannot express such sensitive information or extend compassion or concern through his or her own words, the bond between patient and provider so essential to communication is hampered. Linguistic competence should be emphasized, especially in areas with many special population patients, as a basic element for improving communication.

INADEQUATE INFORMATION PROVIDED TO THE PATIENT

Many professionals have questioned the degree of information that should be conveyed to patients. Moreover, some theorists believe the degree of information that a patient should receive is dependent on culture. For example, providers sometimes tend not to refer to "cancer" in the presence of their terminal Hispanic/Latino patients because of a strong belief by many Latinos that if the patient knows he or she is dying, it will occur sooner (Juarez et al., 1998b).

Research to determine the extent to which patients should be informed has reported that the vast majority of Asian Americans wish to know the diagnosis even if it is poor, and do not agree with the practice of withholding the diagnosis from the patient (Fielding & Hung, 1996). This is in contrast to Taiwanese culture, in which the first person to be notified of a cancer diagnosis is often not the patient, but the head of the family (Tai & Lin, 2001). Many traditional Chinese people feel that it is bad luck to talk about illness or death because it may cause it to happen (McLaughlin & Braun, 1998). Other reasons for withholding a diagnosis are that the family may not want the patient to become dispirited and give up hope or that it is disrespectful to speak of such things to an elder (McLaughlin & Braun, 1998). Health professionals should make every effort to consider these elements of Asian culture when communicating a poor prognosis.

CANCER PREVENTION

Primary Cancer Prevention

Cultural competence in the consumer–provider relationship is vital for improving patient cancer prevention education. Lack of knowledge about cancer causes and risk factors, and lack of awareness about cancer screening are well documented for African-Americans

(Lipkus et al., 1999), Appalachians (Sortet & Banks, 1997), Asian Americans (Facione et al., 2000; Sadler et al., 2001), Hispanic/Latinos (Ramirez et al., 2000b), and Native Americans (Burhansstipanov, 2002). Communication regarding primary prevention, which includes care that minimizes risk factors and incidence of the disease (Fauci et al., 1998), is lacking between providers and their special population patients (Dubé et al., 2000). Improving consumer–provider communications can increase effective patient education and anticipatory guidance based on lifestyle choices, and help reduce risks, exposures, and illnesses in patients (Dubé et al., 2000).

Secondary Cancer Prevention

Efforts to reduce the burden of cancer among special populations have focused largely on early detection and treatment (Gilliland et al., 2000). Studies have clearly cited that minorities do not use cancer screening tests as frequently or as early as Whites and that this may contribute to high cancer morbidity and mortality among special populations (Boyer-Chammard, 1999; Gilliland et al., 2000; Ramirez & Suarez, 2001). In fact, medical research has found that Black and Hispanic/Latino women develop advanced breast cancer at a younger age than Whites, and need screening tests performed earlier (Boyer-Chammard et al., 1999). Special populations would also benefit from early detection strategies available for other cancers. Also, research suggests that participation in cancer screening services by special population patients increases their chances of being retained in the medical system (Gilliland et al, 2000). Therefore, a future focus should be on recruiting special population participants into cancer screening through consumer–provider relationships.

Health providers have the ability to promote cancer prevention in special populations by conveying its significance to their patients. Working in conjunction with patients and providers to strengthen the communication skills necessary to promote cancer prevention will help reduce the disproportionate rates with which disease affects special populations. Patient education is a valuable element of consumer–provider communication, and information provided to special population patients should be presented in a culturally competent manner. To ensure this, more research on communication models for patient education for special populations at the health provider level is needed.

RECOMMENDATIONS TO IMPROVE CONSUMER–PROVIDER COMMUNICATION

Training

Enhancing the ability of health care professionals to communicate both linguistically and culturally with people of special populations is a key component for improving minority cancer care and prevention. This can be accomplished by establishing arenas to improve cultural competency of health care providers.

It is encouraging that efforts to improve physician communication in cancer care have proven successful. For example, interactive training workshops for attending oncologists and fellows to improve communication skills have been shown to increase the participants' confidence in a number of communication areas as well as in managing physician burnout (Baile et al., 1997). Clearly, cultural competency training must be extended to medical students by including it in the curriculum. This is especially important in those regions with heavy concentrations of special populations. Interactive workshops could be introduced to medical students prior to clinical rotations and course refreshers presented throughout residency and fellowship training. Similar tracks for other health professional training also could be useful.

Culturally competent communication with patients also requires that the communication be available in a language that patients can understand. At a minimum, the availability of trained medical translators for non-English-speaking patients is imperative. However, to achieve the goal of strengthening the patient–provider bond, health professionals in special populations regions should be encouraged to learn the language of their patients. This could be promoted by providing continuing education credit for language-related courses.

Additionally, lack of diversity in health care leadership and workforce has been cited as a potential barrier to care (Betancourt et al., 2002). Therefore, a direct way of promoting culturally competent care is to increase the availability of health professionals who are members of special populations groups. To achieve this, the medical education community must support and expand programs that encourage and fund students of special populations to enter the health professions. This will help ensure that providers in areas that serve special populations have, as an adequate proportion of their staff, individuals who can communicate both culturally and linguistically with the consumers they serve.

Research

As previously noted, special populations in consumer–provider research are under-represented. One reason is poor recruitment of minority study participants (Bowen et al., 2000; Saha et al., 1999). Researchers need to be educated about the related sociocultural and linguistic barriers to minority recruitment and encouraged to include special populations in their samples (Bowen et al., 2000). Consequently, research funding for investigators who wish to study consumer–provider communication with special populations should be made available. Also, investigators already working with special populations and who have the expertise in recruiting these participants should be encouraged to explore consumer–provider communication.

Misclassification of ethnicities by physicians and other health care professionals through inaccurate data collection is another concern. To avoid misrepresentation of values, behaviors, and perspectives of specific groups, ethnic classifications are vital to research statistics (Stewart et al., 1999). Despite efforts to improve disease surveillance in the past decade, major gaps exist in current health and cancer data collection and analysis, as has been found for Hispanic/Latinos (Ramirez et al., 1999). The need for accuracy and timeliness in cancer data collection is underscored by the high growth rate of Hispanic/Latino and other special populations (Ramirez et al., 1999).

More research is needed in all areas of consumer–provider communication, with particular emphasis on special populations. We need to explore how racially concordant or discordant consumer–provider relationships affect the quality of consumer–provider communications, consumer satisfaction, and the overall quality of cancer care for special population patients. Additionally, very little is known about the level of participatory interaction preferred by special population patients and how this affects quality of life in cancer care or minority participation in cancer prevention. Because language is a significant barrier for consumer–provider communication with special populations, and translators are often used to overcome this barrier, more needs to be known about how the use of a translator affects the consumer–provider bond, the quality of the medical information received, and the overall quality of cancer care received by non-English-speaking patients. Furthermore, research should focus on identifying and overcoming cultural factors that directly or indirectly influence the quality of consumer–provider communication. For example, given the importance of familial support in the special populations, how does the family influence consumer communication with providers? How does reliance on folk medicine impact consumer-provider relationships? What impact do cultural beliefs about cancer have on consumer–provider communication and compliance with recommended care? What models of consumer–provider communication are most effective with each special population? Additional research questions should focus on identifying existing provider biases and misconceptions about minority patients and how these views of special population patients affect provider communication processes and the resulting quality of care. Overall, although more is known about the Hispanic/Latino and African populations, the amount of research remains inadequate to address consumer–provider communication and, therefore, all special population groups can benefit from further study.

Another troubling factor is the lack of inclusion of recent immigrants in consumer–provider studies. Health care professionals should be aware of the needs and values of this segment of the population. Evaluation of the differences and similarities between the already established groups in the United States and new immigrants is needed. For example, what effects might documented residency status and lack of insurance have on consumer–provider communication? How does acculturation affect the quality of communication with the provider and preference for participatory care? These research questions can be extended to include subgroups of the special populations.

There is also an urgent need for studies using rigorous methods of evaluation to show that training health professionals in key communications skills produces clinically relevant changes in patients and health professionals over time (Maguire, 2000). Existing and newly developed programs should be evaluated to provide evidence that intervention programs with providers to improve their competency in dealing with patients from special populations are effective.

Finally, community leaders and representatives of each special population group need to prioritize the research needs for their population. Too often, the knowledge of the community is underestimated, but it is this very knowledge of their own culture and needs that can be utilized to provide better treatment and care for individuals in the special populations. The prioritization of consumer–provider communication research should focus on addressing the unique needs of each population based on cultural values and nuances that influence health behavior and interactions with health professionals.

As this country becomes more ethnically diverse, health care practitioners must learn about the perspectives and values of a variety of cultural groups (McLaughlin & Braun, 1998). The need to encourage research with special populations to explore consumer–provider communication cannot be overemphasized. Only through increased investigation can we discover the necessary steps for improving the relationship between consumer and provider as it impacts cancer care and prevention. Improved understanding of the special populations can enhance communication and allow health providers to effectively promote a healthier consumer lifestyle.

ACKNOWLEDGMENTS

I wish to express my thanks and appreciation to Fabiola Aparicio-Ting, MPH, Maria D. Chapa, MD, Oscar Perez, Daniel Presswood, and Sandra San Miguel-Majors, MS, in the preparation of this manuscript.

REFERENCES

American Cancer Society. (1997). Cancer Facts and Figures. Accessed August 17, 2004, from http://www.cancer.org.statistics/97cff/97racial.html.

Baile, W. F., Lenzi, R., Kudelka, A. P., Maguire, P., Novack, D., Goldstein, M., Myers, E. G., & Bast, R. C. (1997). Improving physician communication in cancer care: Outcome of a workshop for oncologists. *Journal of Cancer Education, 12*(3), 166-173.

Betancourt, J. R., Green, A. R., & Carrillo, J. E. (2002). Cultural competence in health care: Emerging frameworks and practical approaches. *The Common Wealth Fund, Field Report.* Accessed August 17, 2004, from www.cmwf.org.

Bowen, D., Raczynski, J., George, V., Feng, Z., & Fouad, M. (2000). The role of participation in the Women's Health Trial: Feasibility study in minority populations. *Preventive Medicine, 31,* 474-480.

Boyer-Chammard, A., Taylor, T. H., & Anton-Culver, H. (1999). Survival differences in breast cancer among racial/ethnic groups: A population-based study. *Cancer Detection and Prevention, 23*(6), 463-473.

Brach, C., & Fraser, I. (2000). Can cultural competency reduce racial and ethnic health disparities? A review and conceptual model. *Medical Care Research and Review; 57,* 181-217.

Buck, R. (1984). *Communication of emotion.* New York: Guilford.

Burhansstipanov, L. (1998). Cancer mortality among Native Americans. *Cancer, 83*(11), 2247-2250.

Burhansstipanov, L., Bemis, L. T., & Dignan, M. (2002). Native American recommendations for genetic research to be culturally respectful. *Jurimetrics, 42,* 149-157.

Burhansstipanov, L., & Dresser, C. M. (1993). *Native American Monograph No. 1: Documentation of the Cancer Research Needs of American Indians and Alaska Natives.* Washington DC: National Cancer Institute.

Burhansstipanov, L., & Morris, S. (1998). Breast cancer screening among American Indians and Alaskan Natives. *Federal Practitioner, 15*(1), 12-28.

Cooper-Patrick, L., Gallo, J., Gonzales, J. J., Vu, H. T., Powe, N. R., Nelson, C., & Ford, D. E. (1999). Race, gender, and partnership in the patient-physician relationship. *JAMA, 282*(6), 583-589.

Dillard, J. M. (1983). Southern Appalachian Anglo Americans. In *Multi-cultural counseling* (pp. 229-259). Chicago: Nelson-Hall.

Dubé, C. E., O'Donnell, J., & Novack, D. (2000) Communication skills for preventive interventions. *Academic Medicine, 75*(7), S45-S54.

Facione, N. C., Giancarlo, C., & Chan, L. (2000). Perceived risk and help-seeking behavior for breast cancer: A Chinese American perspective. *Cancer Nursing, 23,* 258-267.

Fauci, A. S., Braunwald, E., Isselbacher, K. J., Wilson, J. D., Martin, J. B., Kasper, D. L., Hauser, S. L., Longo, D. L., & Harrison, T. R. (1998). *Harrison's principles of internal medicine* (14th ed.). New York: McGraw-Hill.

Fielding, R., & Hung, J. (1996). Preferences for information and involvement in decisions during cancer care among a Hong Kong Chinese population. *Psycho-Oncology, 5,* 321-329.

Gilliland, F. D., Rosenberg, R. D., Hunt, W. C., Stauber, P., & Key, C. R. (2000). Patterns of mammography use in Hispanic, American Indian, and non-Hispanic White women in New Mexico, 1994-1997. *American Journal of Epidemiology, 152*(5), 432-437.

Gray, B., & Stoddard, J. J. (1997). Patient–physician pairing: Does racial and ethnic congruity influence selection of a regular physician? *Journal of Community Health, 22*(4), 247-259.

Helton, L. R. (1995). Intervention with Appalachians: Strategies for a culturally specific practice. *Journal of Cultural Diversity, 2*(1), 20-26.

Helton, L. R. (1996). Folk medicine and health beliefs: An Appalachian perspective. *Journal of Cultural Diversity, 3*(4), 123-128.

Henbest, R. J., & Stewart, M. A. (1989). Patient centredness in the consultation 1: A method for measurement. *Family Practice, 6(4),* 249-253

Juarez, G., Ferrell, B., & Borneman, T. (1998a). Influence of culture on cancer pain management in Hispanic patients. *Cancer Practice, 6(5),* 262-269.

Juarez, G., Ferrell, B., & Borneman, T. (1998b). Perceptions of life in Hispanic patients with cancer. *Cancer Practice, 6(6),* 318-324.

Kaplan, S. H., Greenfield, S., Gandek, B., Rogers, W., & Ware, J. E. (1996). Characteristics of physicians with participatory decision-making styles. *Annals of Internal Medicine, 124(5),* 497-504.

Lipkus, I. M., Iden, D., Terrenoire, J., & Feaganes, J. R. (1999). Relationships among breast cancer concern, risk perceptions, and interest in genetic testing for breast cancer susceptibility among African-American women with and without a family history of breast cancer. *Cancer Epidemiology, Biomarkers & Prevention, 8,* 533-539.

Maguire, P. (2000). Improving communication with cancer patients. *European Journal of Cancer Millennium Review, 35(14),* 2058-2065.

McLaughlin, L. A., & Braun, K. L. (1998). Asian and Pacific Islander cultural values: Considerations for health care decision making. *Health & Social Work, 23(2),* 116-127.

Moira, S. A. (1995). Effective physician–patient communication and health outcomes: A review. *Canadian Medical Association Journal, 152(9),* 1423-1433.

Morales, L. S., Reise, S. P., & Hays, R. D. (2000). Evaluating the equivalence of health care ratings by whites and Hispanics. *Medical Care, 38(5),* 517-527.

National Cancer Institute. Special Populations network. Accessed August 18, 2004, from http://crchd.nci.nih.gov/spn/ index.html.

Purnell L. (1999). Culturally competent care for traditional Appalachians. *Imprint, 46(5),* 56-59.

Ramer, L., Richardson, J. L., Cohen, M. Z., Bedney, C., Danley, K. L., & Judge, E. A. (1999). Multimeasure pain assessment in an ethnically diverse group of patients with cancer. *Journal of Transcultural Nursing, 10(2),* 94-101.

Ramirez, A. G., & Suarez, L. (2001). The impact of cancer on Latino populations. In M. Aguire-Molina, C. W. Molina, & R. E. Zambrana (Eds.), *Health issues in the Latino community* (pp. 211-244). San Francisco, CA: Jossey-Bass.

Ramirez, A. G., Suarez, L., McCalister, A., Villareal, R., Trapido, E., Talavera, A. G., Perez-Stable, E., & Marti, J. (2000a). Cervical cancer screening in regional Hispanic populations. *American Journal of Health Behavior, 24(3),* 181-192.

Ramirez, A. G., Suarez, L., Laufman, L., Barroso, C., & Chalela, P. (2000b). Hispanic women's breast and cervical cancer knowledge, attitudes, and screening behaviors. *American Journal of Health Promotion, 14(5),* 292-300.

Ramirez, A. G., Suarez, L., West, D. W., Chalela, P., & Presswood, D. T. (1999). Hispanics: Are we being counted accurately? Challenges and recommendations. *Journal of Registry Management, 26(4),* 142-148.

Ries, L. A. G., Kosary, C. L., Hankey, B. F., Miller, B. A., & Edwards, B. K. (2000). SEER cancer statistics review, 1973-1995. Bethesda, MD: NCI. Accessed August 17, 2004, from http://www.seer.ims.nci.nih.gov/publications/CSR7395.

Rivadeneyra, R., Elderkin-Thompson, V., Silver, R. C., & Waitzkin, H. (2000) Patient centredness in medical encounters requiring an interpreter. *American Journal of Medicine, 108(6),* 470-474.

Sadler, G. R., Dhanjal, S. K., Shah, N. B., Shah, R. B., Ko, C., Anghel, M., & Harshburger, R. (2001). Asian Indian women: Knowledge, attitudes, and behaviors toward breast cancer early detection. *Public Health Nursing, 18,* 357-363.

Saha, S., Komaromy, M., Koepsell, T., & Bindman, A. (1999). Patient-physician racial concordance and the perceived quality and use of health care. *Archives of Internal Medicine, 159(9),* 997-1004.

Saldov, M., Kakai, H., & McLaughlin, L. (1997). *Obtaining informed consent from traditional Japanese elders for treatment in oncology: Final report.* Honolulu: University of Hawaii, School of Social Work.

Savitz Research Solutions. (2001). *Hispanic cancer genetics trial participation.* Hispanic Cancer Genetics Trial Focus Group Project.

Shankar, S., & Figueroa-Valles, N. (1999). Cancer knowledge and misconceptions: A survey of immigrant Salvadorean women. *Ethnicity and Disease, 9(2),* 201-211.

Sortet, J., & Banks, S. (1997). Health beliefs of rural Appalachian women and the practice of breast self-examination. *Cancer Nursing, 20(4),* 231-235.

Stewart, S. L., Swallen, K. C., Glaser, S. L., Horn-Ross, P. L., & West, D. W. (1999). Comparison of methods for classifying Hispanic ethnicity in a population-based cancer registry. *American Journal of Epidemiology, 149(11),* 1063-1071.

Tanjasiri, S., Wallace, S. P., & Shibata, K. (1995). Picture imperfect: Hidden problems among Asian and Pacific Islander elderly. *Gerontologist, 35,* 752-760.

Tai, M. C., & Lin, C. S. (2001). Developing a culturally relevant bioethics for Asian people. *Journal of Medical Ethics, 27(1),* 51-55.

U.S. Census Bureau. Department of Commerce Economics and Statistics Administration. (2001). The Hispanic Population Census 2000 Brief. Washington, DC. Accessed August 18, 2004, from http://www.census.gov /prod/2000pubs.

Wadman, M. (1999). Cancer body "must do more for minorities." *Nature, 397(6717),* 283.

Williams, L. (1985) The vanishing Appalachian: How to "whiten" the problem. In W. Turner & E. Campbell (Eds.), *Blacks in Appalachia* (pp. 201-206). Lexington: University Press of Kentucky.

World Health Organization. (1993). *WHO QOL study protocol: The development of the WHO QOL Assessment Instrument.* Geneva, Switzerland: World Health Organization, Division of Mental Health.

16 Communication and Childhood Cancer

Mary E. Husain
California State University, Fresno

Scott D. Moore
California State University, Fresno

Few, if any, communication contexts carry the emotional weight of sick children, especially the chronic or potentially terminally ill, yet few populations are so understudied in the communication field (Nussbaum, Ragan, & Whaley, 2003). Its social importance and sheer complexity make it one of the more interesting dimensions of communicating with the cancer patient. This chapter tries to make sense out of disparate, complex, and sometimes contradictory bodies of literature that investigate pediatric oncology.

Creating a chapter unique to communication and childhood cancer is challenging. There is a notable absence of literature, and substantial gaps in theory. Likely this is because of both methodological challenges, not the least of which is access to the children and their families, and the emotional nature of the topic itself. By focusing our attention on unique communicative topics, we may, inadvertently, ignore tangential issues salient for future study (such as palliative care for the child). Instead, we have elected to discuss several topics we believe unique to childhood cancer, including developmental identity and emotion/cognition issues, family relational issues, and specialized communication issues. We begin our look at communication and childhood cancer by considering the child's perspective.

Authors Note: In tribute to Ana Cristina (1976-1983)

THE CHILD'S PERSPECTIVE

The diagnosis and treatment of childhood cancer is a traumatic, life-altering experience. Depending on the child's life experiences, there may be significant uncertainty as to the meaning of the increased medical activity. The social world of children who suddenly find themselves in a hospital, interacting in a world of nurses, doctors, and other medical personnel instead of friends and classmates, is dramatically changed. Children face new challenges that encroach on the construction of their social world; interacting with new people, most with whom the child will not develop a relationship. The removal from the normal social relationships has a significant impact on a child's identity and development (Sharf & Vanderford, 2003).

Not only does the child struggle to overcome a potentially fatal disease, the illness creates a biographical disruption. Chronic illness has the capacity to disturb a patient's self-image (Corbin & Strauss, 1988). This is especially true for the child with cancer, because the child's world becomes radically different. A child might not be able to go to school for extended periods of time, play with friends, or participate in activities such as team sports, which were previously enjoyed. Treatment often entails prolonged hospital visits, frequently at out-of-town treatment facilities. A significant impact on the child is not unexpected, when accounting for the malleability of a person's self-concept over time.

A person's self self-concept and identity is developed over the life-span (Nussbaum, 1989). Generally, there are structural and interactional attributes of children's social networks that enhance the development of communication skills; larger social networks typically surround a psychologically competent child (Stohl, 1989). When children are removed from established social networks, their understanding of their world and their body is questioned. The extent to which this happens is likely a function of the child's development and experience with the disease.

Childhood Age and Development

A preponderance of literature suggests that coping with catastrophic illness, like living, evolves through stages. Although stage theory (Bibace & Walsh, 1979, 1980, 1981; Piaget, 1930; Werner, 1948) has dominated the theoretical foundations of pediatric health research, others such as Eiser and colleagues (e.g., Eiser & Eiser, 1987; Eiser, Havermans, & Casas, 1993) have argued that the child's experience and knowledge of his or her disease rather than chronological age or developmental stage more accurately reflect their understanding of disease. In one study of children aged 8–17 and their parents' accounts of cancer communication, Young, Dixon-Woods, Windridge, and Heney (2003) concluded that the child's age did not predict information need. Some of the youngest children requested detailed information, the older, in contrast, wanted only general "basic" information. Indeed, the length of time a child has to understand the nuances of his or her disease is likely as important, if not more important, a marker in understanding childhood oncology as is the child's chronological age. Biological age, however, may protect a child from the emotional weight of surviving cancer. Kazak (1998) reported that parents of child leukemia survivors, who themselves likely suffer from posttraumatic stress, do not necessarily have children who suffer from similar emotional symptoms. In the study, the limited cognitive ability of young children (ages 3–4 at diagnosis), may emotionally protect them from the life-threatening nature of cancer.

Communicating with children with cancer requires specialized strategies, due to their developmental state. Whaley (1994, 2000) detailed interaction strategies for providers centered around cognitive scripts—cognitive expectations that govern the way we anticipate an interaction will progress (O'Hair, Allman, & Moore, 1996), use of topics, and sensitive vocabulary choice. Nussbaum et al. (2003) cautiously suggested the use of metaphors and figurative language when interacting with the pediatric patient. Regardless of the epistemological predisposition for viewing childhood development, communicating with the pediatric patient during diagnosis and treatment is indeed complex.

Voice of the Child in Diagnosis and Treatment

In the 1950s and 1960s, a protective approach toward disclosure with pediatric cancer patients was practiced. This approach typically divorced the child from the dialogue about diagnosis and treatment. However, there is increasing evidence that critically ill children sense both their parents' distress, and their own medical condition despite adult efforts to shelter them. Early disclosure to pediatric cancer patients and open family communication is positively associated with good psychosocial adjustment among long-term survivors (Slavin, O'Malley, Koocher, & Foster, 1982).

Today, the medical interaction with the pediatric patient is typically a triad—the child, the guardian (usually parents), and the physician. In a meta-analysis, Tates and Meeuwesen (2001) explored the state of research concerned with the child's role in the doctor–parent–child interaction. They found that the majority of studies ignored the voice of the child, a position that is antithetical toward the patient-centered trend in health communication.

A common thread running throughout the children's accounts is their reliance on parents to manage communication with health professionals. In a study of 13 families, Young et al. (2003) reported that some young people with cancer still feel marginalized in doctor–parent–patient consultations. Although children varied in their views on disclosing the diagnosis—some children wanted to receive the news at the same time as their parents, others wanted their parents to be told first, and other children did not have a strong preference. Of 19 parents, 17 preferred that the diagnosis be given to them privately, prior to the child being informed. Despite a trend toward increased participation in medical dialogues, many children retain the feeling of being "left out" of doctor–parent–patient communication.

Emotional Issues

There are conflicting reports regarding the degree and extent of psychological and social problems in childhood cancer patients (O'Malley, Koocher, Foster, & Slavin, 1979; Sanger, Copeland, & Davidson, 1999). However, most research indicates that over time, most children adapt in an emotionally healthy manner (Stuber, Kazak, Meeske, & Barakat, 1998). For example, Greenberg, Kazak, and Meadows (1989) compared the psychological adjustment of long-term survivors (5 years since diagnosis or presence of disease) of childhood cancer aged 8 to 16 years with a matched group of healthy children. Most of the survivors, except for those with severe medical late effects, were within normal limits on psychological assessments.

Younger patients have different emotional needs than older patients, including a prefer-ence for affectively positive caregiver communication (Endacott, 1998; O'Hair, Behnke, & King, 1983). It may well be that the need for increased affective support is required by the child to employ a variety of coping strategies. Fritz, Williams, and Amylon (1988) inter-viewed childhood cancer survivors to assess their psychosocial status 2 years after successful malignancy treatment. Results revealed that survivors utilized a diversity of coping styles and that the majority (except for those experiencing residual physical handicaps) were well adjust-ed. For some, an approach style worked well, for others avoidance was effective. Other research suggests that children distract themselves from the illness as a coping strategy (Kameny & Bearison, 1999).

Despite the popularly held belief that severity of the disease influences long-term adjust-ment, research suggests the opposite. Medical severity is the least predictive variable for long-term adjustment, whereas communication patterns during treatment, particularly peer sup-port, are the most predictive of positive psychosocial outcomes (Fritz et al., 1988).

Cognitive Issues

Research has shown that age-dependent developments in cognition change one's ability to effectively communicate (Nussbaum, Hummert, Williams, & Harwood, 1996). Children, like adults, process complex arrays of cognition when interacting with a caregiver. This process involves the use of certain relational knowledge about the caregiver, past memories associat-ed with care delivery, and cognitive scripts—expectations about typical medical procedures, given past experiences (O'Hair et al., 1996). Eiser, Eiser, and Lang (1989) noted that a child's script, despite being limited in experience, is relatively within accord with adults, when pro-cessing the delivery of care. Although not all children experience cognitive difficulties, fully one third of pediatric cancer patients experience a decline in psychosocial adjustment (Sanger et al., 1999).

Treatment for cancer, including the use of radiation, does have some affect on cognitive processing, and therefore communication. Carter, Thompson, and Simone (1991) noted psy-chosocial effects including school problems, particularly in the case of children receiving cra-nial radiotherapy, which can also cause a decline in intellectual performance. Fritz et al., (1988) contended that although overall, long-term psychosocial adjustment is good for child-hood cancer survivors, academic performance declines as a result of the cancer experience. When this leads to school failure, the child may experience poor self-esteem and problemat-ic peer relationships. Sanger et al. (1999) contend that school troubles may stem from absences while undergoing therapy (i.e., children are unable to catch up due to time missed). A decline in cognitive processing of the pediatric cancer patient is likely a result from treat-ments involving the central nervous system. Increased school absences are linked to increased hospital visits and treatment. Emotional repercussions result in cognitive regression that interferes with information processing.

Meadows et al. (1981) noted significant neuropsychological and IQ declines in children with acute lymphocytic leukemia as a result of therapy, and link such a decline directly to the affect of radiotherapy. Of particular concern is that children treated at younger ages (2 to 5) exhibited greater declines than those older than 6.

Peckham, Meadows, Bartel, and Marrero (1988) noted specific cognitive difficulties with "attention/concentration, memory, sequencing, and comprehension" (p. 127) in pediatric oncology patients. Although causality of the impact of treatment options on cognition is still debated, the potential communicative implications are significant. Competent communication presumes a standard level of cognition. Regression in cognitive ability may indeed impact communication, the extent to which is dependent on the type and severity of the regression.

THE FAMILIES' PERSPECTIVE

The impact of childhood cancer on the family is usually felt even before a formal diagnosis is made, when parents first begin to suspect that something is wrong with their child's health. Parents frequently report intuitively sensing something amiss with their child prior to the actual diagnosis (Dixon-Woods, Findlay, Young, Cox, & Heney, 2001; Giammona & Malek, 2002; Levi, Marsick, Drotar, & Kodish, 2000; Young, Dixon-Woods, & Heney, 2002). In their quest to discover the cause of their child's symptoms, parents often request further tests, referrals to specialists, and so forth, which marks the onset of their role as parent advocate (Dixon-Woods et al., 2001; Levi et al., 2000). A prevalent theme in parent accounts is frustration, a result of their concerns not being taken seriously by physicians, and constraint, due to a fear of being mislabeled neurotic (Arksey & Sloper, 1999; Levi et al., 2000; Sloper, 1996). Although the prediagnostic phase has been marginalized in the literature (Arksey & Sloper, 1999), it is during this time that parents' identities shift "from normal parent to parent of a child in crisis" (Dixon-Woods et al., 2001, p. 673). The process of becoming the parent of a child with cancer requires a fundamental redefinition of self. Some of the changes inherent in this process include compromised role functioning, biographical disruption, and reduced quality of life (Young, Dixon-Woods & Heney, 2002).

Young, Dixon-Woods and Heney (2002) pointed out that the parents' caregiving role increases in complexity. As parents of a child with cancer, they are required to perform a range of nursing and emotional tasks, in addition to customary parental duties. These new tasks often involve gaining their child's cooperation with treatment regimes; for example, submission to painful treatments and taking medicines. Because the consequences of noncompliance can be life-threatening, parental pressure increases tremendously, placing new constraints on their identity as a "good parent." Some parents may also experience misplaced guilt, stemming from their inability to protect their child from harm, thus reneging on a fundamental parental responsibility. These feelings may be exacerbated if, in their search for a causal explanation of their child's illness, they blame themselves for difficulties during pregnancy or environmental hazards in early childhood.

Not all changes reported by parents of childhood cancer survivors are negative. According to Van Dongen-Melman, Van Zuuren, and Verhulst (1998), some parents experience positive changes, due to a restructuring of their identity and worldview. These parents cited personal growth and an increased sense of self-reliance as a result of surviving the challenges of parenting a child with cancer. Eiser, Havermans, and Eiser (1995) reported that parents value life more as a result of their child's illness. Nevertheless, even when a child survives, the parents' lives are irreparably altered; their outlook on life will never be quite the same. They will always be the parent of a cancer "survivor" (Young, Dixon-Woods, & Heney, 2002).

Marital and Familial Stress

Not only does the cancer experience impact parents individually, the family unit as a whole is dramatically changed as a result. The postdiagnosis phase is particularly stressful for the family. Dahlquist et al. (1993) noted that in addition to the challenge of their child's illness, parents must deal with peripheral constraints on their time, finances, time together, and physical exhaustion. In their examination of parent interaction patterns approximately 8 weeks after diagnosis (N = 67 marital pairs), 25% of mothers and 28% of fathers reported marital stress. The researchers claimed that the difference between parental anxiety levels, rather than disparate coping style (approach vs. avoidant), was directly related to marital stress. If one partner perceives a high threat level and the other does not, communication difficulties result, which limit the couple's ability to work together and support each other.

Immediately after diagnosis, children with cancer and their families experience significantly high stress levels; however, research seems to support the notion that over time marital stress levels fall within normal parameters. Sawyer, Antoniou, Rice, and Baghurst (2000) reported no significant differences between the emotional distress levels of families of cancer survivors and a cohort in the general community except in the initial assessment. Subsequent annual evaluations conducted over a 4-year period did not reveal a higher incidence of psychological disturbances among families of childhood cancer survivors than in a comparison group. Stable family functioning was also evidenced by marital stability; only one family's marital status changed, and that was from single-parent to married status. Likewise, Speechley and Noh (1992) found no significant differences in depression and anxiety levels between parents of childhood cancer survivors fully 6 months after the cessation of treatment. However, subsamples of parents who experienced low levels of social support did exhibit more depression and anxiety than parents of healthy children. Results indicate that a lack of social support may place families at elevated risk for psychological distress.

Although the impact of childhood cancer extends to the entire family, research on sibling effects is in its early stages (Woodgate & Degner, 2003). Slavin et al. (1982) reported that most siblings (65.5% of 101 interviewed) feel that they should be informed about their brother or sister's diagnosis. Yet frequently, they are excluded from knowledge of the disease (Adams-Greenly, Shiminski-Maher, McGowan, & Meyers, 1986). After diagnosis, the cancer patient may receive more parental attention than other children in the family, which may permanently affect the patient's relationships with siblings (Carter et al., 1991), who may have feelings of abandonment, resentment, sadness, and guilt (Adams-Greenly et al., 1986). However, research indicates that siblings who participate in the care of their ill brother or sister have higher self-esteem, experience less isolation, and improved relationships with their parents than those who were not involved (Woodgate & Degner, 2003).

Although most parents reported stronger marriages and closer families as a result of the cancer experience (Chesler & Parry, 2001), contradictory conclusions regarding long-term negative effects on families exist in the literature. Van Dongen-Melman et al. (1998), in their evaluation of 87 families, reported detrimental marital effects after the completion of treatment (median time off treatment: 4 years and 2 months). These results were attributed to parents' false expectations regarding the cancer experience. Just because parents go through the ordeal of their child's illness together does not necessarily mean that they experience their child's illness the same way or utilize the same coping mechanisms. The consequences of these differences may be increased loneliness and marital friction.

Gendered Parenting

The experience of parenting a child with cancer exacerbates traditional gender-based parenting roles (Brown & Barbarin, 1996; Chesler & Parry, 2001; Young, Dixon-Woods & Heney, 2002). Despite increasingly greater numbers of women in the workforce, women are still socialized to view their primary role in the family as caretakers of children, whereas men's socialization emphasizes the occupational or "breadwinner" role (Brown & Barbarin, 1996; Cook, 1984; Chesler & Parry, 2001). In line with these expectations, mothers are more likely than fathers to assume most of the responsibility for managing the medical aspects of their child's illness (Brown & Barbarin, 1996; Young, Dixon-Woods, Findlay & Heney, 2002). For women, the nursing role is consistent with their prior experiences (Brown & Barbarin, 1996). Logistically, this includes staying with their children during hospitalizations and transporting them to medical appointments. Although some fathers stay with their children in the hospital, sometimes in defiance of their wives' resistance, generally, mothers take a more active role in the care of the sick child in virtually every respect.

Young, Dixon-Woods, Findlay, and Heney (2002) reported that in women, the child's cancer diagnosis generates a need to be physically close to their children in order to protect them physically and emotionally. The obligation of "proximity" impinged on their roles as wives and homemakers in the care of their other children and on their careers. Men expressed frustration over the lack of alone time with their wives, along with the added responsibilities of caring for their other children and additional household tasks during their wife's absence (Brown & Barbarin, 1996).

As a result of spending more time at the hospital and doctors' offices, women function as information brokers for their children and as the primary information liaison between the health care system and the family, a role that leaves many fathers feeling left out of the information loop (Young, Dixon-Woods, Findlay, & Heney, 2002). Because women typically have more interaction with medical staff, they tend to have greater access to medical social support networks than men (Brown & Barbarin, 1996). However, Eiser et al. (1995) pointed out that women's social interactions place them at greater risk to heightened distress through contagion; whereas the tendency of men to withdraw acts as a buffer against stress.

Despite passage of the Family Medical Leave Act, a significant problem families face is employer attitudes toward medical leave (Chesler & Parry, 2001). Although women do maintain employment during the course of a child's illness, they are vulnerable to reduced opportunities in the workplace. According to Overholser and Fritz (1990), women report more frequent career setbacks, 45% of mothers compared to 20% of fathers. Sloper (1996) reported that 50% of mothers and 37% of fathers are negatively impacted professionally. For mothers, this results in decreased employment opportunities and for fathers, stress and tiredness; a consequence of time missed from work and the challenge of trying to "catch up" or not being allowed to take adequate time off. Companies are less likely to accommodate fathers' needs during a child's illness (Chesler & Parry, 2001; Cook, 1984). Typically "lip service" is given to fathers in lieu of specific benefits. For example, Cook (1984) cited a case in which a father was formally given permission for time off but later reprimanded for not completing a task. Although two-income families are the normative, fathers continue to face far greater social pressure and financial obligations as the principal "provider" (Chesler & Parry, 2001).

The Impact of Family Coping on the Child

The child and the family's ability to adjust to living with cancer can significantly affect treatment outcomes (Giammona & Malek, 2002) because the child's resiliency or coping capacity hinges on parental support (Koocher, 1986). Sanger et al. (1999) noted a direct relationship between the child's adjustment and parental coping. Parents's attempts to maintain "family integration, cooperation, and an optimistic definition of the illness" are positively associated with a child's adjustment (p. 472).

Varni, Katz, Colegrove, and Dolgin (1996) evaluated predictive effects of family functioning on newly diagnosed pediatric cancer patients' psychosocial adjustment over time: 1, 6, and 9 months postdiagnosis. Family cohesion and expressiveness typically emerge as significant predictors of the child's adjustment; thus a family environment characterized by support, commitment, and open expression of feelings facilitates the child's adjustment to the cancer diagnosis and treatment. In a comparison of the incidence of posttraumatic stress disorder (PTSD) among children currently on treatment with those who had already completed therapeutic regimes, Butler, Rizzi, and Handwerger (1996) reported that being on treatment or in the preparatory phase of bone marrow transplantation and not having received cranial irradiation are the only significant variables associated with PTSD in the child. Although the incidence of PTSD in the off-treatment group was not greater than in the general community, decreased family cohesiveness was measured. It is speculated that sufficient emotional support over the course of trauma inoculates children.

In a similar study by Kazak (1998), researchers compare anxiety and posttraumatic stress symptoms in childhood leukemia survivors. Posttreatment children (mean time off treatment = 5.79 years) aged 8 to 19 did not exhibit significantly higher symptoms of stress, but their parents did. Among mothers of cancer survivors, 10.2% were in the severe range, compared with 2.8% of mothers of healthy children and 30% fell in the moderate range compared to 19.6% of the comparison group mothers. Although 9.8% of fathers of former leukemia patients fell in the severe range, no fathers of healthy children were in this category and 21.4% were in the moderate range compared with 13% of the comparison group. Some of the symptoms parents reported included intrusion of memories and resurfacing of fears in response to everyday childhood illnesses such as colds. Although parental functioning is not significantly impeded, the effects of parental distress on future family functioning are likely. Similarly, Overholser and Fritz (1990) reported an association between parental coping on both the parents' and the child's long-term adjustment. Families that experience prolonged elevated stress levels may adopt specific coping styles that detrimentally affect positive family communication.

SPECIAL COMMUNICATIVE CIRCUMSTANCES OF CHILDHOOD CANCER

Information Needs of the Parent and Child

Information gathering is a primary function of both the child and the parent (Thompson & Parrott, 2002). As mentioned earlier, the need for information regarding the child's illness may be constrained for both the child and their parents for a variety of factors, such as the child's degree of experience with the disease and the exacerbation of traditional gender-based parenting roles. Nevertheless, the significance of information needs among families of children with cancer cannot be overstated. In Barnhart et al.'s (1994) study, all of the parents surveyed ($N = 77$) expressed a need for information, especially concerning their child's illness. Ljungman et al.'s (2003) interviews with 56 families conclude that parents and adolescents consistently rank the need for information as their most pressing concern, closely followed by the need for social support and self-management therapy.

As mentioned earlier in this chapter, the role of parental advocate which frequently begins during the prediagnostic phase is marked by a quest for information as parents seek an explanation for their child's symptoms. This period in the illness trajectory can be especially problematic. A common theme that emerged in Sloper's (1996) research was the marginalization of parents' special knowledge of their child by health professionals, resulting in diagnostic delays and parental fears that the disease had progressed as a result. Arksey and Sloper (1999) reported similar results among 57% of families ($N = 98$). Parents stated that their doctor told them they were "'neurotic,' 'over-anxious,' or over-reacting'" (p. 490). They attributed diagnostic delays to the discounting of their views by physicians, in addition to system delays. Eiser et al. (1995) reported incidences of parents blaming the family doctor, usually for failing to respond quickly enough to their children's first symptoms of the disease. Especially for fathers, the tendency to blame medical personnel triggered a withdrawal from interaction, which reduced their willingness to utilize medical staff as sources of support and information.

During the diagnostic phase, the initial shock of devastating news may lessen parents' ability to process information due to retention difficulties (Barnhart et al., 1994). Eiser, Parkyn, Havermans, and McNinch (1994) reported that parents' recall of events leading up to the diagnosis is generally good, including symptomatic detail. In contrast, parents experience greater difficulty remembering the actual diagnosis. Apparently, shock impairs one's ability to assimilate the "bad news" (Eiser et al., 1994).

The need for information continues to be extremely important after diagnosis (Barnhart et al., 1994). Parents assume an executive-like role in the management of information (Young et al., 2003). Not only does information gathering contribute to the reduction of uncertainty, it helps parents regain a sense of control, fosters their self-esteem, and contributes to the reduction of negative feelings (i.e., anxiety and fear) they may experience (Van Dongen-Melman, Pruyn, Van Zanen, & Sanders-Woudstra, 1986).

However, information seeking is not limited to parents. Children with cancer also engage in this behavior in order to reduce their uncertainty. Children and their parents utilize both formal and informal sources in their quest for understanding (Levi et al., 2000; Van Dongen-Melman et al., 1986). Ljungman et al. (2003) reported that adolescent cancer patients and their parents prefer written communication if face-to-face contact with health professionals is limited. Although people generally prefer formal sources of information such as doctors, medical personnel, print material, or television programs, when these sources prove inadequate or unavailable, they rely on informal sources; comparing their experience with other parents whose children have had cancer (Van Dongen-Melman et al., 1986). By providing a model, social comparisons are particularly useful for parents struggling with personal issues such as depression. Children also turn to informal sources, especially when they are excluded from the diagnosis. The exclusion of children during the initial diagnostic phase is not unusual. One recent study noted that only 2 out of 13 families received the diagnosis together with their child (Young et al., 2003).

In addition to content, the manner in which information is communicated is extremely important to parents, because coping with a life-threatening illness, along with complex medical terminology and protocols, can be overwhelming, even for highly educated people (Albrecht & Goldsmith, 2003). In Levi et al.'s (2000) study, 27.3% of parents experienced distress as a result of the abrupt delivery of their child's diagnosis, 22.7% felt that their privacy had been violated, and 18.2% claimed that physicians were insensitive to the devastating impact of the diagnosis. Some parents also reported confusion owing to the use of medical jargon by their child's treatment team. In contrast to the prediagnostic phase, Sloper (1996) found that in postdiagnosis 83% of the parents were satisfied with the amount of information they received, 92% felt the information was comprehensible, and the majority, 69% did not want additional information. However, emotional distress (typically measured by the Malaise Inventory) is higher for parents who report that they do not understand the information they received.

Clear and comprehensive information concerning the disease and treatment helps parents make sense of the diagnosis (Sloper, 1996). Reardon and Buck (1989) stressed the importance of information for cancer patients, stating that knowledge of the disease is critical in the construction of coping rules and that the absence of accurate information may result in false and damaging attributions. However, more research is needed concerning the type of information families need. For example, Eiser et al.'s (1994) study challenged assumptions regarding parents' response to "bad news." Even in cases of poor prognosis, parents, particularly fathers, found statistical information encouraging. The researchers claimed that figures may provide a reason for optimism, altering parents' prior conceptions of hopelessness.

Physicians also need to recognize the importance of disclosing diagnostic and treatment information in a manner that will allow parents to risk asking questions without losing face (Sloper, 1996). In a study of 26 parents, 46% reported informational needs they were hesitant to discuss with their child's treatment team (Wells et al., 1990). Therefore, in order to improve parent–physician communication, particularly in the case of chronic or potentially life-threatening diseases such as childhood cancer, the literature reveals that additional physician training in breaking bad news and meeting the ongoing informational needs of families is warranted.

Control

Control is a primary construct in our theoretical understanding of child and adolescent development (Nannis et al., 1982). Loss of control is an overarching theme associated with childhood cancer. For the child, the disease often involves intensive and painful treatments that require ongoing monitoring. Some of the potential consequences of this care include an increased dependency on parents and hospital staff, a loss of privacy, lifestyle restrictions, and parental overprotection (Van Dongen-Melman et al., 1986). In a study that examined control strategies of pediatric oncology patients ages 6 to17 ($N = 52$), Worchel, Copeland, and Barker (1987) noted that behavioral control is the best predictor of emotional adjustment, followed by decisional and cognitive control. The quality of control techniques may be more important than the utilization of multiple techniques. However, confidence in parents, which reduces the amount of control the child must exercise, emerged as a significant predictor of adjustment. Contradictory results regarding the importance of information as a control strategy also exist in the literature. Worchel et al. (1987) reported that for both children and adolescents informational control (as opposed to behavioral control) is not significant. Yet, Nannis et al.'s (1982) study of adolescent cancer patients concluded that knowledge is indeed an important control strategy.

For parents, locus of control may be predictive of long-term psychological functioning. Van Dongen-Melman et al. (1998) stated that parental attribution of control plays an important role in their adjustment. Based on interviews conducted with 85 families of children successfully treated for either leukemia or non-Hodgkin's lymphoma, they concluded that parents with either extreme internal or external control encounter greater negative psychological late effects. Heightened internal control is associated with anxiety, guilt, and depression, whereas extreme external control generates anger and resentment. Parental attribution of control also has the potential to influence parenting style. Parents who attribute their child's recovery largely to their own efforts (exhibiting a strong internal locus of control), frequently adopt an overly protective parenting style.

Control may be related to the illness trajectory. Nannis et al. (1982) stated that as perceptions of disease severity increases, parental perceptions of control declines. For adolescents, including those with a poor, possibly terminal prognosis, the ability to engage in the routine daily activities of life and make plans for the future, however fantastical, is associated with a sense of control. Although, the literature does not recommend a return to the antiquated medical model of sheltering the child from knowledge regarding their disease, research does support the need for families to maintain, as much as possible, their normal behaviors and lifestyles during the course of the child's cancer treatment.

Loss of One's Assumptive World: Bereavement Without Death

Childhood cancer challenges the family's assumptive world as family members struggle to deal with a new, unexpected reality brought on by the disease (Giammona & Malek, 2002). Initially, the shock may be overwhelming; especially because there is a societal expectation that old people get cancer, not children. In Van Dongen-Melman et al.'s (1998) study ($N = 85$ families), all but one parent of childhood cancer survivors report negative changes. These negative effects are described as either losses or a continuation of uncertainty and increased anxiety. The first category of loss concerns a change in life outlook. Parents are less optimistic about the future and experience feelings of increased vulnerability. In addition, the illness period is described as a lost time period in their lives due to the practical demands of caring for their ailing child.

The second loss category concerns marital relationships. Although marital stress as a late effect was only reported in one marriage, relational friction during the treatment phase is common. Partners' different coping styles may constrain relational closeness during this time. Some parents deal with the loss of their image of a healthy child as a result of medical aftereffects. Even if their child recovers, minor residual disabilities serve as a permanent reminder of the cancer experience.

Another category of negative changes impacting the family is the continuation of uncertainty and anxiety owing to the fear of relapse in a child. In families whose children experience physiological and/or psychological late effects, extra caregiving demands are placed on parents. These parents tended to view their child as vulnerable and fragile. Although parents of childhood cancer survivors do not typically describe their feelings in terms of mourning, the disease triggers profound losses that inalterably change their assumptive world (Van Dongen-Melman et al., 1998) and may be quite similar to the psychological process of grief. The unique circumstances of pediatric oncology are not limited to psychological dimensions; there are profound personal and professional changes that occur with frequency.

Personal and Professional Costs

Health care costs and associated non-medical expenses are a significant concern among families facing a life-threatening illness (Overholser & Fritz, 1990). Loss of insurance or increased policy restrictions are commonly faced by pediatric cancer survivors and their families (Carter et al., 1991). Lansky et al. (1979) reported that the financial burden of cancer ranks second to the disease itself as a source of anxiety. In fully half of families surveyed ($N = 70$), monetary losses topped 25% or more of the family income. As Barnhart et al. (1994) noted, the costs of non-medical household expenses include increased child care and the need for specialized medical equipment. Financial strain among families is also related to career loss associated with having a child with cancer (Overholser & Fritz, 1990). As mentioned earlier, although mothers are impacted to a greater extent than fathers, the family unit is potentially impacted by the reduced income of both parents at a time of increased expenses.

Not only does the experience of having childhood cancer impact the parents' professional lives, but former pediatric patients may encounter obstacles acquiring health and life insurance and later employment (Carter et al., 1991; Green, 1989). In addition, their personal lives may be adversely affected. Although child/adolescent cancer survivors do not have a higher divorce rate than the general population, their long-term marital relationships may be negatively impacted by stress stemming from uncertainty regarding disease recurrence, long-term therapy complications, and the inability to have children (Green, 1989).

CONCLUSION

The health concerns of children and their unique communication issues have been marginalized in health communication research (Nussbaum et al., 2003). Despite the decline in childhood cancer mortality rates and improved prognoses in recent years (Sawyer et al., 2000; Van Dongen-Melman et al., 1998), receiving a cancer diagnosis creates a cataclysmic rift in the lives of these children and their families. Its impact on the family is monumental, resulting in far-reaching effects: physically, psychologically, and socially. Despite the profound and pervasive effects of childhood cancer, the communication literature has paid scant attention to the views and experiences of children with cancer and their families. Consequently, we have drawn primarily from research across multiple disciplines in order to present an overview of the multifaceted psychological and social communicative problems presented by childhood cancer.

Significant challenges lie ahead for future researchers if we are to unearth the complex communicative challenges faced by children with cancer, their families, and their health care providers. Existing bodies of literature are fragmented, and much of the research is either atheoretical (cf. Van Dongen-Melman et al., 1986) or lacks a unifying theory from which to study communication and pediatric oncology. There is a compelling need for broad-based studies from which generalized theories concerning health communication can be derived. Studies have frequently utilized either convenience (e.g., Pyke-Grimm, Degner, Small, & Mueller, 1999; Wells et al., 1990) or opportunistic samples (e.g., Young et al., 2003).

Researchers also face significant methodological challenges. Much of the research has been plagued by the lumping of age definitions (Butler et al., 1996; Kazak, 1998; Kameny & Bearison, 1999; Levi et al., 2000; Meadows et al., 1981; Sanger et al., 1999; Sawyer et al., 2000; Slavin et al., 1982; Young et al., 2003), an overrepresentation of Caucasian families coupled with a glaring omission of diverse ethnic groups (e.g., Barnhart et al., 1994; Cook, 1984; Dahlquist et al., 1993; Kazak, 1998; Levi et al., 2000; Woodgate & Degner, 2003; Young et al., 2003), and the exclusion of non-English-speaking subjects (e. g., Butler et al., 1996; Dahlquist et al., 1993; Kazak, 1998; Ljungman et al., 2003; Varni et al., 1996; Worchel et al., 1987). Patients from different ethnic backgrounds than the provider frequently report the medical interaction as less participative (Cooper-Patrick et al., 1999). Examination of single-parent families of children with cancer is absent from the literature. According to Brown and Barbarin (1996), "Caring for a child with cancer is likely qualitatively different and potentially more stressful for single parents" (p. 57). Research is needed that will incorporate the needs of diverse families. Finally, more longitudinal studies are necessary in order to predict and prevent long-term distress in childhood cancer survivors and their parents (Stuber et al., 1998), along with research based on observable versus reported behaviors (Worchel et al., 1987).

Another problematic issue in the literature is the potential misrepresentation of parental experiences due to the preponderance of female representation in the research (Chesler & Parry, 2001). For example, in Levi et al.'s (2000) study ($N = 22$), 73% of participants were mothers. This is echoed by Barnhart et al. (1994), whose survey of 77 parents showed 82% were mothers or female caregivers. Nannis et al.'s (1982) interview of 15 parents included 13 female subjects. In Sanger et al.'s (1991) study ($N = 48$ pediatric patients), each assessment was completed by one parent, 92% of whom were mothers. In Cook's (1984) research ($N = 145$ parents) on the influence of gender on parents of children with cancer, 62% of the participants were mothers. Women are the usual respondents in surveys because they are more accessible owing to the primacy of their role as caregiver—mothers are more likely to accompany their sick children to medical appointments. As a result, the father's voice is frequently underrepresented or lost in the literature. The views of fathers need to be examined in order to gain a more complete understanding of family communication when a child has cancer.

The lack of attention to triadic communication is another weakness in the research. Typically, either one or both parents function as intermediaries or advocates for their children during doctor and treatment visits (Arksey & Sloper, 1999). Because interactional dynamics in triads are fundamentally different from dyadic communication, further research is needed to illuminate the parents' role and especially the voice of the child, whose presence has generally been ignored in medical encounters (Tates & Meeuwesen, 2001). Children's accounts in cancer communication have largely been discounted (Arksey & Sloper, 1999). Most likely, incorporating children's perspectives will continue to be a problem owing to the difficulty of gaining access to the somewhat elusive populations of pediatric patients, their families, and caregivers.

Finally, more attention needs to be paid to discrete stages in the illness trajectory, especially the process of obtaining a diagnosis of childhood cancer. Although parents' expert knowledge of their child plays a pre-eminent role in arriving at a diagnosis (Arksey & Sloper, 1999), a recurrent theme in the literature is the marginalization by doctors of their special knowledge of the child. Future research should examine the long-term treatment and compliance consequences of unsatisfactory parent–physician communication during the prediagnosis phase. The implications for future parent–physician interactions have not as yet been addressed.

Understanding the communicative impact of cancer on children, families, and caregivers is a daunting task. Literature hides in a multitude of disciplines, with differing methodologies, and differing theoretical grounding. Because of the multitude of challenges, communication and pediatric oncology provides significant opportunities for communication researchers, not the least of which is integrating information and generating theory. As we continue to unravel the mysteries of communication and childhood cancer, we find more questions than answers; however, the answers are both academically and emotionally rewarding.

REFERENCES

Adams-Greenly, M., Shiminski-Maher, J., McGowan, N., & Meyers, P. A. (1986). A group program for helping siblings of children with cancer. *Journal of Psychosocial Oncology, 4*(4), 55-67.

Albrecht, T. L., & Goldsmith, D. J. (2003). Social support, social networks, and health. In T. L. Thompson, A. M. Dorsey, K. I. Miller, & R. Parrott (Eds.), *Handbook of health communication* (pp. 263-284). Mahwah, NJ: Erlbaum.

Arksey, H., & Sloper, P. (1999). Disputed diagnoses: The cases of RSI and childhood cancer. *Social Science & Medicine, 49,* 438-497.

Barnhart, L. L., Fitzpatrick, V. D., Sidell, N. L., Adams, M. J., Shields, G. S., & Gomez, S. J. (1994). Perception of family need in pediatric oncology. *Child and Adolescent Social Work Journal, 2*(2), 137-148.

Bibace, R., & Walsh, M. E. (1979). Developmental stages of children's conceptions of illness. In G. Stone, F. Cohen, & N. Adler (Eds.), *Health psychology: A handbook* (pp. 285-301). San Francisco: Jossey-Bass.

Bibace, R., & Walsh, M. E. (1980). Development of children's conceptions of illness. *Pediatrics, 66,* 912-917.

Bibace, R., & Walsh, M. E. (1981). Children's conceptions of illness. In R. Bibace & M. E. Walsh (Eds.), *Children's conceptions of health, illness, and bodily functions* (pp. 31-48). San Francisco: Jossey-Bass.

Brown, K. A., & Barbarin, O. A. (1996). Gender differences in parenting a child with cancer. *Social Work in Health Care, 22*(4), 53-71.

Butler, R. W., Rizzi, L. P., & Handwerger, B. A. (1996). Brief report: The assessment of posttraumatic stress disorder in pediatric cancer patients and survivors. *Journal of Pediatric Psychology, 21,* 499-504.

Carter, M. C., Thompson, E. I., & Simone, J. V. (1991). The survivors of childhood solid tumors. *Pediatric Clinics of North America, 38,* 505-526.

Chesler, M. A., & Parry, C. (2001). Gender roles and/or styles in crisis: An integrative analysis of the experiences of fathers of children with cancer. *Qualitative Health Research, 11*(3), 363-384.

Cook, J. A. (1984). Influence of gender on the problems of parents of fatally ill children. *Journal of Psychosocial Oncology, 2*(1), 71-91.

Cooper-Patrick, L., Gallo, J. J., Gonzales, J. J., Vu, H. T., Powe, N. R., Nelson, C., & Ford, D. E. (1999). Race, gender, and partnership in the patient-physician relationship. *Journal of the American Medical Association, 282,* 583-589.

Corbin, J., & Strauss, A. (1988). *Unending work and care: Managing chronic illness at home.* San Francisco: Jossey-Bass.

Dahlquist, L. M., Czyzewski, D. I., Copeland, K. G., Jones C. L., Taub E., & Vaughan J. K. (1993). Parents of children newly diagnosed with cancer: Anxiety, coping, and marital distress. *Journal of Pediatric Psychology, 18*, 365-376.

Dixon-Woods, M., Findlay, M., Young B., Cox H., & Heney D. (2001). Parents' accounts of obtaining a diagnosis of childhood cancer. *The Lancet, 357*, 670-674.

Eiser, C., & Eiser, J. (1987). Explaining illness to children. *Communication and Cognition, 20*, 277-290.

Eiser, C., Eiser, J. R., & Lang, J. (1989). Scripts in children's reports of medical events. *European Journal of Psychology of Education, 4*, 377-384.

Eiser, C., Havermans, T., & Casas, R. (1993). Healthy children's understanding of their blood: Implications for explaining leukaemia to children. *British Journal of Educational Psychology, 63*, 528-537.

Eiser, C., Havermans, T., & Eiser, J. (1995). Parents' attributions about childhood cancer: Implications for relationships with medical staff. *Child: Care, Health and Development, 21*(1), 31-42.

Eiser, C., Parkyn, T., Havermans, T., & McNinch, A. (1994). Parents' recall on the diagnosis of cancer in their child. *Psycho-Oncology, 3*, 197-203.

Endacott, R. (1998). Needs of the critically ill child: A review of the literature and report of a modified Delphi study. *Intensive and Critical Care Nursing, 14*, 66-73.

Fritz, G. K., Williams, J. R., & Amylon, M. (1988). After treatment ends: Psychosocial sequelae in pediatric cancer survivors. *American Journal of Orthopsychiatry, 58*, 552-561.

Giammona, A. J., & Malek, D. M. (2002). The psychological effect of childhood cancer on families. *The Pediatric Clinics of North America, 49*, 1063-1081.

Green, D. M. (1989). *Long-term complications of therapy for cancer in childhood and adolescence.* Baltimore, MD: Johns Hopkins University Press.

Greenberg, H. S., Kazak, A. E., & Meadows, A. T. (1989). Psychological functioning in 8-16-year-old cancer survivors and their parents. *The Journal of Pediatrics, 114*, 488-493.

Kameny, R. R., & Bearison, D. J. (1999). Illness narratives: Discursive constructions of self in pediatric oncology. *Journal of Pediatric Nursing, 14*(2), 73-79.

Kazak, A. E. (1998). Posttraumatic distress in childhood cancer survivors and their parents. *Medical and Pediatric Oncology Supplement 1*, 60-68.

Koocher, G. P. (1986). Psychosocial issues during the acute treatment of pediatric cancer. *Cancer, 58*, 468-472.

Lansky, S. B., Cairns, N. U., Clark, G. M., Lowman, J., Miller, L., & Trueworthy, R. (1979). Childhood cancer: Nonmedical costs of the illness. *Cancer, 43*, 403-408.

Levi, R. B., Marsick, R., Drotar, D., & Kodish, E. D. (2000). Diagnosis, disclosure, and informed consent: Learning from parents of children with cancer. *Journal of Pediatric Hematology/Oncology, 21*(1), 3-12.

Ljungman, G., McGrath, P. J., Cooper, E., Widger, K., Ceccolini, J., Fernandez, C., Frager, G., & Wilkins, K. (2003). Psychosocial needs of families with a child with cancer. *Journal of Pediatric Hematology/Oncology, 25*(3), 223-231.

Meadows, A. T., Massari, D. J., Fergusson, J., Gordon, J., Littman, P., & Moss, K. (1981). Declines in IQ scores and cognitive dysfunctions in children with acute lymphocytic leukaemia treated with cranial irradiation. *The Lancet, 2*, 1015-1018.

Nannis, E. D., Susman, E. J., Strope, B. E., Hersh, S. P., Levine, A. S. & Pizzo, P. A., (1982). Correlates of control in pediatric cancer patients and their families. *Journal of Pediatric Psychology, 7*(1), 75-84.

Nussbaum, J. F. (1989). Life-span communication: An introduction. In J. F. Nussbaum (Ed.), *Life-span communication: Normative processes* (pp. 1-4). Hillsdale, NJ: Erlbaum.

Nussbaum, J. F., Hummert, M. L., Williams, A., & Harwood, J. (1996). Communication and older adults. In B. Burleson (Ed.), *Communication yearbook* (Vol. 19, pp. 1-47). Thousand Oaks, CA: Sage.

Nussbaum, J. F., Ragan, S., & Whaley, B. (2003). Children, older adults, and women: Impact on provider-patient interaction. In T. L. Thompson, A. M. Dorsey, K. I. Miller, & R. Parrott (Eds.), *Handbook of health communication* (183-204). Mahwah, NJ: Erlbaum.

O'Hair, D., Allman, J., & Moore, S. D. (1996). A cognitive-affective model of relational expectations in the provider–patient context. *Journal of Health Psychology, 1*, 307-322.

O'Hair, D., Behnke, R., & King, P. (1983). Age related patient preferences of physician communication behavior. *Educational Gerontology, 9*, 147-158.

O'Malley, J. E., Koocher, G., Foster, D., & Slavin, L. (1979). Psychiatric sequelae of surviving childhood cancer. *American Journal of Orthopsychiatry, 49*, 608-616.

Overholser, J. C., & Fritz, G. K. (1990). The impact of childhood cancer on the family. *Journal of Psychosocial Oncology, 8*(4), 71-85.

Peckham, V. C., Meadows, A. T., Bartel, N., & Marrero, O. (1988). Educational late effects in long-term survivors of childhood acute lymphoncytic leukemia. *Pediatrics, 81*(1), 127-133.

Piaget, J. (1930). *The child's conception of physical causality*. London: Kagan Paul.

Pyke-Grimm, K. A., Degner, L., Small, A., & Mueller, B. (1999). Preferences for participation in treatment decision making and information needs of parents of children with cancer: A pilot study. *Journal of Pediatric Oncology Nursing, 16*(1), 13-24.

Reardon, K. K., & Buck R. (1989). Emotion, reason, and communication in coping with cancer. *Health Communication, 1*, 41-54.

Sanger, M. S., Copeland, D. R., & Davidson, E. R. (1999). Psychosocial adjustment among pediatric cancer patients: A multidimensional assessment. *Journal of Pediatric Psychology, 16*(4), 463-474.

Sawyer, M., Antoniou, G., Rice, M., & Baghurst, P. (2000). Childhood cancer: A 4-year prospective study of the psychological adjustment of children and parents. *Journal of Pediatric Hematology/Oncology, 22*(3), 214-220.

Sharf, B. F., & Vanderford, M. L. (2003). Illness narratives and the social construction of health. In T. L. Thompson, A. M. Dorsey, K. I. Miller, & R. Parrott (Eds.), *Handbook of health communication* (pp. 9-34). Mahwah, NJ: Erlbaum.

Slavin, L. A., O'Malley, J. E., Koocher, G. P., & Foster, D. J. (1982). Communication of the cancer diagnosis to pediatric patients: Impact on long-term adjustment. *American Journal of Psychiatry, 139*(2), 179-183.

Sloper, P. (1996). Needs and responses of parents following the diagnosis of childhood cancer. *Child, Health and Development, 22*(3), 187-202.

Speechley, K. N., & Noh, S. (1992). Surviving childhood cancer, social support and parents' psychological adjustment. *Journal of Pediatric Psychology, 17*(1), 15-31.

Stohl, C. (1989). Children's social network and the development of communicative competence. In J. F. Nussbaum (Ed.), *Life-span communication: Normative processes* (pp. 53-77). Hillsdale, NJ: Erlbaum.

Stuber, M. L., Kazak, A. E., Meeske, K., & Barakat, L. (1998). Is posttraumatic stress a viable model for understanding responses to childhood cancer? *Child and Adolescent Psychiatric Clinics of North America, 7*(1), 169-182.

Tates, K., & Meeuwesen, L. (2001). Doctor–parent–child communication: A (re)view of the literature. *Social Science & Medicine, 52*, 839-851.

Thompson, T. L., & Parrott, R. (2002). Interpersonal communication and health care. In M. L. Knapp & J. A. Daly (Eds.), *Handbook of interpersonal communication* (3rd ed., pp. 680-725). Thousand Oaks, CA: Sage.

Van Dongen-Melman, J.E.W.M., Pruyn, J. F. A., Van Zanen, G. E., & Sanders-Woudstra, J. A. R. (1986). Coping with childhood cancer: A conceptual view. *Journal of Psychosocial Oncology, 4*, 147-161.

Van Dongen-Melman, J.E.W.M., Van Zuuren, F. F., & Verhulst, F. C. (1998). Experiences of parents of childhood cancer survivors: A qualitative analysis. *Patient Education and Counseling, 34*, 185-200.

Varni, J. W., Katz, E. R., Colegrove, R., & Dolgin, M. (1996). Family functioning predictors of adjustment in children with newly diagnosed cancer: A prospective analysis. *Journal of Child Psychology/Psychiatry, 37*(3), 321-328.

Wells, L. M., Heiney, S. P., Swygert, E., Troficanto, G., Stokes, C., & Ettinger, R. S. (1990). Psychosocial stressors, coping resources, and information needs of parents of adolescent cancer patients. *Journal of Pediatric Oncology Nursing, 7*(4), 145-148.

Werner, H. (1948). *Comparative psychology of mental development.* New York: Science Editions.

Whaley, B. B. (1994). "Food is to me as gas is to cars?": Using figurative language to explain illness to children. *Health Communication, 11,* 185-193.

Whaley, B. B. (2000). Explaining illness to children: Theory, strategies, and future inquiry. In B. Whaley (Ed.), *Explaining illness: Research, theory and strategies* (pp. 195-207). Mahwah, NJ: Erlbaum.

Woodgate, R. L., & Degner, L. F. (2003). Expectations and beliefs about children's cancer symptoms: Perspectives of children with cancer and their families. *Oncology Nursing Forum, 30*(3), 479-491.

Worchel, F. F., Copeland, D. R., & Barker, D. G. (1987). Control-related coping strategies in pediatric oncology patients. *Journal of Pediatric Psychology, 12*(1), 25-38.

Young, B., Dixon-Woods, M., Findlay, M., & Heney, D. (2002). Parenting in a crisis: Conceptualizing mothers of children with cancer. *Social Science & Medicine, 55,* 1835-1847.

Young, B., Dixon-Woods, M., & Heney D. (2002). Identity and role in parenting a child with cancer. *Pediatric Rehabilitation, 5*(4), 209-214.

Young, B., Dixon-Woods, M., Windridge, C., & Heney, D. (2003). Managing communication with young people who have a potentially life threatening chronic illness: Qualitative study of patients and parents. *British Medical Journal, 326,* 305-308.

.

V

TREATMENT ISSUES

17 | Narrative Research in Palliative Care

Exploring the Benefits

Elaine M. Wittenberg-Lyles
University of Texas

Sandra L. Ragan
University of Oklahoma

Although "to palliate" literally means to comfort, to reduce the intensity of, to control the violence of, "palliative care," in medical parlance, has frequently been equated with hospice care. "Hospice" enjoys a more concrete, less ambiguous set of practices, in that is it reserved for patients with 6 months or less to live: If they wish to receive Medicare benefits, patients can be provided with hospice services only if certified as "terminally ill with a life expectancy of six months or less if the disease runs its normal course" (Golth, 1998, p. 21). Thus, palliative or comfort care (i.e., pain and symptom management, along with attention to the patient's emotional, psychological, and spiritual needs) can and does occur with hospice care, yet it also can be administered to patients at any stage of disease, whether terminal or not. Nonetheless, both lay and medical personnel often use the terms *hospice* and *palliative care* synonymously, and most of the research literature in palliative care concerns care given at end of life.

Several researchers have begun to advocate that palliative care include the addressing of a patient's needs in their entirety, from the time of diagnosis of cancer to disease recurrence and throughout the entire disease process, even if the result is survival and not death (Balfour, 1995). Because of the complexities for physicians in both accurately forecasting end of life and also in communicating that prognosis to patients and their loved ones, some suggest the assignment of a palliative care team at the time of diagnosis (Ackerman & Oliver, 1997;

Morris & Christie, 1995). Even more recently, a palliative care team comprised of MDs, PhDs, and RNs state: "There is a growing consensus that in patients with life-threatening illnesses, palliative care should be integrated early and concurrent with treatment of the underlying disease" (Wolfe et al., 2000, p. 2474).

This chapter deals with palliative care as the overarching system of care that medical caregivers, family members, and friends can provide patients during any stage of a serious illness. Because such care is not limited to end-of-life hospice services, the argument that we develop—that patients' stories or narratives are pivotal to palliative care—is one that is germane for patients and caregivers throughout the course of serious illness, from diagnosis to (potential) death.

One of the primary barriers to palliative care at end of life and throughout the progress of disease is the acknowledgment of the boundaries of medicine (Janssens, Zylicz, & Have, 1999). The medical profession's focus on cure frequently results in the patient's prolonged suffering as continued attempts to prolong life fail. This medicalization of death has resulted in increasing numbers of people dying in pain and in hospitals. Whereas more than 90% of U.S. adults claim a preference for dying at home, 52% die in hospitals and 24% in nursing homes (von Gunten, 2002). An earlier article by Holstein (1997) reported that almost 80% will die in institutional settings where death is public and, more importantly, under the control of medical specialists. A similarity can be seen in the medicalization of childbirth: Whereas women had traditionally given birth at home, by 1940, 50% of U.S. women gave birth in hospitals, and by 1996, 97% to 99% did (Nelson, 1996).

The acceptance of death by the health care staff and medical community as an inevitable aspect of life must take place in order for palliative care to be implemented throughout the course of a life-threatening disease and at end of life. Unfortunately, Western civilization's approach to health care projects a dichotomy between the disease and the person, wherein one reality is objective and the other is subjective (Kane & Primomo, 2001). This limited view of health care, in which death is not considered part of the care process, impedes the practice of palliative care. Health care staff fail to acknowledge that curative treatment co-exists with other facets of health care that contribute to the well-being of the patient (Janssens, Zylicz, & Have, 1999). Consequently, this fixation on cure leaves patients' psychosocial needs unmet as they move from living to dying.

Even more problematic is that there is no common definition of palliative care in the health care industry (Abma, 2001) and consequently, the practice of palliative care has not been enthusiastically adopted by the medical community. A simple database search of Article1st (FirstSearch), which indexes articles from January 1, 1990 to the present was used to search the *Journal of the American Medical Association (JAMA)* for the keyword "palliative care." The search resulted in 20 articles that included the keyword (see Appendix A for a summary of article findings). Overall, 10 of the 20 articles focused specifically on providing an explication of palliative care and what it involves for medical education, the medical staff for the dying, and for patients. Three articles centered around legal issues that affected palliative care, and one article evaluated medical education in palliative care.

It appears that there is growing interest in palliative care from the medical community. Initially, articles on palliative care were published in special sections of the journal. Dating back to the first referenced article ("Palliative care code," 1996), palliative care was being discussed merely in commentaries, letters to the editor, and from a legal perspective. Although only one article was published in 1996, there were 10 articles published on the topic in 2000. More recently, palliative care has been discussed more regularly in a section titled Medical

News and Perspectives and has even garnered a special section on the topic entitled "Perspectives on Care at the Close of Life," which is sponsored with a grant by the Robert Wood Johnson Foundation.

However, palliative care is defined differently, depending on who is writing about it. Most definitions of palliative care focus on providing comfort care only when dealing with a dying or seriously ill patient or on controlling the patient's pain. The definition that we most like is von Gunten's (2002): "palliative care may be defined as the interdisciplinary care of patients and families focused on the relief of suffering and improving quality of life" (p. 876). The lack of a consensual definition of palliative care is one of the barriers to making palliative care more prominent among hospitals as well as hospital staff. Inevitably, patients won't receive the most beneficial kinds of palliative care if the medical staff is not knowledgeable about what it is and how it deviates from hospice care or if the medical care team cannot arrive at a common definition.

Holstein (1997) and others argued that death needs to be considered an important part of the human condition in order for palliative care to be advanced by medical care providers. As such, the dying process requires a paradigm shift from the standpoint of health care—a shift that moves the focus from curing to healing and is characterized by a loss of control by all involved; that is, neither doctors nor other caregivers nor the patients themselves are able to keep the patient from an inevitable demise (Kane & Primomo, 2001).

Further education about the dying process is needed in order to inform the medical community about palliative care and why it is so important in health care practice. We propose that narrative research can provide such insight into three main areas of palliative care: the coping needs of terminally ill patients, their families, and their health care staff; as a pedagogical tool in teaching health care staff about patients' needs in the dying process; and as a means to evaluating current palliative care practices. We further note that narrative research could benefit the extension of palliative care as a practice throughout the course of life-threatening illness and not just at its end stages.

A NARRATIVE APPROACH TO ILLNESS

Janssens, Zylicz, and Have (1999) surmised that palliative care is total care that includes the medical, psychosocial, and spiritual. Predominantly centered around pain management among medical health care providers, the focus of palliative care is decision making with an emphasis on quality rather than quantity of life (Janssens et al., 1999). Kane and Primomo (2001) argued that palliative care involves the care of the patient in the "context of the patient's life and interconnectedness with the world around him or her" (p. 166).

One of the ways in which this interconnectedness can best be understood is through the telling of personal narratives. Ragan, Wittenberg, and Hall (2003) noted that much of the literature on palliative care focuses exclusively on a biomedical approach to care—the relief of pain and symptom management. Yet when the patient's voice is heard and considered, as in Margaret Edson's (1993) remarkable play, "W;t," or in the real stories of patients filmed for Bill Moyers's (2000), televised documentary, "On Our Own Terms: Moyers on Dying," concerns other than physical relief emerge as patients share their personal narratives. Burton (1998) posited that narratives are the result of people's multiple relationships in community.

As such, she concluded: "narrative themes are expressions of meaning-making stemming from the interaction of cultural factors, family structure, and life cycle events" (p. 124). The life cycle provides a context for understanding meaning and includes predictable developmental crises such as birth, marriage, and death as well as unpredictable life crises such as a terminal illness diagnosis. Vanderford, Jenks, and Sharf (1997), in a special issue of the journal *Health Communication* which deals with patient-centered approaches to health care, maintained that patients are "active interpreters, managers, and creators of the meaning of their health and illness" (p. 14).

Telling personal narratives allows people to formulate new meanings concerning illness as well as death (Holstein, 1997). In *The Wounded Storyteller*, Frank (1995) posited that illness is a call for stories. Moreover, these stories function to repair the individual's sense of self as well as to let others know what is happening. "Disease happens in a life that already is a story, and this story goes on, changed by illness but also affecting how the illness story is formed" (Frank, 1995, p. 54). The contextual aspects of these stories typically include fatigue, pain, and uncertainty.

Illness interrupts life and narratives thus function to make sense of life. Although these narratives are "uncomfortable" in the telling, Frank (1995) argued that they are necessary in dealing with death. Frank also identified illness as a crisis of self wherein stories function to reaffirm an ill person's own sense of self as well as the individual's relationship with others. Thus, illness stories function to redefine/identify the ill person. "The self is being formed in what is told" in three ways: (a) with ourselves, (b) reaffirming relationships with others, and (c) reaffirming that the story is worth listening to (Frank, 1995).

Frank identified three types of illness narratives that are told by patients. He believes that some of these narratives are told in combination. First is the *restitution narrative* ("Yesterday I was healthy, today I'm sick, tomorrow I'll be healthy again"). The focus of such narratives is on tests, treatments, and possible outcomes. This is a learned narrative as patients learn about how illness is told through the media as well as the brochures published from health care institutions (Frank, 1995).

Second is the *chaos narrative*, which is the opposite of the restitution narrative ("Life never gets better, I'm doomed"). These particular narratives are absent of any order with no coherent sequence, and the majority of the narrative is spent cursing god and dying. "The person living the chaos story has no distance from her life and no reflective grasp on it. Lived chaos makes reflection, and consequently storytelling, impossible" (Frank, 1995, p. 98).

Third is the *quest narrative* wherein the patient accepts illness and seeks to use it to advantage. It is within these types of narratives that the patient believes that something will be gained through the storytelling experience. Furthermore, patients are able to fend off chaos and position themselves as persons with stories to tell. It is these types of stories that are most often shared with the public, such as celebrity stories of illness.

Overall, each narrative encompasses cultural and personal preferences: "in both listening to others and telling our own stories, we become who we are." (Frank, 1995, p. 77). Illness stories thus overlap with and are bounded by spiritual autobiographies, survivor stories, and stories of gender identity. Moreover, with a terminal illness diagnosis a sense of temporality is lost as the future is uncertain. As such the preparation for death can include looking back and summarizing life (Benzein, Norberg, & Saveman, 2001). Frank (1995) concluded that such self-stories proliferate, and it is possible that they serve as a coping mechanism for patients, family members, and health care staff.

COPING

Terminal illness forces an individual to rethink his or her personal sense of meaning in life (Boston, Towers, & Barnard, 2001). Burton (1998) proposed that spiritual narratives are a result of an amalgamation of life-cycle events, cultural factors, and family structure. As such, these narratives center around three basic themes: explanation (in defining the illness and in defining what life means), power (in terms of autonomy), and connection (in terms of relationships with others). These three themes are examined as they relate to palliative care.

Explanation of Pain

Palliative care researchers conceptualize pain as a culmination of four elements: physical, psychological, social, and spiritual (Ohlen, Bengtsson, Skott, & Segesten, 2002). Ohlen et al., proposed that narratives allow expression of suffering and management of suffering. In a study of personal narratives by 16 palliative care patients, the authors found meanings of experiencing alleviation of suffering to include an endurable body, being independent and feeling at home, feelings of connectedness, and an inner peace. They concluded that personal reflection facilitates the alleviation of suffering by allowing the individual to reconcile oneself with one's life as it has become.

Caregivers of the terminally ill are also affected by the patient's pain, especially if those they are caring for are family members. Ersek and Ferrell (1994) investigated the meaning of cancer pain from the perspective of the patient as well as the caregiver. Attempts for the patient to create meaning from pain include making causal attributions, identifying the benefits of the disease (such as getting closer to others), making social comparisons, and viewing the cancer experience from a higher force (Ersek & Ferrell, 1994). They also found that patients reflected on their lives as a way of dealing with pain. However, caregivers regarded pain as causing suffering, grief, and as a challenge to hope. Together, patients and caregivers are faced with negotiating pain and its meaning. Ersek and Ferrell (1994) noted that these communicative strategies in such negotiations may include avoidance as well as illusions about control. Narratives may facilitate a negotiated coping process that is beneficial to both parties.

Chochinov (2002) proposed a model of palliative care that he termed "dignity-conserving care." It is a model that employs narrative to help conserve or bolster the dignity of dying patients. *Dignity* is defined as "the quality or state of being worthy, honored, or esteemed" (p. 2254). Chochinov noted that without examining what "satisfaction, psychological comfort, or feeling in control and supported means to the dying patient . . . achieving them as therapeutic outcomes remains challenging, and all too often beyond reach" (p. 2254). He then said that these features need to be studied from the vantage point of patients themselves and explained dignity psychotherapy as a way of eliciting patients' life histories, their stories.

Holstein (1997) also discussed the concept of *death with dignity*. To her, this involves the recognition of the ill person as fully human as well as recognizing the ramifications of the disease for significant others. Moreover, Holstein asserted that although the primary goal of palliative care is pain control, "attention to suffering means active talk about death" (p.

851). Such talk allows the health care staff to become aware of the individual patient's needs as well as garner a better understanding of the patient's awareness/acceptance of death. For example, Menard and Saucier (2000) set out to improve palliative care by applying an intervention model. Through a particular case study, the authors' brief intervention involved four meetings with the patient and his significant others. Menard and Saucier concluded that these forums provided an opportunity for much needed dialogue that facilitated more successful coping.

Power (Decision Making)

Coping patterns of patients are a fundamental aspect of decision making, particularly as it relates to pain management. Research supports that changes in social relationships, psychological moods, and spiritual attitudes all contribute to medical decisions (see Janssens et al., 1999). Moreover, Ersek and Ferrell (1994) noted that cancer patients' and caregivers' fears of addiction affected decision making in end-of-life care.

However, the role of the physician proves to be the pivotal determinant in palliative care practice. The physician is the one who not only delivers the prognosis but also determines when palliative care is offered or whether it is offered at all. Holstein (1997) argued that this position allows doctors to say things that others cannot say, especially when it comes to making end-of-life decisions. Doctors initiate or fail to initiate talk about palliative care; patients are generally unwilling to broach the topic, particularly in the context of a compliant/submissive patient and an authoritative/controlling doctor. Unfortunately, therefore, physicians are solely responsible for beginning the discussion of and implementation of palliative care. Given their role in initiating palliative care, it is particularly critical that physicians realize that they are not always able to cure their patients. This is a struggle for many doctors who, because of their medical school socialization (Harter & Kirby, in press; Ragan, Mindt, & Wittenberg, 2005) and their insistence on the biomedical approach of "fixing" the patient, perceive that they are failures when a patient succumbs to disease (O'Hair, Scannell, & Thompson, 2005).

Doctor–patient communication inhibits a patient's ability to assume responsibility, as the diagnosis is the primary source of the patients' identity and it is given by the doctor (Frank, 1995). Moreover, Abma (2001) argued that physicians do not recognize patients as those with a story to tell. Frank (1995) concurred, positing that when physicians interrupt patient history the hidden message is "your story is not worthy of being told." Rather, the physician focuses on the illness and not the patient as a person. In this manner, patients do not have a chance to adequately participate in the decision-making process. In order for doctors to take an active role in the palliative care process, they must be willing to listen to the patient's narrative concerning their views of their illness as well as its profound effect on their lives. Only in this manner can doctors fully provide the regimen necessary to treat the patient as a whole person on a physical as well as spiritual level.

Connection (Hope)

Palliative care patients experience the dialectical tension of living in the world of the living and healthy and living in the world of the sick and dying (Benzein et al., 2001). Consequently, hope becomes a way of life as "the experience of living with a terminal illness grows to be more personal and subjective and the need to have a sense of integrity and wholeness becomes essential" (Kane & Primomo, 2001, p. 165). Benzein et al. (2001) conducted a study of palliative home-care patients with cancer using narrative research. Many of the patients told the interviewer that they felt better after sharing their story and that the interview helped them formulate their own thoughts and feelings.

"Dying persons say that dying is a personal living experience" (Boston et al., 2001, p. 250). For a terminally ill patient, hope is experienced in many ways. Benzein et al. explored the meaning of lived experience of hope in cancer patients receiving palliative care at home. Their findings suggest that hope consists of four dimensions. The most prevalent aspect of hope expressed was a hope for being cured and it was especially related to palliative care treatment. A second dimension of hope included the desire to live as normally as possible, free from the stigma of illness, and typically involved setting goals for oneself. A third dimension of hope was characterized by the presence of confirmative relationships with self, others, and pets. Finally, hope was expressed through the reconciliation with life and death that often took the form of personal narratives (Benzein et al., 2001). Thus, in terms of palliative care, narratives could possibly serve as a juncture between hoping for a cure and living with the hope for comfort with life and death.

Health Care Staff and Coping

Nurses and other health care staff are an important part of palliative care. Boston et al. (2001) proposed that palliative caretakers are faced not only with the physical aspects of care but also with the emotional aspects of caring for the dying. Empathy and good listening are often viewed as necessary skills for caring for the dying. Typically, the health care staff/team spends 40 hours or more a week with a dying patient and through assistance and care develops interpersonal relationships with the patient and his or her family. It is inevitable that the death of a patient takes a toll on the staff. Yang and Mcilfatrick (2001) proposed that the primary stressors on palliative care staff include the relationship dynamics between the physician and the nurse, the family's emotional reactions, concealing illness or prognosis from the patient, and do not resuscitate orders for patients.

Evans, Bibeau, and Conley (2001) examined coping strategies used by hospice workers. More than 45% of the health care staff questioned reported that they were satisfied with their coping; however, the remainder of the participants was only slightly satisfied to completely dissatisfied. Evans et al. (2001) found that those who were dissatisfied engaged in confrontative strategies (hostile/aggressive efforts to alter the situation), accepted responsibility (acknowledging one's role in the problem), and escaped avoidance (efforts to escape or avoid the problem).

DiTullio and MacDonald (1999) also examined the stress associated with hospice work. Participants responded that the most stressful aspect about hospice work is time cramping (not enough time to do everything) and emotional cramping (a lack of time for one's emotional self-care). On an organizational level, participants reported that "inadequate communication" was a major source of stress. DiTullio and MacDonald found that the primary coping strategy included relaxation, meditation, and self-soothing behavior, such as smoking and overeating. As might be anticipated due to the nurturing roles that women have been taught to play in our culture, the large majority of hospice staff is female.

In a comparison of death anxiety between hospice and emergency nurses, Payne, Dean, and Kalus (1998) found that hospice nurses had lower death anxiety. Moreover, the hospice nurses in their study all reported that they were able to talk to their colleagues at work. It is possible that being able to talk about death contributed to lower death anxiety. Thus, narratives about death and dying by health care staff could facilitate better coping and consequently better work performance. That is, talking about their job experiences could serve as a coping mechanism for dealing with job stress.

NARRATIVES AS A PEDAGOGICAL TOOL

The patient–caregiver relationship is an important aspect of palliative care. Boston et al. (2001) suggested that this relationship is so strong that it impacts the patient's decisions concerning end-of-life care, as well as the decisions of family members. The majority of palliative care comes from nurses; especially in palliative home care, the nurse is seen and functions as a solo practitioner (Aranda & Kelso, 1997).

Aranda and Kelso proposed that it is the nurse who facilitates dying in palliative home care. They reason that the role of the nurse is seen as routine in any health care setting, the nurses' job is to provide explanation and information about health care happenings, and nurses are skilled at reducing embarrassment as the body is no longer able to take care of itself. In this manner, the nurse develops relationships with the patient as well as the family. Aranda and Kelso (1997) found that family members of palliative patients viewed the nurse as an extension of their own family, as they too lived the "dying" experience, and in that capacity the nurse serves to reassure family members that they did a good job. These findings suggest that there is more to be learned from the nurses' experiences that could enhance palliative care altogether.

Durgahee (1997) posited that narratives and other reflective practices function as a teaching and learning tool for the medical community. The author examined storytelling (which included talking and writing in a personal diary) of working nurses who were taking a course in the care of the dying. The overall conclusion was that reliving clinical experiences through storytelling enhances self-concept, increases communication skills, and increases insight development. Moreover, the act of keeping a personal diary promoted purposeful observation, awareness of experience, and insight into communication practices. Durgahee argued that reflective processes enhance communication skills as they make individuals aware of what they are saying and how they say it.

Moreover, James, Jones, Rodin, and Catton (2001) found that frontline oncology professionals do prefer case presentations and discussions that address the development of communication skills as a way of continuing education in psychosocial care. The authors also found that nonpsychosocial professionals prefer to learn communication skills, whereas psychosocial professionals prefer to learn counseling skills, coping with life-threatening illness, and then communication skills. In any case, pedagogical practices that involve narratives, such as storytelling and personal diaries, allow palliative care professionals to become more aware of their communication skills.

NARRATIVE AS AN EVALUATIVE TOOL

One approach to examining communication and death is through problematic integration theory (Hines, Babrow, Badzek, & Moss, 2001). PI theory proposes that individuals conceptualize their experiences through the integration of probabilistic and evaluative orientations, which is frequently problematic. The resulting dilemma creates alternatives in which information taken in forces an individual to shift from one experience to another. Consequently, communication is seen as a way of dealing with life experience and a vital aspect in the journey from life to death.

Naturally, this type of communication is contextual and recalling such experiences can provide a means to evaluating such experiences. Narratives, which are embedded in situations, thus become a worthwhile examination (Abma, 2001). Abma advocated a responsive evaluation approach to palliative care. According to Abma, the responsive approach assumes that "human beings actively interpret their past or anticipated experience by developing narratives" (p. 263). These narratives give order and meaning to events we often don't understand (Abma, 2001). Thus, narratives operate as a way of understanding our reality as they reflect human intention and action as well as providing meaning (Abma, 2001).

A poignant example of this can be seen in the narrative shared by a 75-year-old man who had been volunteering for hospice for 10 years:

> [In] my first 2 or 3 years with hospice, there was a patient who came up that was a retired Colonel and he had worked at the ROTC up in [name of town] and had been a customer of mine and he always had me fix his mother's (television) set. And I saw his name come up and I didn't act on it right away. Back then I was more . . . well I was young enough it didn't bother me back then. So after IDT [hospice meeting], I called his wife from the office and told her who I was and uh I guess she said something to him if he would like me to come out and he said yes. And I went out there and that guy was sitting up, propped up in bed just as chipper as you would want anybody to be and he had pancreatic cancer which usually is a fast moving one. And I had a heck of a nice visit with that old guy. I set up with his wife that I would come back in a week and she was going to go do her shopping and uh when I called to make sure it was alright for me to come she said that he was so bad that she didn't want to leave him. And he died a couple of days later. You know I wish now . . . why didn't I get on this right away when I saw [his name on the list]? I may have had a patient [then] . . . I don't know. But I feel it is a privilege to do what I can for those people that I know.

Reflection of his decision allows him to evaluate the experience. Consequently, the volunteer concluded that he no longer waits to contact a person he knows when he sees one on the patient list.

Narratives also provide a means to evaluating medical decisions. For example, Durgahee (1997) found that clinical experiences shared through storytelling aid nurses in ethical decision making. Through reflection, nurses are better able to analyze the "interactions and needs of the parties involved, leading to new understandings" (p. 136). Durgahee posited that narrative reasoning is part of the process of ethical decision making.

Moreover, Jones (1999) offered three ways in which narratives are important in developing medical ethics. First, narratives can provide case examples for teaching principle-based professional ethics. Second, narratives can provide moral guides for living a "good life." Finally, in providing their readers with experiential truth and passion, narratives "compel re-examination of accepted medical practices and ethical precepts" (Jones, 1999, p. 253).

Recognizing that different people produce different narratives about a program or practice, Abma (2001) argued that the focus of narratives should involve what people say, the structure of the experience, how they communicate their ideas, and the kind of narrative form chosen. This type of data would provide valuable insight into current palliative care practices and is sure to dictate a direction for future palliative care practices.

CONCLUSION

Narrative research about the cancer experience can be beneficial in promoting and learning more about palliative care. Narratives function to help patients and their families accept the reality of their prognosis, to garner further understanding about dying and about the care of the dying, and to serve as a means for evaluating palliative care practices. Limited social science studies of death and dying have utilized narrative research, with some of our best contemporary stories of dying patients coming from fiction (e.g., Margaret Edson's play, "W;t") or from documentaries on death and dying (e.g., Bill Moyers' PBS television documentary). Yet a significant strain of research by social psychologist James Pennebaker points to the medical and therapeutic benefits of patients' stories and self-disclosures (Pennebaker, 1993; Pennebaker & Beall, 1986; Pennebaker, Kiecolt-Glaser, & Glaser, 1988). Pennebaker's (1995) research indicates that talking about a traumatic event positively affects health outcomes, whereas not talking about it can promote negative health outcomes. Currently, a clinical trial is underway at M.D. Anderson Cancer Center in Texas, which utilizes Pennebaker's findings in assessing the medical and psychological benefits of cancer patients' self-disclosures in written journal recordings. Other social psychologists are also turning to journal writing as a means of gathering narratives concerning death. Durgahee (1997), for example, employed journal writing as a pedagogical tool in teaching others how to care for the dying. The results from the study suggest that personal diaries improve overall communication and lead to better assessment, care planning, and interactions. Perhaps richer meaning and data regarding palliative care can be found in narratives that are written rather than orally communicated. At any rate, both oral and written narratives require further investigation as effective therapeutic tools for the palliative care provider.

On a final note, we argue once again that the narratives or life stories of patients facing life-threatening illness, whether or not that illness culminates in death, need to be told and need to be heard. One of the functions of social support suggested by Geist-Martin et al. (2003) is unconditional listening; giving voice to a person's story—the person's uncertainties, anxieties, and fears—in a way that validates the individual as fully human, even when, particularly when he or she is confronting serious or fatal disease. "Being heard and validated, talking about our uncertainties and fears, often provides much comfort when we are in situations where we feel powerless or frightened. It allows us to write—and revise—our story in our own way and to have that story heard" (p. 222). Talk about death persists as one of our culture's worst taboos. Yet, talk about one's own inevitable or imminent demise is paradoxically healing. Valuing our own and others' stories as we confront our mortality may help us to fully embrace our humanity.

APPENDIX
JAMA Overview

DATE/ AUTHOR(S)	DEFINITION OF PALLIATIVE CARE	FOCUS OF PATIENT	TOPIC/ISSUE	SPECIAL AUDIENCE/ FOCUS	TYPE OF ARTICLE/ SECTION PUBLISHED
December 18, 1996 JAMA 276;1	"the care of dying patients in hospitals" (p. 1864).	**Dying**	Palliative Care Code (V66.7) included in the International Classification of Diseases, 9th Rev., Clinical Modification	New code Update	Health Agencies Communication
September 3, 1997 JAMA 278;9 Billings & Block	"the study and management of patients with active, progressive, far-advanced disease for whom the prognosis is limited and the focus of care is the quality of life." (p. 733).	**Seriously-Ill**	Formal evaluation of Under-graduate Medical Education	Medical education	Review
January 7, 1998 JAMA 279;1 Sapir, M.	"focuses on comfort, alleviation of pain, and emotional support in coping with dying, death, and loss . . . " (p. 21).	**Dying**	Defining palliation in terms of medical education	Medical education	Letter to editor
January 7, 1998 JAMA 279;1 Fox, E.	"the palliative care model is applied most appropriately to patients who are entering the final phase of a predictably progressive course toward death." (p. 21).	**Dying**	Defining palliation model and curative model	Medical education	In reply to Letter to the Editor
January 5, 2000 JAMA 283;1 Magid	"to relieve physical and psychological suffering" (p. 114).	**Pain**	Pain, suffering, and meaning	Pain	Editor's Note
January 5, 2000 JAMA 283;1 Foley	"palliative care offers pain control, symptom management, and psychological and existential support to maximize patients' quality of life." (p. 115).	**Pain**	Pain Care	Pain	Commentary

DATE/ AUTHOR(S)	DEFINITION OF PALLIATIVE CARE	FOCUS OF PATIENT	TOPIC/ISSUE	SPECIAL AUDIENCE/ FOCUS	TYPE OF ARTICLE/ SECTION PUBLISHED
January 5, 2000 JAMA 283;1 Abrahm	World Health Organization definition of palliative care—"we physicians must expand our focus of care beyond the disease to encompass all dimensions of the patient's distress." (p. 116).	Pain	The role of the clinician in palliative medicine	Doctor-patient communication	Essay
January 12, 2000 JAMA 283;2 Orentlicher & Caplan	"treatment of pain and other physical suffering in dying patients." (p. 255).	Dying	The Pain Relief Promotion Act of 1999	Legal issues affecting palliative care	Policy Perspectives
November 15, 2000 JAMA 284;19 Zerzan, Stearns, & Hanson	"Palliative care is comprehensive inter-disciplinary care designed to promote quality of life for patients and families living with a terminal or incurable illness." (p. 2489).	Dying	Access to palliative care and hospice in nursing homes	Nursing Home Patients/Staff	Special Communication
November 15, 2000 JAMA 284;19 Crawley et. al.	"end-of-life care" (p. 2518).	Dying	Palliative and end-of-life care in the African American Community	African-American community	Commentaries
November 15, 2000 JAMA 284;19 Wolfe, et.al.	"communication about end-of-life issues" (p. 2470).	Dying	Understanding of prognosis among parents of children who died of cancer	Children/ Doctor-Patient communication of prognosis	Original Contribution/ Research Study– Survey and Interview
November 15, 2000 JAMA 284;19 Stephenson	"Such care not only addresses the physical needs ... such as managing pain and other symptoms, but also brings together a team of physicians, nurses, social workers, therapists, clergy, volunteers, and others to provide psycho-logical, social, and spiritual support." (p. 2437).	Pain	Palliative care needed for children	Children	Medical News and Perspectives

DATE/ AUTHOR(S)	DEFINITION OF PALLIATIVE CARE	FOCUS OF PATIENT	TOPIC/ISSUE	SPECIAL AUDIENCE/ FOCUS	TYPE OF ARTICLE/ SECTION PUBLISHED
November 15, 2000 JAMA 284;19 Mitka	"end-of-life care" (p. 2441).	**Dying**	Practice (7 promises a physician SHOULD make to a dying patient); Local initiatives (hospitals with palliative care programs); Nursing care	Medical/ Healthcare staff	Medical News and Perspectives
November 15, 2000 JAMA 284;19 Phillips	"end-of-life care" (p. 2442).	**Dying**	Growth of end-of-life care–promoting knowledge of	Medical/ Healthcare staff	Medical News and Perspectives
August 15, 2001 JAMA 286;7 Vastag	"palliative care for pain, nausea, fatigue, and other debilitating symptoms." (p. 778).	**Pain**	NCI to lead palliative care improvements	Palliative care improvements	Medical News and Perspectives
February 20, 2002 JAMA 287;7 Von Gunten	"goal is comfort and quality of life." (p. 875). Author further defines primary palliative care, secondary palliative care, and tertiary palliative care.	**Pain**	Use of secondary and tertiary palliative care in US hospitals	Evaluation of palliative care practices	Perspectives on Care at the Close of Life
May 1, 2002 JAMA 287;17 Chochinov	"The basic tenets of palliative care, including symptom control, psychological and spiritual well-being, and care of the family, may all be summarized under the goal of helping patients to die with dignity." (p. 2253).	**Dying**	Providing dignity-conserving care	Medical staff of the dying	Perspectives on Care at the Close of Life
February 20, 2002 JAMA 287;7 Stevens	"therapy that focuses on decreasing pain and suffering by providing patients with medication for relief of their symptoms and with comfort and support." (p. 938).	**Pain**	Explication of palliative care	Information for patients	Patient Page

DATE/ AUTHOR(S)	DEFINITION OF PALLIATIVE CARE	FOCUS OF PATIENT	TOPIC/ISSUE	SPECIAL AUDIENCE/ FOCUS	TYPE OF ARTICLE/ SECTION PUBLISHED
August 28, 2002 JAMA 288;8 Lamberg	"sometimes called comfort care, goes beyond pain relief to embrace emotional, social, and spiritual needs of seriously ill patients . . . " (p. 943).	**Seriously-Ill**	Explication of palliative care	Medical staff of the dying	Medical News and Perspectives
September 11, 2002 JAMA 288;10 McPhee & Markowitz	"to provide comfort and quality of life as death approaches." (p. 1279).	**Dying**	Reflections at a palliative care unit	Experiences of palliation	Perspectives on Care at the Close of Life: CODA

REFERENCES

Abma, T. A. (2001). Evaluating palliative care: Facilitating reflexive dialogues about an ambiguous concept. *Medicine, Health Care and Philosophy, 4,* 261-276.

Ackerman, G. M., & Oliver, D. J. (1997). Psychosocial support in an outpatient clinic. *Palliative Medicine, 11,* 167-168.

Aranda, S. K., & Kelso, J. (1997). The nurse as coach in care of the dying. *Contemporary Nurse, 6,* 117-122.

Balfour, H. M. (1995). When does palliative care begin? A needs assessment of cancer patients with recurrent diseases. *Journal of Palliative Care, 11,* 53.

Benzein, E., Norberg, A., & Savemna, B. (2001). The meaning of the lived experience of hope in patients with cancer in palliative home care. *Palliative Medicine, 15,* 117-126.

Boston, P., Towers, A., & Barnard, D. (2001). Embracing vulnerability: Risk and empathy in palliative care. *Journal of Palliative Care, 17,* 248-253.

Burton, L. A. (1998). The spiritual dimension of palliative care. *Seminars in Oncology Nursing, 14,* 121-128.

Chochinov, H. M. (2002). Dignity-conserving care—A new model for palliative care: Helping the patient feel valued. *JAMA, 287*(17), 2253-2260.

DiTullio, M., & MacDonald, D. (1999). The struggle for the soul of hospice: Stress, coping, and change among hospice workers. *American Journal of Hospice & Palliative Care, 16,* 641-655.

Durgahee, T. (1997). Reflective practice: Nursing ethics through story telling. *Nursing Ethics, 4,* 135-146.

Edson, M. (1993). *W;t.* New York: Farrar, Straus & Giroux.

Ersek, M., & Ferrell, B. R. (1994). Providing relief from cancer pain by assisting in the search for meaning. *Journal of Palliative Care, 10,* 15-22.

Evans, W. M., Bibeau, D. L., & Conley, K. M. (2001). Coping strategies used in residential hospice settings: Findings from a national study. *American Journal of Hospice and Palliative Care, 18,* 102-110.

Frank, A. W. (1995). *The wounded storyteller: Body, illness, and ethics.* Chicago: University of Chicago Press.

Geist-Martin, P., Berlin Ray, E., & Sharf, B. F. (2003). *Communicating health: Personal, cultural, and political complexities.* Belmont, CA: Wadswoth.

Golth, F. M. (1998). Foreword. *Hospice care: A physician's guide.* National Hospice Organization.

Harter, L. M., & Kirby, E. (in press). Socializing medical students in an era of managed care: The ideological significance of standardized and virtual patients. *Communication Studies.*

Hines, S. C., Babrow, A. S., Badzek, L., & Moss, A. (2001). From coping with life to coping with death: Problematic integration for the seriously ill elderly. *Health Communication, 13,* 327-342.

Holstein, M. (1997). Reflections on death and dying. *Academic Medicine, 72,* 848-855.

James, J., Jones, J. M., Rodin, G., & Catton, P. (2001). Can assessment of psychosocial orientation assist continuing education program development in psychosocial oncology? *Journal of Cancer Education, 16,* 24-28.

Janssens, R., Zylicz, Z., & Have, H. (1999). Articulating the concept of palliative care: Philosophical and theological perspectives. *Journal of Palliative Care, 15,* 38-44.

Jones, A. (1999). Narrative based medicine: Narrative in medical ethics. *British Medical Journal, 318,* 253-256.

Kane, J. R., & Primomo, M. (2001). Alleviating the suffering of seriously ill children. *American Journal of Hospice & Palliative Care, 18,* 161-169.

Menard, D., & Saucier, A. (2000). John's story: An application of the Calgary Family Intervention Model. *Canadian Oncology Nursing Journal, 10,* 64-68.

Morris, R. I., & Christie, K. M. (1995). Initiating hospice care. *Home Healthcare Nurse, 13*, 21-26.

Moyers, B. (2000). *On our own terms: Moyers on dying* (Produced and directed by G. Pellett). Public Affairs Television, Inc.

Nelson, E. J. (1996). The American experience of childbirth: Toward a range of safe choices. In R. L. Parrott & C. M. Condit (Eds.), *Evaluating women's health messages: A resource book* (pp. 109-123). Thousand Oaks, CA: Sage.

O'Hair, H. D., Scannell, D., & Thompson, S. (2005) Agency through narrative: Patients managing cancer care in a challenging environment. In L. M. Harter, P. Japp, & C. S. Beck (Eds.), *Narratives, health, and healing: Communication theory, research, and practice* (pp. 413-432). Mahwah, NJ: Erlbaum.

Ohlen, J., Bengtsson, J., Skott, C., & Segesten, K. (2002). Being in a lived retreat—embodied meaning of alleviated suffering. *Cancer Nursing, 25*, 318-325.

Palliative care code. (1996). *JAMA, 276*(23), 1864.

Payne, S. A., Dean, S. J., & Kalus, C. (1998). A comparative study of death anxiety in hospice and emergency nurses. *Journal of Advanced Nursing, 28*, 700-706.

Pennebaker, J. W. (1993). Putting stress into words: Health, linguistic, and therapeutic implications. *Behavior Research & Therapy, 31*, 539-548.

Pennebaker, J. W. (1995). Emotion, disclosure and health: An overview. In J. W. Pennebaker (Ed.), *Emotion, disclosure, and health* (pp. 3-10). Washington, DC: American Psychological Association.

Pennebaker, J. W., & Beall, S. K. (1986). Confronting a traumatic event: Toward an understanding of inhibition and disease. *Journal of Abnormal Psychology, 95*, 274-281.

Pennebaker, J. W., Kiecolt-Glaser, J. K., & Glaser, R. (1988). Disclosure of traumas and immune function: Health implications for psychotherapy. *Journal of Counseling and Clinical Psychology, 56*, 239-245

Ragan, S. L., Mindt, T., & Wittenberg-Lyles, E. (2005). Narrative medicine and education in palliative care. In L. M. Harter, P. Japp, & C. S. Beck (Eds.), *Narratives, health, and healing: Communication theory, research, and practice* (pp. 259-276). Mahwah, NJ: Erlbaum.

Ragan, S. L., Wittenberg, E., & Hall, H. T. (2003) The communication of palliative care for the elderly cancer patient. *Health Communication, 15*, 219-226.

Vanderford, M. L., Jenks, E.G., & Sharf, B.F. (1997). Exploring patients' experiences as a primary source of meaning. *Health Communication, 9*, 13-26.

Von Gunten, C. F. (2002). Secondary and tertiary palliative care in US hospitals. *JAMA, 287*(7), 875-881.

Wolfe, J., Klar, N., Grier, H. E., Duncan, J., Salem-Schatz, S., Emanuel, E. J., & Weeks, J. C. (2000). Understanding of prognosis among parents of children who died of cancer: Impact on treatment goals and integration of palliative care. *JAMA, 284*(19), 2469-2475.

Yang, M., & Mcilfatrick, S. (2001). Intensive care nurses' experiences of caring for dying patients: A phenomenological study. *International Journal of Palliative Nursing, 7*, 435-441.

18 | Communication and Cancer Hospice Care

Toward Negotiating Attitudinal and Research Obstacles

Jim L. Query, Jr.
University of Houston

Kevin B. Wright
University of Oklahoma

Eileen S. Gilchrist
University of Oklahoma

Arguably, some of the most significant conversations in which individuals engage in during their lifetime will occur in a health context. Often, the first and final conversations that we experience are health-related. Across the life span, inevitably, most individuals will be compelled to make critical health care decisions, and the information on which those decisions are based stem from health information messages. As early as 1963, with the publication of a special issue of the *Journal of Communication* focusing on mental health and selected messages, communication scholars have recognized the inextricable association among health, health communication, and a wide array of health outcomes (for reviews, see Kreps, Bonaguro, & Query, 1998; Kreps & O'Hair, 1995; Kreps, O'Hair, & Clowers, 1994; Kreps, Query, & Bonaguro, in press). In the subsequent 40 years, the emerging field of health communication inquiry and theory has developed as a vibrant and important area of study focused on the roles performed by human and mediated communication in health care delivery and promotion (Kreps et al., 1998; Kreps et al., in press). In addition to now having two journals devoted to health communication inquiry—*Health Communication* and the *Journal of Health Communication: International Perspectives*—in 2004, health communication courses are now being offered at 77 universities and colleges across the United States (Query, Wright, Bylund, & Mattson, in press).

Despite a 5-year average survival rate for all cancers at 62% (ACS, 2003), the American Cancer Society (ACS) recently reported that about 556,500 individuals would die from cancer, or 1,500 per day (http://www.cancer.org/downloads/STT/CAFF2003PWSecured.pdf, p. 2). And it is this context, end-of-life (EOL) care, that has received scant attention in health communication inquiry and pedagogy, particularly communication issues related to the advanced stages of distinct cancer types and hospice care. As O'Hair et al. (2003) reported:

> Theoretically driven, empirical research is desperately needed in such postdiagnostic communication processes as survivorship, quality of life, palliative and hospice care, and loss, bereavement, and grief for those millions of people who have been diagnosed with the second leading cause of death in our nation. (p. 193)

The sparse communication-based research that does examine hospice interaction has assessed team member outcomes, volunteer outcomes, and communication practices (see Coopman, 2001; Coopman & Applegate, 2000; Egbert & Parrott, 2003; Zimmerman, 1994; Zimmerman & Applegate, 1992). What has been noticeably absent, however, is a systematic examination of interpersonal communication in providing cancer patients and their loved ones with social support (Kreps, 2003), especially in hospice contexts. To help provide a heuristic springboard for additional work in this challenging arena, this chapter provides a brief overview of Western views of death and dying, examines decision-making and referral processes; explains key definitions; offers a précis of the history of hospice care; assesses communication issues surrounding the caregiver–patient relationship and their implications for individuals with cancer and their caregivers; and identifies future research directions.

END-OF-LIFE CARE

Western Views and Impediments to Death and Dying

Death is an experience that all people share since the inception of time. Within medical institutions, the manner in which individuals succumb, however, is an evolving and changing process, made so by modern sterile environments and complex medical treatments. In many Western societies, despite the groundbreaking of work of Kubler-Ross (1969), discussing issues of death and dying among providers and patients still frequently creates powerful feelings such as rampant uncertainty and intense emotional discomfort. Wilkinson, Bailey, Aldridge, and Roberts (1999) aptly captured the nature of this fluid and arduous process: "Conversations with patients facing life-threatening illnesses are not easy, and the demands on health care professionals are immense as they endeavor to deliver care that meets the patients' differing physical and psychological needs" (p. 342). Another contributing factor to such emotionally laden and complex interaction resides in the advent of life-prolonging technology.

Randall and Downie (1996), for example, noted that medical technology has made it possible to prolong life far beyond the point at which death would naturally occur. In contemporary times, many individuals die at the time they do because technological interventions have been withheld, thereby "allowing" them to succumb to their illnesses, or "letting die." Advance directives, such as do not resuscitate orders, and health power of attorney designations can ensure that such decisions are consistent with the prior wishes of the dying persons.

The Choice Between Passing Away at a Traditional Health Care Facility or Home

Notwithstanding a century of unprecedented medical advancements, the overwhelming preference regarding EOL care is the desire of most patients with serious, incurable diseases to die at home, a death that has been associated with greater satisfaction by bereaved family members (Ratner, Norlander, & McSteen, 2001). Lynn (2001) poignantly described the import of a death with dignity: "most people want more than just longer life; they want the end of life to be meaningful, comfortable, and supportive to loved ones" (p. 926). A "driving force" that has enabled many individuals to realize a "good death" has been the increasing visibility, prevalence, and legitimatization of palliative and hospice care options.

Since the 1980s, palliative and hospice care have grown from alternative health care movements to accepted options within the U.S. health care system. The World Health Organization (WHO, 2002) defines *palliative care* as "an approach which improves the quality of life of patients and their families facing life-threatening illness, through the prevention, assessment and treatment of pain and other physical, psychosocial and spiritual problems." The U.S. Department of Health and Human Services defines *hospice* as "a public agency or private organization or subdivision of either of these that—is primarily engaged in providing care to terminally ill individuals." Ragan, Wittenberg, and Hall (2003) noted the difference between these two forms of care, "In contrast to hospice care, which precludes the use of any curative treatment at life's end stages, PC [palliative care] seeks primarily to comfort patients and to keep them pain free, yet it does not necessarily preclude medical treatment" (p. 219). Although hospice care is now widely accepted by the medical community and third-party payers, the option is underutilized. As Chen, Haley, Robinson, and Schonwetter (2003) reported:

> Despite the rapid growth in the number of hospice patients served and the acceptance of hospice as a legitimate healthcare provider for patients near the end of life, it was estimated that, of 2.4 million Americans who died in 2000, only one of every four was under hospice care at the time of death. (p. 789)

Hospice care is now facing several challenges, including stagnant referral patterns (Rhymes, 1990).

History of Hospice

Although there are records of hospices as early as the fourth century, Cicely Saunders' approach to care for the dying is regarded as the foundation of the modern hospice movement (Thoresen, 2003). In the 1940s, Saunders originally studied to be a nurse, but was motivated by the pain and loneliness of the dying to become a physician. In 1957, she began her first job as a physician investigating terminal pain and its relief. As a result of her ideas, strategies, alliances, team building, and compassion, in 1967, St. Christopher's Hospice was opened in Sydenham, London (Howarth & Leaman, 2001). In 1998, Saunders, who was nearly 80 years old, continued to work full-time as St. Christopher's chair (Moore, 1998). In 1974, hospice arrived in the United States with the opening of Hospice Inc. in Connecticut, a hospice home services-only organization. In 1975, the first modern use of the term, *palliative care*, occurred when Palliative Care Service began in Royal Victoria Hospital in Montreal to care for patients with advanced disease. Hospice Inc. opened its first residential unit in 1978.

The hospice movement and organizations that provide hospice care have grown exponentially since the late 1970s. As noted in the Medicare Payment Advisory Commission report to Congress (2002), Medicare hospice development and participation has grown, largely as a result of a 1989 Congressional mandate to increase reimbursement rates by 20% to organizations providing hospice care. The number of hospices participating in Medicare increased from 31 in 1984 to 2,273 in 2000. This number consisted of 739 home health agency-based hospices, 554 hospital-based hospices, 20 skilled nursing facility-based hospices, and 960 freestanding hospices. In 2000, Medicare hospices served 474,408 people with each person receiving an average of 47 days of care each. More than 90% of hospice care was provided in patients' homes and 78% of hospice care was for cancer patients (Moore, 1998). However, 30% of patients died within 1 week of admission when using Medicare, perhaps due to difficulty in accessing benefits. Hospice care providers often label this "brink-of-death" care, as compared to genuine EOL care (Nicoll, 2002). Such services are also pejoratively described as "drive-by-hospice care" because hospice team members often move from one patient to the next, rushing to complete visits, documentation, and follow-up only to learn of the death the next morning before "care" could be provided (see Nicoll, 2002).

In light of the preceding paradox—increasing institutional participation coupled with fleeting service provision—a "burning" question then surfaces: Who is being referred to hospice care? Hongbin, Haley, Robinson, and Schonwetter (2003) studied 234 adult patients diagnosed with advanced lung, breast, prostate, or colon cancer with a life expectancy of less than 1 year. Of the participants, 173 received hospice care and 61 received traditional hospital care. Assessing the demographic, clinical, and other patient-related characteristics, it was discovered that "patients receiving hospice care were significantly older (average age 69 vs. 65 years), less educated (average 11.9 vs. 12.9 years), and had more people in their households (average 1.66 vs. 1.16 persons)" (p. 789). Similar research compared 121 patients with cancer who were referred to hospice with 206 nonreferred patients (Grande, McKerral, & Todd, 2002). Their findings revealed that older patients and those with lower socioeconomic status were less likely to be referred. Another study of 352,000 cancer deaths in Nova Scotia between 1992 and 1997 showed similar findings (Burge, Johnston, Lawson, Dewar, & Cummings, 2002).

Who Decides?

Scant research has been conducted regarding why and how patients with terminal illness, such as cancer, make EOL decisions. Hines, Babrow, Badzek, and Moss (1997) defined EOL decisions as, "one in which a patient (or legally authorized surrogate) facing the progression of an incurable medical condition (a) refuses or consents to or (b) withdraws from or continues a life-sustaining treatment that may result in or perpetuate a significant reduction in the patient's quality of life" (p. 200).

Chen et al. (2003) noted that discussions regarding hospice care "often include such factors as perceptions of hospice as 'medical failure', denial by patients, families, and healthcare providers, poor communication about hospice options, and patient values" (p. 789). Lynn (2001) explained that "enrollment in a hospice program requires that decision-makers confront the prognosis and their uncertainties about it, consider the desirability of other services, recognize variations among available hospice programs, address financial issues, and weigh the distress of patients and loved ones at being labeled as 'dying'" (p. 925).

Is it then the patient who makes the decision to enter hospice? If a patient is unconscious, confused, or unable to assimilate information, then it is reasonable that the next of kin be given information to help make that decision. As alluded to previously, advance directives and health power of attorney assignments can aid in this decision-making process. Concerning "competent" and sapient patients, Wilkes (1984) found that many physicians frequently give information to family members first, even when patients are able to understand. This practice has raised some ethical issues when some relatives do not want that information shared with the patient. Competent and lucid patients are morally, ethically, and legally entitled to their medical information.

Physician Referral. Researchers estimate that between 15 and 16 million referrals are made each year in the U.S. health care system (Forrest & Reid, 1997). Referrals are made from one provider to another because providers have different areas of expertise, and because increasingly, specialized medical care has created segregated knowledge and procedures practiced by distinct types of providers (Anthony, 2003). Before the arrival of medical financial gatekeepers, such as managed care, insurance companies, primary care providers, and Medicare/Medicaid, physician referrals were primarily based on referral networks. The referring process has changed from a professional decision delivered via professional networks to a more bureaucratic process. Irrespective of restrictive changes, however, Anthony noted that physicians still "describe the process of making referrals as a two-part decision: (1) whether to refer, and (2) to whom to refer" (p. 2034).

Chen et al. (2003) conducted research between December 1995 and September 1997, that studied 173 hospice patients in Tampa, Florida. Findings of that research indicated that "the final decision to enter hospice was described as being made by families in more than 41% cases, followed by patients themselves (27.7%), and physicians (26.6%)" (p. 793). Navari (2000) surveyed 173 patients with advanced cancer, 7 to 10 days after they received a recommendation for palliative care only, without further interventional treatment. The results found only 27% of respondents chose hospice. Those who did choose hospice indicated that their decision was influenced by their physician (88%), their caregiver (47%), and knowledge of hospice programs (44%).

Describing a hospice referral conversation, Sawyers (2002) explained how after telling a young woman that no additional treatment would slow the growth of her cancer, the patient became distraught. The physician then suggested she bring her husband to the next visit so they could discuss her options. The third author recently discussed the hospice referral process with Dr. Russell Postier, a surgeon at the University of Oklahoma Health Science Center. Dr. Postier indicated that during the referral conversation, it was essential to have the decision maker present. He believed this role was not often held by the patient, but by one or two family members. Dr. Postier noted that he determined who the decision maker was by who the patient made the most eye contact with and then he would direct the majority of his comments to that person. He concluded that if the decision maker was absent when discussing hospice, the patient would rarely make the decision to accept the hospice referral. Although anecdotal, the preceding observation supports the role of family members as the decision makers when contemplating hospice use (personal communication).

Many of the elderly, who are disproportionately heavy users of health care, typically allow a companion to interact with their physicians (Beisecker, 1989). These companions are often family members who also serve as caregivers. Their presence in medical encounters may be necessary to comply with doctor's recommendations and to make decisions for the patient. Research conducted to determine the influence of a companion in elderly physician visits (Beisecker, 1989) found that 57% of the comments were exchanges between physician–patient, while physician–companion exchanges composed 38% of the interaction. This study found the companion to be most active during the history and feedback segments of the medical encounter, during which the companion directed more comments to the physician than the physician directed to the companion. The companion was categorized as playing one of three roles during the encounter: (a) the watchdog, who provided or elaborated on information shared by the patient and who obtained information from the physician; (b) the significant other, who provided the physician with information about his or her caregiving role; or (c) the surrogate patient, who assumed the patient's role by answering questions for and providing unrequested information about the patient's health, behavior, and/or emotions.

It was found that when companions acted as a significant other, physicians typically switched their focus from the patient and directed comments to the companion: "The companion indeed became the significant other for the doctor, and the doctor altered his or her behavior to acknowledge the presence of the companion" (Beisecker, 1989, p. 63). During interviews conducted after the medical encounters, patients and companions discussed their roles. Companions indicated that they spoke on behalf of patients due in part to patients' memory problems, or before the visit the patient had told the companion about the medical problem so that the companion could inform the physician. Several patients indicated that they were not comfortable discussing their medical problems with a physician and one patient indicated he/she did not wish to appear foolish to the physician. Summing up the study's findings, "the doctor can, and often does, alter his behavior to coincide with the expectations and behavior of the companion" (Beisecker, 1989, p. 66).

Chen et al. (2003) reported that more than half the participants in their study of the hospice referral process first learned about hospice services from their physicians. Although this information was usually discussed with others, nearly one third of patients did not have further discussions with anyone else before the decision was made. This high level is troubling when considered with Morrison, Morrison, and Glickman's (1994) findings that physicians identified barriers to communication about EOL care including discomfort talking about death and dying, lack of knowledge, difficulty determining appropriateness, and time constraints. Although access to inpatient hospice care for a large population of persons dying may be desirable, in terms of pain management for example, referral to hospice shortly before death often requires another site than what is preferred by the patient and/or their decision makers due in part to bed availability and other contextual constraints (Miller, Kinzbrunner, Pettit, & Williams, 2003).

McGorty and Bornstein (2003) reported that more than 90% of physicians are aware of hospice, yet only 75% of physicians discussed hospice options with patients. Concerning the latter group, only 75% of those doctors discussed hospice "selectively," noting that they waited until they thought their patients were prepared to accept such options. They cited the following reasons for lack of hospice care referrals: lack of experience with hospice; negative perceptions of hospice; uncomfortable communicating a poor prognosis; fear of losing control of patients' medical care; overestimating life expectancy, and complicated admission criteria.

HOSPICE CAREGIVER–PATIENT COMMUNICATION ISSUES

Role of Caregivers

Caregivers for individuals with cancer play an important role in hospice programs in terms of meeting patient needs (Andrews, 2001; Meyers & Gray, 2001; Siegel, Raveis, Houts, & More, 1991; Weitzner, McMillan, & Jacobson, 1999), and they often contend with a number of communication-related issues that have far-reaching implications for the physical and psychological well-being of patients and caregivers. According to Allen, Haley, Small, and McMillan (2002), "prior research suggests that the quality of communication among terminally ill individuals, their caregivers, and hospice staff influences patient and caregiver outcomes" (p. 508). Although some researchers have identified communication as an integral part of the process of providing hospice care (Bakas, Lewis, & Parsons, 2001; Martinez, 1996; Zamborsky, 1996), few studies have examined specific communication variables and how they may be related to health outcomes.

Some of the many responsibilities hospice patient caregivers must cope with include the following: (a) providing physical assistance and emotional support to patients, (b) being a liaison between patients and an interdisciplinary team of providers, (c) handling financial and social affairs for patients, and (d) monitoring and communicating symptoms for providers. These responsibilities present numerous and formidable communication challenges for caregivers of individuals with cancer enrolled in hospice programs, and we examine these in greater detail next.

Challenges of Providing Care and Caregiver Communication. Most primary caregivers for individuals with cancer are family members (even among patients enrolled in hospice programs) and many are ill-equipped to manage the physical and emotional stress of caregiving duties (Andrews, 2001; Rusinak & Murphy, 1995; Sarna & McCorkle, 1996). Although trained hospice workers provide support in terms of providing medical care and taking care of a variety of physical needs of patients, family caregivers must handle a variety of tasks, including providing emotional support, transportation, managing finances, monitoring symptoms, coordinating schedules, increased housework, as well as running errands, and caregiver burden has been found to increase as patients enter into later stages of the disease (Andrews, 2001; Laizner, Yost, Borg, & McCorkle, 1993). These activities, coupled with the stress of coming to grips with the imminent death of a loved one, can lead to physical and emotional exhaustion for many caregivers.

Although many hospice programs have made great efforts to target the needs of caregivers, most hospice and palliative care researchers have argued that more attention needs to address caregiver burden (Andrews, 2001; Bakas et al., 2001). Communication among the caregiver, his or her social network members, the hospice team, and patient may play a paramount role in helping the individual to cope effectively with the stress of caregiving. Unfortunately, however, caregivers for individuals with cancer often lack the diverse communication skills necessary to effectively meet the needs of the patient and their own needs (Andrews, 2001; Bakas et al., 2001). The caregivers communication competence may play an important role in terms of mobilizing social support from his or her social network.

For example, in a recent study, Query and Wright (2003) found that older adults with cancer and their caregivers with higher communication competence scores had lower perceived stress levels and higher satisfaction with their support networks than those individuals who had lower communication competence scores. This study supports Kreps' (1988a) relational health communication model, which argues that communication competence is the central variable in terms of influencing perceptions of social support and perceived stress. Although future intervention research is needed, communication competence training may help caregivers and individuals with cancer to better mobilize support from their social networks, and it could help to reduce caregiver stress. Key parts of Kreps' model have also been confirmed among nontraditional students, elders residing in retirement communities, and caregivers for individuals with Alzheimer's disease (Query & James, 1989; Query & Kreps, 1996; Query, Parry, & Flint, 1992).

Communication Issues Surrounding Symptom Management

Hospice researchers have found that caregivers and individuals with cancer influence each other through interaction in terms of psychological and physical outcomes. For example, several researchers have found a relationship between patient symptom distress and caregiver depression and/or perceptions of caregiver burden (Andrews, 2001; Foxall & Gaston-Johansson, 1996; B. Given, Given, Helms, Stommel, & DeVoss, 1997; Kurtz, Kurtz, Given, & Given, 1995; Sarna & Brecht, 1997). Increased patient symptom distress can increase the number of tasks in the hospice caregiver's daily schedule as well as add to his or her stress level. Although hospice care is typically provided by an interdisciplinary team that attempts to relieve symptom distress and promote quality of life, much of the day-to-day care burden falls on family caregivers. Individuals with cancer may experience a number of symptoms associated with the disease and its treatment, including pain (Allen et al., 2002; Donnelly, Walsh, & Rybicki, 1994), fatigue and dyspnea (Nail, 2002). According to Bakas et al. (2001), "family caregivers must be able to not only recognize these symptoms, but also assist patients in managing them" (p. 849).

The need to alleviate pain is a common aspect of caring for individuals with cancer (Brescia, Portenoy, Ryan, Krasnoff, & Gray, 1992). However, adequate pain relief among hospice patients with cancer has been found to be a significant problem across studies (McMillan, 1996), and many of the problems related to pain control are associated with communication issues experienced by the patient or between patients and caregivers (Panke, 2002). According to Allen et al. (2002), "the treatment of pain is a primary goal of hospice care, but enactment of this goal can be complicated by communication breakdown between care recipients, caregivers, and hospice staff" (p. 512). For instance, the inability of some hospice patients to provide caregivers with verbal cues, such as the ability to verbally report pain in late stages of cancer, or the difficulty that caregivers may have interpreting nonverbal or behavioral cues that a patient is in pain, can lead to situations where individuals with cancer are not receiving adequate pain relief (Panke, 2002).

Pain is a multidimensional concept that is experienced distinctly, and often idiosyncratically, by individuals and cultures. Varying experiences and perceptions of pain often increase the difficulty for individuals with cancer and caregivers to assess the degree to which people are in pain and how pain should be treated. According to Panke (2002), "patients who aren't able to communicate verbally are at risk for underassessment and inadequate pain relief, those at highest risk being patients with cognitive impairment, intubated patients, infants, and patients older than 85" (p. 28). Verbal and nonverbal communication play a pivotal role in the assessment and control of pain. And most studies have concluded self-reports of pain are the most reliable indicator of the pain a terminally ill patient is experiencing. According to Allen et al., (2002), "the presence of cognitive and sensory deficits, however, may hamper an individual's ability to communicate painful experiences" (p. 508). In addition, the authors reported, "given that cognitive functioning and gender differences may affect a person's self-report of pain, caregivers are commonly used as proxies for obtaining pain reports in clinical settings" (p. 508). Despite caregivers commonly acting as liaisons between patients and hospice staff in terms of reporting pain, family caregiver reports of pain tend to have a low correspondence with patient self-reports (Allen et al., 2002; Elliot, Elliot, Murray, Braun, & Johnson, 1996). Nonverbal and behavioral cues indicating pain are often used by caregivers as a sign of whether to increase pain medications; however, it can be difficult for caregivers and hospice staff to "recognize that a particular behavior indicates pain, especially if they are unfamiliar with how the patient usually behaves" (Panke, 2002, p. 28).

Family caregivers are important sources of information about patient behaviors, and they are often crucial in terms of communicating information about pain to hospice staff and other providers. Effective assessment of pain is imperative in terms of its control, and information about pain needs to be effectively communicated to achieve the balance among adequate pain control and over- or undermedication (Panke, 2002). Overmedicating patients can lead to numerous problems, such as the accumulation of toxins associated with pain medications, renal dysfunction, decreased cognitive functioning, and organ failure. Undermedication can lead to inadequate pain control and unnecessary suffering for patients.

Communication Problems Associated With Caregiving

Willingness to Communicate Concerns. Many family caregivers are reluctant to communicate problems they encounter during the caregiving process to the people they are caring for, or others within their social network, because they do not want to burden them with the added stress of thinking about these concerns (Bakas et al., 2001; Laizner et al., 1993). This finding is consistent with other research on social support and caregivers that has found that family member caregivers often avoid communicating about their problems with others as they do not want to overstep interpersonal boundaries, or add stress to lives of others by raising concerns about caregiving (Chesler & Barbarin, 1984; Flint, Query, & Parrish, 2005; Query & Flint, 1996).

By not communicating their concerns to others, however, caregivers do not give themselves the opportunity to vent their frustrations or to receive advice or other offers of assistance from their social network. In addition, professional hospice staff may experience stress due to the caregiving process, but they often lack the resources to talk about their concerns (Zamborsky, 1996). Caregivers may experience added stress when they do not have the opportunity to express their concerns, and this deficit can lead to depression, burnout, anxiety, social withdrawal, and reduced quality of life (Bakas et al., 2001; C. Given et al., 1993). In addition, according to Bakas et al. (2001), "the reluctance of caregivers to communicate their needs and concerns may also affect their ability to provide care" (p. 847). As a result, patients and caregivers may be negatively affected by the caregiver's reluctance to communicate his or her needs and concerns.

Communication of Emotional Support. Researchers have found that the provision of emotional support is one of the most time-consuming and challenging aspects of caring for hospice patients, often requiring more of a caregiver's time and effort than other daily caregiving tasks (Bakas et al., 2001; Carey, Oberst, McCubbin, & Hughes, 1991; Toseland, Blanchard, & McCallion, 1995). This result has been found to apply to both lay caregivers and professional hospice staff. According to Andrews (2001), "because the caregiver is the center of support for the needs of the patient with cancer, if the caregiver fails, the patient suffers" (p. 1469). Given the high uncertainty and pervasive fear associated with coming to terms with one's own mortality among individuals with cancer, it is not surprising that emotional support is a common need among hospice patients. Listening to patient concerns and providing empathic responses to patients is a hallmark of providing holistic hospice care, however, it can be very time consuming for caregivers (professional and family), especially when faced with accomplishing multiple tasks while providing daily care to patients. Patient irritability, confusion, and aggressive behaviors during late-stage cancer may make it even more difficult and exhausting for caregivers to provide emotional support. Moreover, professional hospice staff and family caregivers often have little training regarding providing emotional support, and there is a need for education and training about how to recognize, manage, and cope with these issues to effectively provide emotional support (Bakas et al., 2001).

SPECIAL ISSUES AND FUTURE RESEARCH DIRECTIONS

Internet Sources and Hospice Organizations

Families and loved ones of patients needing hospice services, as well as patients, often turn to the Internet and hospice organizations for information. The overwhelming growth of the Internet and hospice programs in the past decade has lead to the creation of numerous Web sites and organizations designed to provide information and support for hospice patients, their families, caregivers, and health professionals. The appendix provides a list of several examples of these organizations and their corresponding Web sites.

Researching Difficulties

As has been well established, the goal of EOL care is to meet the physical, emotional, and spiritual needs of patients facing a terminal prognosis. The question must then be asked if it is morally ethical to research that population. Adelman and Frey (2001), as well as Frey (2004) confronted such issues arguing for a balancing of interests and compassion. Robbins (1998) asked the following questions: Will research determine whether those patients who receive palliative care experience a "better" death than those who do not? And perhaps more importantly, Who defines a "good death" and how different is that definition for each individual? As is true for much of communication research, EOL care studies are often of a qualitative nature, whereas health care providers typically want "numbers" to determine effectiveness of treatments. As the outcome—death—will be the same for all EOL care patients, research must address if quality of life is improved by palliative care. Because patients most often receive palliative care for such a limited number of days and often while experiencing debilitating symptoms and distress, it becomes even more imperative that scholars use great prudence in establishing research agendas and methods.

Children

The death rate of children has fallen considerably since the turn of the century when influenza and pneumonia were the leading causes of death. In the case of childhood cancer, although these are generally rare, the ACS estimated that some 9,000 children between the ages of 0 and 14 would die in 2003 (http://www.cancer.org/downloads/STT/CAFF2003PWSecured.pdf, p. 10). The ACS (2003) also stated that notwithstanding its relative infrequency, "cancer is the chief cause of death by disease in children between ages 1–14" (http://www.cancer.org/downloads/STT/CAFF2003PWSecured.pdf, p. 10).

Relative to hospice care, the Institute of Medicine (2003) reported that although a number of children's hospitals have palliative care or hospice programs, it is often assumed that parents will provide most care at home for dying children. Because causes of death in children are often different from the causes of death in adults, palliative care guidelines that are appropriate for adults are often inappropriate for children.

When inpatient EOL care is required or requested for pediatric patients, one objective noted by the Institute of Medicine is rooms with home-like features. Although these rooms may be equipped with medical devices, the focus of service and environment should be on peace and comfort. The American Academy of Pediatrics (2000) reported the following:

> in addition to alleviating pain and other physical symptoms, physicians must provide access to therapies that are likely to improve the child's quality of life. Such therapies may include education, grief and family counseling, peer support, music therapy, child life intervention or spiritual support for both the patient and siblings, and appropriate respite care. (p. 351)

Clearly, the physician referral process is fundamental to providing these services to perhaps the most tender and vulnerable of EOL patients.

Cultural differences

Cultural experience has a significant impact on the ways individuals experience, react to, and interpret health care delivery, including death and the process leading to a long-term illness death (Geist-Martin, Ray, & Sharf, 2003; Kreps & Kunimoto, 1994). Most of the EOL care literature was based in the United Kingdom as hospice originated there. Although researchers in the United States have finally begun to conduct EOL studies, the literature regarding hospice care for those of other cultural backgrounds is almost nonexistent. One study of Chinese hospice care (Smith & Smith, 1999) provided a narrative approach to experiences by patients and nurses in a Hong Kong hospice and concluded that hospice in China is considered a place to rest rather than to die. Because cultural populations vary, EOL care also needs to be researched from varying cultural perspectives. Poulson (1998) identified several salient cultural issues to be considered, including the possible need for translators, varying religious traditions, differing communication patterns, diverse social customs, familial hierarchies, and death rituals. Also related to cultural differences is the lack of research of minorities' experiences with EOL care. Karim, Bailey, and Tunna (2000) found that Black/minority ethnic populations are referred to hospice less often than White populations. In the study, many physicians stated that they believed minority families preferred to provide palliative care for their ill family members; yet, they also conceded that this impression was not based on any empirical basis.

Theory-Based Research

Few theory-based studies have been conducted regarding physician referrals in general, and to hospice care in particular (O'Hair et al., 2003). Problematic integration (PI) is one theory that has been used. PI is based on the underlying premises that human experience is shaped and forged by probability estimates of risk, value orientations concerning desired levels of uncertainty, and that these orientations are inextricably tied to decision-making and interaction patterns (Babrow, Hines, & Kasch, 2000). The theory further explains that integration can be problematic when expectations and desire conflict: "The theory of problematic integration (PI) suggests that illness is essentially the ongoing experience of interwoven problematic integrations and that communication is essential to the experience of illness, for patients, friends and loved one, and health care providers" (Brashers & Babrow, 1996, p. 246).

PI theory has also been employed to research how decisions are made by and for elderly patients near death (Hines, Babrow, Badzek, & Moss, 1997, 2001). In particular, examining the communication between dialysis patients and unit nurses revealed that patients sought information that enabled them to cope with treatment rather than information that nurses thought was critical to the patients' ability to make decisions about whether to continue treatment. Hines (2001) further developed PI theory by suggesting that it be used in an effort to improve communication about EOL issues to ensure that patient's EOL preferences are expressed, understood, and respected.

It also seems that communication accommodation theory (CAT) can be used to study the physician referral process. CAT states that when engaged in a conversation, people modify their communication to either increase or decrease the differences between themselves and their conversational partner. CAT provides a theoretical framework to study the role of this cognitive process (Hummert, Shaner, & Garstka, 1995). The original aim of CAT was to specify the attuning processes of convergence and divergence. A third process has since been added to account for linguistic maintenance (Coupland, Coupland, & Giles, 1991). CAT is a vibrant theory in the study of health communication in general, and in particular, within the context of elderly populations. Moreover, CAT is essential to understanding elderly health processes as attuning is a core component of many supportive encounters (Williams, Giles, Coupland, Dalby, & Manasse, 1990).

Based on previous CAT research and the literature regarding physicians, the referral process, and hospice care, future research can address questions such as: To what extent will physicians assume the patient lacks the ability to comprehend effectively and therefore use interpretability (i.e., speaking louder or slower, when addressing the patient but not when addressing the companion/decision maker)? To what degree will physicians overaccommodate by using patronizing speech when talking to patients based on a stereotypically notions of a "dying person"? To what degree will physicians underaccommodate patients to avoid addressing them directly and instead communicate primarily with companions/decision makers? To what extent do companions participate in the communication process during the referral discussion? What percentage of companions' comments are directed toward the physician and patient? What percentage of comments is directed to the companions, by the physician and by the patient?

The Institute of Medicine (2003) noted the following challenges in researching this rightfully protected population: (a) obtaining information from the perspective of the person dying, their loved ones, and health providers; (b) coping with the variations in the quality of existing data; (c) coping with the difficulties in collecting data from dying people and their loved ones; (d) characterizing the quality of EOL care; and (e) defining the period to be considered "end of life."

SUMMARY

Although this population may seem to pose insurmountable obstacles precluding health communication research, health communication researchers have a moral and ethical imperative to assist the dying, their family members, and their professional caregivers to the best of our abilities. The prognosis cannot be altered by such research; however, caring, well-trained, and empathic health communication scholars can help facilitate the final journey that all of us will ultimately experience. Such a lofty goal can only be achieved through rigorous, sensitive, and empowering research designs that have the potential to inform health care policies, practices, and interventions, as well as provide a catalyst for the development of training programs that address pressing social, health-related problems (Kreps, 1989).

Many individuals will die from the degenerating consequences of chronic disease (Lynn, 2000). And most types of cancer are chronic, although all are not fatal, especially if caught early in stage I or II. Death is not an easy subject for most people to discuss, yet the uncertainties of death demand sensitive and caring communication (Kreps, 1988b). A recent survey found that 93% of Americans believe improving EOL care is important. EOL care and its planning by healthcare providers, patients and their families, as well as loved ones present pressing social, legal and ethical issues. Hopefully, this chapter serves to help others contemplate and address some of these "thorny" issues in subsequent investigations.

APPENDIX

http://www.acponline.org/public/h_care/: American College of Physicians Home Care Guide for Advanced Cancer
This guide is for the family, friends, and hospice workers caring for those patients with advanced cancer who are living at home. It provides the information they need to deal with caregiving problems while working cooperatively with a team of health professionals, such as nurses, physicians, and social workers who are members of a hospice, home health, or oncology care team.

http://www.lastacts.org/: Last Acts
Last Acts is a campaign to improve end-of-life care by a coalition of professional and consumer organizations. Last Acts believes in palliative care, focused on managing pain and making life better for individuals and families facing death. Last Acts envisions a world in which dying people and their loved ones receive excellent care and are honored and supported by their community. This site is for professionals and volunteers working to improve care of the dying.

http://www.aahpm.org/: American Academy of Hospice and Palliative Medicine (AAHPM)
AAHPM is an organization of physicians and other medical professionals dedicated to excellence in palliative medicine, the prevention and relief of suffering among patients and families by providing education and clinical practice standards, fostering research, facilitating personal and professional development of its members, and public policy advocacy.

http://www.growthhouse.org/: Growth House
Growth House provides a portal or international gateway to resources for life-threatening illness and end-of-life care. Its primary mission is to improve the quality of compassionate care for people who are dying through public education and global professional collaboration.

http://www.hospicefoundation.org/: Hospice Foundation of America
This is a not-for-profit organization that provides leadership in the development and application of hospice and its philosophy of care. Through programs of professional development, research, public education and information, Hospice Foundation of America assists those who cope either personally or professionally with terminal illness, death, and the process of grief.

http://www.hpna.org/: Hospice and Palliative Nurse Association (HPNA)
The purpose of the HPNA is to exchange information, experiences, and ideas; to promote understanding of the specialties of hospice and palliative nursing; and to study and promote hospice and palliative nursing research.

http://www.nhpco.org/templates/1/homepage.cfm: The National Hospice and Palliative Care Organization (NHPCO)
NHPCO is the largest nonprofit membership organization representing hospice and palliative care programs and professionals in the United States. The organization is committed to improving end-of-life care and expanding access to hospice care with the goal of profoundly enhancing quality of life for people dying in America and their loved ones.

http://www.hospiceinfo.org/: The National Hospice Foundation (NHF)
NHF is a charitable organization created in 1992 to broaden America's understanding of hospice through research and education. Its mission is to expand America's vision for end-of-life care. In doing so, it engages and informs the public about the quality end-of-life care that hospice provides.

http://www.capcmssm.org/: The Center to Advance Palliative Care (CAPC)
CAPC is dedicated to increasing the availability of quality palliative care services in hospitals and other health care settings for people with life-threatening illnesses, their families, and caregivers. A national initiative supported by the Robert Wood Johnson Foundatic:, with direction and technical assistance provided by the Mount Sinai School of Medicine (NY), CAPC provides health care professionals with the tools, training, and technical assistance necessary to start and sustain successful palliative care programs.

http://www.hospicenet.org/: Hospice Net
Hospice Net provides information and support to patients and families facing life-threatening illnesses. Hospice Net is an independent, nonprofit organization working exclusively through the Internet.

http://www.abhpm.org/: The American Board of Hospice and Palliative Medicine (ABHPM)
ABHPM was formed in 1995 to establish and implement standards for the certification of physicians practicing hospice and palliative medicine. ABHPM creates and administers the certifying examination, works to implement high standards for training, and contributes to setting the standards for excellence in palliative medicine.

http://www.abcd-caring.com: Americans for Better Care of the Dying (ABCD)
ABCD is a Washington, DC-based organization dedicated to ensuring that all Americans can count on good end of life care. Its goals are to build momentum for reform, explore new methods and systems for delivering care, and shape public policy through evidence-based understanding. ABCD aims to accomplish these goals by focusing its efforts on fundamental reforms; such as, improved pain management, better financial reimbursement systems, enhanced continuity of care, support for family caregivers, and changes in public policy.

http://www.compassionindying.org: Compassion in Dying Federation
This Group provides national leadership for client service, legal advocacy, and public education to improve pain and symptom management, increase patient empowerment and self-determination and expand end-of-life choices to include aid-in-dying for terminally ill, mentally competent adults.

http://www.npha.org: The National Prison Hospice Association
This organization promotes hospice care for terminally ill prisoners. Its purpose is to assist corrections and hospice professionals in their continuing efforts to develop high-quality patient care procedures and management programs. The group provides a network for the exchange of information between corrections facilities, community hospices, and other agencies about existing programs, best practices, and new developments in the prison hospice field.

http://www.hospiceweb.com: Hospice Web
Hospice Web provides a link to general hospice Web sites as well as state-specific hospice care providers.

REFERENCES

Adelman, M. B., & Frey, L. R. (2001). Untold tales from the field: Living the autoethnographic life in an AIDS residence. In S. L. Herndon & G. L. Kreps (Eds.), *Qualitative research: Applications in organizational life* (2nd ed., pp. 205-226). Cresskill, NJ: Hampton Press.
Allen, R. S., Haley, W. E., Small, B. J., & McMillan, S. C. (2002). Pain reports by older hospice cancer patients and family caregivers: The role of cognitive functioning. *The Gerontologist, 42,* 507-514.
American Academy of Pediatrics. (2000). Palliative care for children. *Pediatrics, 106*(2), 351-357.

American Cancer Society. (2003). Cancer facts and figures, 2003. Available at http://www.cancer.org/downloads/STT/CAFF2003PWSecured.pdf. Accessed March 22, 2004.

Andrews, S. C. (2001). Caregiver burden and symptom distress in people with cancer receiving hospice care. *Oncology Nursing Forum, 28,* 1469-1474.

Anthony, D. (2003). Changing the nature of physician referral relationships in the US: The impact of managed care. *Social Science and Medicine, 56,* 2033-2044.

Babrow, A. S., Hines, S. C., & Kasch, C. R. (2000). Managing uncertainty in illness explanations: An application of problematic integration theory. In B. B. Whaley (Ed.), *Explaining illness: Research, theory, and strategies* (pp. 41-67). Mahwah, NJ: Erlbaum.

Bakas, T., Lewis, R. R., & Parsons, J. (2001). Caregiving tasks among family caregivers of patients with lung cancer. *Oncology Nursing Forum, 28,* 847-854.

Beisecker, A. E. (1989). The influence of a companion on the doctor-elderly patient interaction. *Health Communication, 1*(1), 55-70.

Brashers, D. E., & Babrow, A. S. (1996). Theorizing communication and health. *Communication Studies, 47*(3), 243-251.

Brescia, F. J., Portenoy, R. K., Ryan, M., Krasnoff, L., & Gray, G. (1992). Pain, opioid use, and survival in hospitalized patients with advanced cancer. *Journal of Clinical Oncology, 10,* 149-155.

Burge, F., Johnston, G., Lawson, B., Dewar, R., & Cummings, I. (2002). Population-based trends in referral of the elderly to a comprehensive palliative care programme. *Palliative Medicine, 16,* 255-256.

Carey, P. J., Oberst, M. T., McCubbin, M. A., & Hughes, S. H. (1991). Appraisal and caregiving burden in family members caring for patients receiving chemotherapy. *Oncology Nursing Forum, 18,* 1341-1348.

Chen, H., Haley, W. E., Robinson, B. E., & Schonwetter, R. S. (2003). Decisions for hospice care in patients with advanced cancer. *Journal of the American Geriatrics Society, 51*(6), 789-797.

Chesler, M. A., & Barbarin, O. A. (1984). Difficulties of providing help in a crisis: Relationships between parents of children with cancer and their friends. *Journal of Social Issues, 40,* 113-134.

Coopman, S. (2001). Democracy, performance and outcomes in interdisciplinary health care teams. *Journal of Business Communication, 38,* 261-284.

Coopman, S., & Applegate, J. (2000). Social-cognitive influences on the use of persuasive message strategies among health care team members. *American Communication Journal, 3(2)*. Available at www.acjournal.org.

Coupland, N., Coupland, J., & Giles, H. (1991). *Language, society and the elderly: Discourse, identity and aging.* Oxford, UK: Blackwell.

Donnelly, S., Walsh, D., & Rybicki, L. (1994). The symptoms of advanced cancer in 1,000 patients. *Journal of Palliative Care, 10,* 57.

Egbert, N., & Parrott, R. (2003). Empathy and social support for the terminally ill: Implications for recruiting and retaining hospice and hospital volunteers. *Communication Studies, 54,* 18-34.

Elliot, B. A., Elliot, T. E., Murray, D. M., Braun, B. L., & Johnson, K. M. (1996). Patients and family members: The role of knowledge and attitudes in cancer pain. *Journal of Pain and Symptom Management, 12,* 209-220.

Flint, L. J., Query, J. L., & Parrish, A. (2005). Negotiating communication obstacles while experiencing Alzheimer's disease: The case of one family. In E. B. Ray (Ed.), *Case studies in health communication* (2nd ed.). Mahwah, NJ: Erlbaum.

Forrest, C., & Reid, R. (1997). Passing the baton: HMOs' influence on referrals to specialty care. *Health Affairs, 16*(6), 157-162.

Foxall, M. J., & Gaston-Johansson, F. (1996). Burden and health outcomes of family caregivers of hospitalized bone marrow transplant patients. *Journal of Advanced Nursing, 24,* 915-923.

Frey, L. R. (2004, April). *Researcher greed: The difficulties of dialoguing about death.* Paper presented at the annual conference of the Central States Communication Association, Cleveland, OH.

Geist-Martin, P., Ray, E. B., & Sharf, B. F. (2003). *Communicating health: Personal, cultural, and political complexities.* Belmont, CA: Wadsworth.

Given, B. A., Given, C. W., Helms, E., Stommel, M., & DeVoss, D. N. (1997). Determinants of family caregiver reaction: New and recurrent cancer. *Cancer Practice, 5,* 17-24.

Given, C. W., Stommel, M., Given, B., Osuch, J., Kurtz, M. E., & Kurtz, J. C. (1993). The influence of cancer patients' symptoms and functional states on patients' depression and family caregivers' reaction and depression. *Health Psychology, 19,* 771-777.

Grande, G. E., McKerral, A., & Todd, C. J. (2002). Which cancer patients are referred to hospital at home for palliative care? *Palliative Medicine, 16,* 115-123.

Hines, S. C. (2001). Coping with uncertainties in advance care planning. *Journal of Communication, 51*(3), 498-513.

Hines, S. C., Babrow, A. S., Badzek, L., & Moss, A. H. (1997). Communication and problematic integration in end-of-life decisions: Dialysis decisions among the elderly. *Health Communication, 9,* 199-217.

Hines, S. C., Babrow, A. S., Badzek, L., & Moss, A. H. (2001). From coping with life to coping with death: Problematic integration for the seriously ill elderly. *Health Communication, 13*(3), 327-342.

Hongbin, C., Haley, W. E., Robinson, B. E., & Schonwetter, R. S. (2003). Decisions for hospice care in patients with advanced cancer. *Journal of the American Geriatrics Society, 51*(6), 789-799

Howarth, G., & Leaman, O. (Eds.). (2001). *Encyclopedia of death and dying.* London: Routledge.

Hummert, M. L., Shaner, J. L., & Gartska, T. A. (1995). Cognitive processes affecting communication with older adults: The case for stereotypes, attitudes, and beliefs about communication. In J. F. Nussbaum & J. Coupland (Eds.), *Handbook of communication and aging research* (pp. 105-131). Mahwah, NJ: Erlbaum.

Institute of Medicine. (2003). *When children die: Improving palliative and end-of-life care for children and their families.* Washington, DC: The National Academies Press.

Karim, K., Bailey, M., & Tunna, K. (2000). Nonwhite ethnicity and the provision of specialist palliative care services: Factors affecting doctors' referral patterns. *Palliative Medicine, 14,* 471-478.

Kreps, G. L. (1988a). Communicating about death. *Journal of Communication Therapy, 4,* 2-13.

Kreps, G. L. (1988b). Relational communication in health care. *Southern Speech Communication Journal, 53,* 344-359.

Kreps, G. L. (1989). Setting the agenda for health communication research and development: Scholarship that can make a difference. *Health Communication, 1*(1), 11-15.

Kreps, G. L. (2003). Opportunities for health communication scholarship to shape public health policy and practice: Examples from the National Cancer Institute. In T. L. Thompson, A. M. Dorsey, K. I. Miller, & R. Parrott (Eds.), *Handbook of health communication* (pp. 609-624). Mahwah, NJ: Erlbaum.

Kreps, G. L., Bonaguro, E. W., & Query, J. L. (1998). The history and development of the field of health communication. In L. D. Jackson & B. K. Duffy (Eds.), *Health communication research: A guide to developments and directions* (pp. 1-15). Westport, CT: Greenwood Press.

Kreps, G. L., & Kunimoto, E. (1994). *Effective communication in multicultural health care settings.* Newbury Park, CA: Sage.

Kreps, G. L., & O'Hair, D. (Eds.). (1995). *Communication and health outcomes.* Cresskill, NJ: Hampton Press.

Kreps, G. L., O'Hair, D., & Clowers, M. (1994). The influence of human communication on health care outcomes. *American Behavioral Scientist, 38,* 248-256.

Kreps, G. L, Query, J. L., & Bonaguro, E. W. (in press). The interdisciplinary study of health communication and its relationship to communication science. In A. Schorr (Ed.), *Gesundheits-Kommunikation* [Health communication]. Göttingen, Germany: Hogrefe-Huber Publishers.

Kubler-Ross, E. (1969). *On death and dying.* New York: Collier Books, MacMillan.

Kurtz, M. E., Kurtz, J. C., Given, C. W., & Given, B. (1995). Relationship of caregiver reactions and depression to cancer patients' symptoms, functional states, and depression—a longitudinal view. *Social Science and Medicine, 40,* 837-846.

Laizner, A. M., Yost, L. M., Borg, F. K., & McCorkle, R. (1993). Needs of family caregivers of persons with cancer: A review. *Seminars in Oncology Nursing, 9,* 114-120.

Lynn, J. (2000). Learning to care for people with chronic illness facing the end of life. *Journal of the American Medical Association, 284*(19), 2508-2511.

Lynn, J. (2001). Serving patients who may die soon and their families: The role of hospice and other services. *Journal of the American Medical Association, 285*(7), 925-932.

Martinez, J. M. (1996). The interdisciplinary team. In D. C. Sheehan & W. B. Forman (Eds.), *Hospice and palliative care: Concepts and practices* (pp. 21-29). Sudbury, MA: Jones & Bartlett.

McGorty, E. K., & Bornstein, B. H. (2003). Barriers to physicians' decisions to discuss hospice: Insights gained from the United States hospice model. *Journal of Evaluation in Clinical Practice, 9*(3), 363-372.

McMillan, S. C. (1996). Pain and pain relief experienced by hospice patients with cancer. *Cancer Nursing, 19*(4), 298-307.

Medicare Payment Advisory Commission. (2002). Report to the Congress: Medicare beneficiaries access to hospice. Accessed December 7, 2003, from http://www.medpac.gov/publications/congressional_reports/may 2002_HospiceAccess.pdf.

Meyers, J. L., & Gray, L. N. (2001). The relationships between family primary caregiver characteristics and satisfaction with hospice care, quality of life, and burden. *Oncology Nursing Forum, 28,* 73-82.

Miller, S. C., Kinzbrunner, B., Pettit, P., & Williams, J.R. (2003). How does the timing of hospice referral influence hospice care in the last days of life? *Journal of the American Geriatrics Society, 51,* 798-806.

Moore, A. (1998). Hospice care hijacked? *Christianity Today, 42*(3), 38-41.

Morrison, R. S., Morrison, E. W., & Glickman, D. F. (1994). Physician reluctance to discuss advance directives. *Archives of Internal Medicine, 154,* 2311-2318.

Nail, L. M. (2002). Fatigue in patients with cancer. *Oncology Nursing Forum, 29,* 537-546.

Navari, R. M. (2000). Preferences of patients with advanced cancer for hospice care. *Journal of the American Medical Association, 284*(19), 2449.

Nicoll, L. H. (2002). When there's little time left. *Journal of Hospice and Palliative Nursing, 4*(1), 4-5.

O'Hair, D. et al., (2003). Cancer survivorship and agency model: Implications for patient choice, decision making, and influence. *Health Communication, 15,* 193-202.

Panke, J. T. (2002). Difficulties in managing pain at the end of life. *American Journal of Nursing, 102,* 26-33.

Poulson, J. (1998). Impact of cultural differences in care of the terminally ill. In N. MacDonald (Ed.), *Palliative medicine: A case-based manual* (pp. 244-252). New York: Oxford University Press.

Query, J. L., & Flint, L. J. (1996). The caregiving relationship. In N. Vanzetti & S. Duck (Eds.), *A lifetime of relationships* (pp. 455-483). Pacific Grove, CA: Brooks/Cole.

Query, J. L., & James, A. C. (1989). The relationship between interpersonal communication competence and social support among elderly support groups in retirement communities. *Health Communication, 1(3),* 165-184.

Query, J. L., & Kreps, G. L. (1996). Testing a health communication model among caregivers for individuals with Alzheimer's disease. *Journal of Health Psychology, 1(3),* 335-351.

Query, J. L., Parry, D., & Flint, L. J. (1992). The relationship among social support, communication competence, and cognitive depression for non-traditional students. *Journal of Applied Communication Research, 20(1),* 78-94.

Query, J. L., & Wright, K. B. (2003). Assessing communication competence in an on-line study: Toward informing subsequent interventions among older adults with cancer, their lay caregivers, and peers. *Health Communication, 15,* 205-219.

Query, J. L., Wright, K. B., Bylund, C., & Mattson, M. (in press). Health communication instruction: Towards identifying common learning goals, course content, and pedagogical strategies. *Health Communication.*

Ragan, S. L., Wittenberg, E., & Hall, H. T. (2003). The communication of palliative care for the elderly cancer patient. *Health Communication, 15,* 219-226.

Randall, F., & Downie, R. S. (1996). *Palliative care ethics: A good companion.* New York: Oxford University Press.

Ratner, E., Norlander, L., & McSteen, K. (2001). Death at home following a targeted advanced-care planning process at home: The kitchen table discussion. *Journal of the American Geriatrics Society, 49,* 778-781.

Robbins, M. (1998). *Evaluating palliative care: Establishing the evidence base.* New York: Oxford University Press.

Rhymes, J. (1990). Hospice care in America. *Journal of the American Medical Association, 264*(3), 369-372.

Rusinak, R. L., & Murphy, J. F. (1995). Elderly spousal caregivers: Knowledge of cancer care, perceptions of preparedness, and coping strategies. *Journal of Gerontological Nursing, 21,* 33-41.

Sarna, L., & Brecht, M. (1997). Dimensions of symptom distress in women with advanced lung cancer: A factor analysis. *Heart and Lung, 26,* 23-30.

Sarna, L., & McCorkle, R. (1996). Burden of care and lung cancer. *Cancer Practice, 4,* 245-251.

Sawyers, M. (2002). Care, not cure: What to say when treatment fails. *Journal of Hospice and Palliative Nursing, 4*(3), 133-134.

Siegel, K., Raveis, V. H., Houts, P., & More, V. (1991). Caregiver burden and unmet patient needs. *Cancer, 68,* 1131-1140.

Smith., S. J., & Smith, D. J. (1999). Evaluating Chinese hospice care. *Health Communication, 11*(3), 223-235.

Thoresen, L. (2003). A reflection of Cicely Saunders' views of a good death through the philosophy of Charles Taylor. *International Journal of Palliative Nursing, 9*(1), 19-23.

Toseland, R. W., Blanchard, C. G., & McCallion, P. (1995). A problem solving intervention for caregivers of cancer patients. *Social Science in Medicine, 40,* 517-528.

U.S. Department of Health and Human Services. (2000). Hospice care. Retrieved November 24, 2003, from http://www.access.gpo.gov/nara/crf/waisidx_00/42cfr418_00.html

Weitzner, M. A., McMillan, S. C., & Jacobson, P. B. (1999). Family caregiver quality of life: Differences between curative and palliative cancer treatment settings. *Journal of Pain and Symptom Management, 17,* 418-428.

Wilkes, E. (1984). Dying now. *Lancet, 1*(8383), 950-952.

Wilkinson, S., Bailey, K., Aldridge, J., & Roberts, A. (1999). A longitudinal evaluation of a communication skills programme. *Palliative Medicine, 13,* 341-348.

Williams, A., Giles, H., Coupland, N., Dalby, M., & Manasse, H. (1990). The communicative contexts of elderly social support and health: A theoretical model. *Health Communication, 2*(3), 123-143.

World Health Organization. (2002). Palliative care: What is it? Retrieved November 24, 2003, from http://www.who.int/hiv/topics/palliative/PalliativeCare/en/

Zamborsky, L. J. (1996). Support groups for hospice staff. In D. C. Sheehan & W. B. Forman (Eds.), *Hospice and palliative care: Concepts and practices* (pp. 131-137). Sudbury, MA: Jones & Bartlett.

Zimmerman, S. (1994). Social cognition and evaluations of health care team communication effectiveness. *Western Journal of Communication, 58,* 116-141.

Zimmerman, S., & Applegate, J. L. (1992). Person-centered comforting in the hospice interdisciplinary team. *Communication Research, 19,* 240-263.

19 | Care Not Cure

Dialogues at the Transition

Geoffrey H. Gordon
Oregon Health & Science University

People living with cancer face multiple communication challenges, including receiving the diagnosis, choosing and starting initial treatment, completing treatment and following up, responding to treatment failure or recurrent disease, and arranging end of life care. Materials are available to help clinicians with some of these challenges, including giving bad news, (Buckman & Baile, 2002; Girgis & Sanson-Fisher, 1995), choosing initial treatment (Ellis, Butow, & Tattersall, 2002; Kunkel, Myers, Lartey, & Oyesanmi, 2000), coaching survivors (Walsh-Burke & Marcusen, 1999), discussing advance directives (Emanuel, Danis, & Pearlman, 1995; Roter et al., 2000), and providing end of life care (Larson & Tobin, 2000; von Gunten, Ferris, & Emanuel, 2000). However, few guidelines exist to help clinicians talk with patients and families when the current treatment is not working and no other anticancer treatment is available. This conversation may take place over several encounters until the patient, family, and medical team are all in agreement regarding the goals, methods, and expected results of treatment.

The goal of this chapter is to highlight some challenges to effective communication at transitions to palliative care, review communication skills training for cancer physicians, and raise questions for further research.

313

COMMUNICATION CHALLENGES AT THE TRANSITION

Conversations about care when no further disease-specific treatment is available can be extraordinarily difficult for both doctor and patient. Up to 20% of oncologists have low self-rated communication competence in this area. Compared with their peers, they are more likely to experience patient death as a personal failure and to find these conversations to be the worst part of being an oncologist (Mayer, Cassel, Emanuel, & Schnipper, 1998). Some principles of giving bad news apply, including eliciting the full range of patient concerns related to the diagnosis and treatment, expressing empathy verbally and nonverbally, assessing patient preferences for information and decision making, and giving information in simple language, with pauses to assess understanding and to answer questions (Baile, Glober, Lenzi, Beale, & Kudelka, 1999; Friedrichsen, Strang, & Carlsson, 2000; Lo, Quill, & Tulsky, 1999).

The news of progressive disease and no further treatment options to cure or control it is particularly devastating. Immediate and urgent issues for communication include (a) prognostic uncertainty ("How much time do I have?"), (b) death and dying ("Where and how will I die?"), and (c) the meaning of hope ("I can't lose hope—but what am I hoping for?").

Discussing prognostic uncertainty is a major communication challenge in conversations at the transition. A third or more of patients undergoing cancer treatment with palliative intent erroneously believe that they are being treated for cure (Quirt et al., 1997). There are several layers of uncertainty at play. First, physicians (with or without clinical prediction instruments) are not very good at estimating when an individual patient will die (Finucane, 1999). Second, they may be reluctant to communicate their estimate to the patient. For example, physicians referring terminally ill patients to hospice intentionally gave them an overly optimistic prognosis almost a third of the time (Lamont & Christakis, 2001). Third, the limitations of language, both qualitative and quantitative, make it very difficult for physicians to explain probabilistic information without bias (Mazur & Merz, 1994; O'Connor, 1989). Fourth, the patient may misinterpret or reject the physician's estimate due to fear, denial, or grief (Quill & Townsend, 1991). Use of written treatment plans that include information about the extent of disease, goals of treatment, and expected results may be useful in getting medical teams, patients, and families "on the same page" (Butow, Dunn, Tatersall, & Jones, 1994; Smith, 2000).

A second challenge is our inability in Western culture to talk comfortably about death. Most deaths now occur in medical facilities rather than patients' homes, and death has become a medical problem rather than a natural event. Clinicians and medical facilities are not well prepared to provide end-of-life care. Many symptoms and needs (physical, psychological, socioeconomic, and spiritual) are unmet, and much of the care provided is "high burden, low benefit ." (Nelson et al., 2001; SUPPORT, 1995). Many factors contribute to this problem. As patients get sicker, they are more willing to undergo greater treatment burdens for smaller possibilities of benefit (Finucane, 1999). Physicians (by selection or training) may endorse roles, relationships, and rewards that put them in conflict with the goals of palliative care (Haidet et al., 1998; Quill & Suchman, 1993). They may also lack skills for effective communication. For example, physician misunderstanding of patient preferences for end-of-life care are common, even for patients with metastatic cancer with whom they have discussed end of life care (Barasso, Osura, & Luna, 1992). Finally, health care institutions are organized and financed around delivery of episodic, highly technical tests and treatments rather than palliative care (Lynn, 2001).

A third challenge is our lack of understanding of the definition and dynamics of hope. When hope is narrowly focused on disease response, honest disclosure of treatment failure can be seen as "taking away the patient's hope" (Lee, Fiarclough, Antin, & Weeks, 2001; Steinhauser et al., 2000). However, cancer patients may find new objects and sources of hope as the disease progresses (Herth, 1990). For example, initial hope for cure may be modified to hope for a pain free day, a sense of control over the dying process, or attending a special event like a wedding or graduation. Patients lose hope when they feel abandoned or isolated ("there is nothing more we can do for you") or when they suspect their doctors or families are withholding information (Fallowfield, Jenkins, & Beveridge, 2002; Weissman, 2001).

When these communication challenges converge, a "recovery plot" may result (The, Hak, Loeter, & van der Wal, 2000). For example, a physician sees a patient with small cell lung cancer and little chance of cure and describes an overall poor but uncertain prognosis. The physician then quickly states that prognoses are only statistics and that the patient might do much better than predicted. The two embark on a course of aggressive treatment. The tumor shrinks but never disappears, or reappears quickly. Treatment is continued but never discussed again—the patient assumes that the doctor would not give a useless treatment, and the doctor does not want to take away the patient's hope by stopping treatment. In the end, both doctor and patient admit that they never thought the disease was curable, and the patient regrets losing valuable time to pursue the treatment.

In an alternative (and more satisfactory) scenario the physician: (a) asks what the patient understands about the nature and extent of the disease and the goals and results of treatment; (b) allows the patient to express feelings; and (c) asks about specific concerns such as anticipated physical symptoms, loss of function, mood changes, or impact on the family (Baile et al., 1999; Friedrichsen et al., 2000; Lo et al., 1999; von Gunten et al., 2000). The physician explicitly acknowledges that the disease is progressing and no further anticancer treatments are available and expresses the wish that things were different (Quill, Arnold, & Platt, 2001). The physician then reassures the patient that care will continue, with the aim of clarifying and achieving their hopes and goals within the constraints of progressive disease (Friedrichsen et al., 2000; Lo et al., 1999; Steinhauser et al., 2000). The physician and medical team shift attention and language away from the disease process and toward relief of suffering and maintaining function (Norton & Bowers, 2001). Finally, the physician and team might reflect, individually or together, on their reactions to the treatment failure and how it affects their roles and relationships with the patient, family, and each other (Block, 2001; Coulehan, 1995; Meier, Back, & Morrison, 2001; Novack et al., 1997).

COMMUNICATION SKILLS TRAINING FOR CANCER CLINICIANS

Communication skills are linked to important outcomes such as greater satisfaction (patient and physician), greater patient understanding and acceptance of treatment plans, reduced patient distress, and fewer lawsuits (Hall, Roter, & Katz, 1988; Levinson et al., 1997; Stewart et al., 1999). Interventions to improve physician-patient communication improve patient outcomes in hypertension, diabetes, and postoperative recovery (Gittell et al., 2000; Kaplan, Greenfield, & Ware, 1989; Rost, Flavin, Cole, & McGill, 1991). In oncology, benefits of effective communication include improved patient coping, quality of life, and distress, and reduced clinician fatigue, emotional exhaustion, and burnout (Fallowfield, Hall, Maguire, & Baum, 1990; Maguire, 1999).

Common communication deficiencies include interrupting patients early in the encounter (Beckman & Frankel, 1984; Maguire, Faulkner, Booth, Elliott, & Hillier, 1996), failing to elicit the full range of patient concerns (Beckman & Frankel, 1984; Stewart, McWhinney, & Buck, 1979), missing opportunities to express understanding of the patient's ideas and feelings (Eisenthal, Koopman, & Stoeckle, 1990; Suchman, Markakis, Beckman, & Frankel, 1997), and minimizing the patient's role in treatment planning (Gaudagnoli & Ward, 1998; Waitzkin, 1984). However, communication skills can be taught, learned, and maintained for physicians at all levels of training (Bowman, Goldberg, & Millar, 1992; Maguire, 1990; Maguire, Fairbairn, & Fletcher, 1986; Putnam, Stiles, Jacob, & James, 1988; Roter et al., 1995; Stillman, Sabars, & Redfield, 1976), including skills for giving bad news (Baile et al., 1999; Jewett et al., 1982; Vetto, Elder, Toffler, & Fields, 1999). Workshops for practicing oncologists can improve self-rated communication skills (Baile et al., 1999; Parle, Maguire, & Heaven, 1997) as well as skills with simulated (Maguire, Booth, Elliott, & Jones, 1996) and actual (Fallowfield et al., 2002) patients. These latter workshops include essential elements of skills-based learning such as (a) a supportive learning climate, (b) negotiated goals with the learner, (c) clear description and demonstration of the desired skills, (d) practice with observation and feedback, (e) periodic review and application of the skills to situations of increasing complexity, and (f) opportunities for personal reflection on one's experiences as a learner and clinician (Kurtz, Silverman, & Draper, 1998; Lipkin et al., 1995; Novack, Volk, Drossman, & Lipkin, 1993).

COMMUNICATION SKILLS AT THE TRANSITION: AREAS FOR RESEARCH

Teaching

What is the "dose-response" effect for communication skills training? What kind of teaching, for how long, is optimal for improving clinicians' communication skills? Medical student and resident programs last 2-4 hours; residential workshops for practitioners last 2-3 days. Both have shown lasting improvement in skills with simulated and actual patients, respectively. Workshops of several sessions followed by ongoing coaching may be more effective than single-training events. We need to know more about the optimal "dose" (amount and frequency) of teaching, the impact of "boosters" to revisit and reinforce learning, and appropriate outcome measures for learners at different levels of expertise.

What is the best method of delivering communication skills training? The knowledge base and concepts underlying communication skills can be presented in writing, lecture, or online. Learners can use computer-based programs to observe skills and to distinguish effective from ineffective ones (Buckman & Baile, 2002). However, communication skills are best learned through practice with direct observation and feedback. Some faculty training may be necessary because faculty who teach communication vary widely in the issues they identify and teach about (Buyck & Lang, 2002). Real-time observation and feedback on communication skills by trained simulated patients is available online (Novack, personal communication).

How do you measure success of teaching? Success has many levels, including acquiring a skill, using it in practice, and affecting patient outcome. A variety of communication skill-assessment instruments are available but only a few have been studied extensively (Boon & Stewart, 1998). Currently there is no "gold standard" that is widely accepted and applicable across a wide spectrum of clinical encounters. Communication skills and impact of training may be best assessed in a 360 degree fashion with ratings by self, patients (real or simulated), and observers (faculty, staff, peers) (Accreditation Council, 2002).

Practice

What is the best way for oncologists to discuss prognostic uncertainty with patients? Traditionally, physicians view disclosing uncertainty as potentially damaging to the doctor-patient relationship. However, empirical studies refute this (Gordon, Joos, & Byrne, 2000). Aids to shared decisions in cancer and other areas are available but not widely used (O'Connor et al., 2001). Qualitative analysis of comments by individual physicians and patients as they review videotapes of actual decision-making conversations could provide new directions for research.

What is the impact of electronic communication on physician-patient communication at the transition? A significant percentage of the population uses the Internet and the most common reason for accessing the Internet is for health-related concerns. Patients with cancer can find information, support, and advice. A growing number of physicians communicate with their patients electronically. The impact of electronic communication on the doctor-patient relationship and on interdisciplinary communication remains unclear.

Systems

What is the relative importance of system effect versus training effect in changing physician behavior? The SUPPORT (1995) study indicated that there is a limit to the effectiveness of physician-patient communication skills training on practice habits in end-of-life care. Determining the relative impact of changes in leadership, policies, resources, and training on the quality of end-of-life care is an important research area (Lynn et al., 2000).

What are the characteristics of physicians who obtain additional training in communication skills? What are the characteristics of systems that encourage or mandate this training? Physicians who voluntarily enroll in 2-5 day communication skills training programs are usually already aware of the importance of these skills to their work. Some have additional interests in psychosocial medicine, or in experiential, interactive teaching methods. Physicians enrolling in workshops on specific topics (e.g., taking a sexual history or giving bad news) want practical tips and updates because they encounter the problem frequently, or find it interesting or difficult. Health care systems that encourage or mandate communication skills training want to maintain high patient satisfaction scores to retain patients in the system and to reduce malpractice risk.

CONCLUSION

Communication is a set of skills that can be taught, learned, and maintained, and which have a clear impact on healthcare outcomes. Training programs are effective in improving communication skills of cancer clinicians at various levels of training.

Medical education is implementing competency-based assessment and certification of individuals and training programs, including communication and interpersonal skills (Accreditation Council, 2002). At the same time, healthcare organizations increasingly view communication as an essential element of patient safety and quality of care (Berwick, 2002). These initiatives will provide new opportunities for collaborative research on patient-centered and systems-based teaching and practice, including communication around management of cancer and other serious progressive diseases (Weissman et al., 1999).

REFERENCES

Accreditation Council for Graduate Medical Education. (2002). Outcomes project: Enhancing residency education through outcomes assessment. Available at http://www.acgme.org/outcome/comp/compFull.asp. Accessed May 7, 2002

Baile, W. F., Glober, G. A., Lenzi, R., Beale, E. A., & Kudelka A. P. (1999). Discussing disease progression and end-of-life decisions. *Oncology, 13*, 1021-1035.

Baile, W. F., Kudelka, A. P., Beale, E. A., Glober, G. A., Myers, E. G., Greisinger, A. J., Bast, R. C. Jr., Goldstein, J. B., Novack, D., & Lenzi, R. (1999). Communication skills training in oncology. Description and preliminary outcomes of workshops on breaking bad news and managing patient reactions to illness. *Cancer, 86*, 887-897.

Barroso, P., Osuna, E., & Luna, A. (1992). Doctors' death experience and attitudes towards death, euthanasia, and informing terminal patients. *Medicine & Law, 11*, 527-533.

Beckman, H.B., & Frankel, R.M. (1984). The effect of physician behavior on the collection of data. *Annals of Internal Medicine, 101*, 692-696.

Berwick, D. M. (2002). A user's manual for the IOM's "Quality Chasm" report. *Health Affairs (Millwood), 21*, 80-90.

Block, S. D. (2001). Perspectives on care at the close of life. Psychological considerations, growth, and transcendence at the end of life: The art of the possible. *JAMA, 285*, 2898-2905.

Boon, H., & Stewart M. (1998). Patient-physician communication assessment instruments: 1986 to 1996 in review. *Patient Education and Counseling, 35*, 161-176.

Bowman, F. M., Goldberg, D. P., & Millar, T. (1992). Improving the skills of established general practitioners: The long-term benefits of group teaching. *Medical Education, 26*, 63-68.

Buckman, R., & Baile, W. F. (2002). *A practical guide to communication skills in cancer care* (3 CD disk set). Toronto: Medical Audio Visual Communications.

Butow, P. N., Dunn, S. M., Tattersall, M. H. N., & Jones, Q. J. (1994). Patient participation in the cancer consultation: Evaluation of question prompt sheet. *Annals of Oncology, 5*, 199-204.

Buyck, D., & Lang, F. (2002). Teaching medical communication skills: A call for greater uniformity. *Family Medicine, 34*, 337-343.

Coulehan, J. L. (1995). Tenderness and steadiness: Emotions in medical practice. *Literature and Medicine, 14*, 222-236.

Eisenthal, S., Koopman, C., & Stoeckle, J. D. (1990). The nature of patients' requests for physicians' help. *Academic Medicine, 65*, 401-405.

Ellis, P. M., Butow, P. N., & Tattersall, M. H. (2002). Informing breast cancer patients about clinical trials: A randomized clinical trial of an educational booklet. *Annals of Oncology, 13,* 1414-1423.

Emanuel, L. L., Danis, M., Pearlman, R., & Singer P. (1995). Advance care planning as a process: Structuring the discussions in practice. *Journal of the American Geriatric Society, 43,* 440-446.

Fallowfield, L. J., Hall, A., Maguire, G. P., & Baum, L. (1990). Psychological outcomes of different treatment policies in women with early breast cancer outside a clinical trial. *British Medical Journal, 301,* 575-580.

Fallowfield, L. J., Jenkins, V. A., & Beveridge, H. A. (2002). Truth may hurt but deceit hurts more: Communication in palliative care. *Palliative Medicine, 16,* 297-303.

Fallowfield, L., Jenkins, V., Farewell, V., Saul, J., Duffy, A., & Eves, R. Efficacy of a cancer research UK communication skills training model of oncologists: A randomized controlled trial. *Lancet, 359,* 650-656.

Finucane, T. E. (1999). How gravely ill becomes dying: A key to end-of-life care. *JAMA, 282,* 1670-1672.

Friedrichsen, M. J., Strang, P. M., & Carlsson, M. E. (2000). Breaking bad news in the transition from curative to palliative cancer care—patient's view of the doctor giving the information. *Supportive Care in Cancer, 8,* 472-478.

Gaudagnoli, E., & Ward, P. (1998). Patient participation in decision-making. *Social Science & Medicine, 47,* 329-339.

Girgis, A., & Sanson-Fisher, R. W. (1995). Breaking bad news: Consensus guidelines for medical practitioners. *Journal of Clinical Oncology, 13,* 2449-2456.

Gittell, J. H., Fairfield, K. M., Bierbaum, B., Head, W., Jackson, R., Kelly, M., Laskin, R., Lipson, S., Siliski, J., Thornhill, T., & Zuckerman, J. (2000). Impact of relational coordination on quality of care, postoperative pain and functioning, and length of stay: A nine-hospital study of surgical patients. *Medical Care, 38,* 807-819.

Gordon, G. H., Joos, S. K., & Byrne, J. (2000). Physician expressions of uncertainty during patient encounters. *Patient Education and Counseling, 40,* 59-65.

Haidet, P., Hamel, M. B., Davis, R. B., Wenger, N., Reding, D., Kussin, P. S., Connors, A. F. Jr., Lynn, J., Weeks, J. C., & Phillips, R. S. (1998). Outcomes, preferences for resuscitation, and physician-patient communication among patients with metastasis colorectal cancer. SUPPORT Investigators. Study to Understand Prognoses and Preferences for Outcomes and Risks of Treatments. *American Journal of Medicine, 105,* 222-229.

Hall, J. A., Roter, D. L., & Katz, N. R. (1988). Meta-analysis of correlates of provider behavior in medical encounters. *Medical Care, 26,* 657-675.

Herth, K. (1990). Fostering hope in terminally ill people. *Journal of Advanced Nursing, 15,* 1250-1259.

Jewett, L. S., Greenberg, L. W., Champion, L. A., Gluck, R. S., Leikin, S. L., Altieri, M. F., & Lipnick, R. N. (1982). The teaching of crisis counseling to pediatric residents: A one-year study. *Pediatrics, 70,* 907-911.

Kaplan, S. H., Greenfield, S., & Ware, J. E., Jr. (1989). Assessing the effects of physician-patient interactions on the outcomes of chronic disease. *Medical Care, 27,* S110-127.

Kunkel, E. J., Myers, R. E., Lartey, P. L., & Oyesanmi, O. (2000). Communicating effectively with the patient and family about treatment options for prostate cancer. *Seminars in Urologic Oncology, 18,* 233-240.

Kurtz, S., Silverman, J., & Draper J. (1998). The "how": Principles of how to teach and learn communication skills. In S. Kurtz, J. Silverman, & J. Draper (Eds.), *Teaching and learning communication skills in medicine* (pp. 33-50). Abingdon UK; Radcliffe Medical Press.

Lamont, E. B., & Christakis, N. A. (2001). Prognostic disclosure to patients with cancer near the end of life. *Annals of Internal Medicine, 134,* 1196-1205.

Larson, D. G., & Tobin, D. R. (2000). End-of-life conversations: Evolving practice and theory. *JAMA, 284,* 1573-1578.

Lee, S. J., Fiarclough, D., Antin, J. H., & Weeks, J. C. (2001). Discrepancies between patient and physician estimates for the success of stem cell transplantation. *JAMA, 285,* 1034-1038.

Levinson, W., Roter, D. L., Mullooly, J. P., Dull, V. T., & Frankel, R. M. (1997). Physician-patient communication. The relationship with malpractice claims among physicians and surgeons. *JAMA, 277,* 533-539.

Lipkin, M. Jr., Kaplan, C., Clark, W., & Novack, D. H. (1995). Teaching medical interviewing: The Lipkin model. In M. Lipkin, Jr., S.M. Putnam, & A. Lazare (Eds.), *The medical interview: Teaching, research, and practice* (pp. 422-435). New York: Springer-Verlag.

Lo, B., Quill, T., & Tulsky, J. (1999). Discussing palliative care with patients. *Annals of Internal Medicine, 13,* 744-749.

Lynn, J. (2001). Serving patients who may die soon and their families: The role of hospice and other services. *JAMA, 285,* 925-932.

Lynn, J., DeVries, K. O., Arkes, H. R., Stevens, M., Cohn, F., Murphy, P., Cinvinsky, K. E., Hamel, M. B., Dawson, N. Y., & Tsevat, J. (2000). Ineffectiveness of the SUPPORT intervention: Review of explanations. *Journal of the American Geriatric Society, 48,* S206-213.

Maguire P. (1990). Can communication skills be taught? *British Journal of Hospital Medicine, 43,* 215-216.

Maguire P. (1999). Improving communication with cancer patients. *European Journal of Cancer, 35,* 1415-1422.

Maguire, P., Booth, K., Elliott, C., & Jones, B. (1996). Helping health professionals involved in cancer care acquire key interviewing skills—the impact of workshops. *European Journal of Cancer, 32A,* 1486-1489.

Maguire, P., Fairbairn, S., & Fletcher, C. (1986). Consultation skills of young doctors: I-Benefits of feedback training interviewing as students persist. *British Medical Journal, 292,* 1573-1576.

Maguire, P., Faulkner, A., Booth, K., Elliott, C., & Hillier, V. (1996). Helping cancer patients disclose their concerns. *European Journal of Cancer, 32A,* 78-81.

Mayer, R. J., Cassel, C., Emanuel, E., & Schnipper, L. (1998, May). *Report of the task force on end of life issues.* Paper presented at Presidential Symposium, 34th Annual Meeting of the American Society of Clinical Oncology, Los Angeles, CA.

Mazur, D. J., & Merz, J. F. (1994). Patients' interpretations of verbal expressions of probability: Implications for securing informed consent to medical interventions. *Behavioral Science and Law, 12,* 417-426.

Meier, D. E., Back, A. L., & Morrison, R. S. (2001). The inner life of physicians and care of the seriously ill. *JAMA, 286,* 3007-3014.

Nelson, J. E., Meier, D. E., Oei, E. J., Nierman, D. M., Senzel, R. S., Manfredi, P. L., Davis, S. M., & Morrison, R. S. (2001). Self-reported symptom experience of critically ill cancer patients receiving intensive care. *Critical Care Medicine, 29,* 277-282.

Norton, S. A., & Bowers, B. J. (2001). Working toward consensus: Providers' strategies to shift patients from curative to palliative treatment goals. *Research in Nursing & Health, 24,* 258-269.

Novack, D. H., Suchman, A. L., Clark, W., Epstein, R. M., Najberg, E., & Kaplan, C. (1997). Calibrating the physician: Personal awareness and effective patient care. *JAMA, 278,* 502-509.

Novack, D. H., Volk, G., Drossman, D. A., & Lipkin, M., Jr. (1993). Medical interviewing and interpersonal skills teaching in US medical schools. Progress, problems, and promise. *JAMA, 269,* 2101-2105.

O'Connor, A. M. (1989). Effects of framing and level of probability on patients' preferences for cancer chemotherapy. *Journal of Clinical Epidemiology, 42,* 119-126.

O'Connor, A. M., Stacey, D., Rovner, D., Holmes-Rovner, M., Tetroe, J., Llewellyn-Thomas, H., Entwistle, V., Rostom, A., Fiset, V., Barry, M., & Jones, J. (2001). Decision aids for people facing health treatment or screening decisions. *Cochrane Database Systematic Review, 3,* CD001431

Parle, M., Maguire, P., & Heaven, C. (1997). The development of a training model to improve health professionals' skills, self-efficacy and outcome expectancies when communicating with cancer patients. *Social Science & Medicine, 44,* 231-240.

Putnam, S. M., Stiles, W. B., Jacob, M. C., & James S. A. (1988). Teaching the medical interview: An intervention study. *Journal of General Internal Medicine, 3,* 38-47.

Quill, T. E., Arnold, R. M., & Platt, F. (2001). "I wish things were different." Expressing wishes in response to loss, futility, and unrealistic hopes. *Annals of Internal Medicine, 135,* 551-555.

Quill, T. E., & Suchman, A. L. (1993). Uncertainty and control: Learning to live with medicine's limitations. *Humane Medicine, 9,* 109-120.

Quill, T. E., & Townsend, P. (1991). Bad news: Delivery, dialogue, and dilemmas. *Archives of Internal Medicine, 151,* 463-468.

Quirt, C. F., Mackillop, W. J., Ginsburg, A. D., Sheldon, L., Brundage, M., Dixon, P., & Ginsburg, L. (1997). Do doctors know when their patients don't? A survey of doctor-patient communication in lung cancer. *Lung Cancer, 18,* 1-20.

Rost, K. M., Flavin, K. S., Cole, K., & McGill, J. B. (1991). Change in metabolic control and function status after hospitalization. Impact of patient activation intervention in diabetic patients. *Diabetes Care, 14,* 881-889.

Roter, D. L., Hall, J.A., Kern, D. E. et al. (1995). Improving physicians' interviewing skills and reducing patients' emotional distress. A randomized clinical trial. *Archives of Internal Medicine, 155,* 1877-1884.

Roter, D. L., Larson, S., Fischer, G. S., Arnold, R. M., & Tulsky, J. A. (2000). Experts practice what they preach: A descriptive study of best and normative practices in end of life discussions. *Archives of Internal Medicine, 60,* 3477-3485.

Smith, T. J. (2000). Tell it like it is. *Journal of Clinical Oncology, 18,* 3441-3445.

Steinhauser, K. E., Clipp, E. C., McNeilly M., Christakis, N., Parker, J., & Tulsky, J. A. (2000). In search of a good death: Observations of patients, families, and providers. *Annals of Internal Medicine, 132,* 825-832.

Stewart, M., Brown, J. B., Boon, H., Galajda, J., Meredith, L., & Sangster, M. (1999). Evidence on doctor-patient communication. *Cancer Prevention Control, 3,* 25-30.

Stewart, M. A., McWhinney, I. R., & Buck, C. W. (1979). The doctor/patient relationship and its effect upon outcome. *Journal of the Royal College of General Practitioners, 29,* 77-82.

Stillman, P. L., Sabars, D. L., & Redfield, D. L. (1976). The use of para-professionals to teach interviewing skills. *Pediatrics, 57,* 769-774.

Suchman, A. L., Markakis, K., Beckman, H. B., & Frankel R. A. (1997). Model of empathic communication in the medical interview. *JAMA, 277,* 678-682.

SUPPORT Principal Investigators, The. (1995). A controlled trial to improve care for seriously ill hospitalized patients. The study to understand prognoses and preferences for outcomes and risks of treatments (SUPPORT). *JAMA, 274,* 1591-1598.

The, A., Hak, T., Loeter, G., & van der Wal, G. (2000). Collusion in doctor-patient communication about imminent death: An ethnographic study. *British Medical Journal, 321,* 1376-1381.

Vetto, J. T., Elder, N. C., Toffler, W. L., & Fields, S. A. (1999). Teaching medical students to give bad news: Does formal instruction help? *Journal of Cancer Education, 14,* 13-17.

von Gunten, C. F., Ferris, F. D., & Emanuel, L. L. (2000). Ensuring competency in end-of-life care: Communication and relational skills. *JAMA, 284,* 3051-3057.

Waitzkin, H. (1984). Doctor-patient communication. Clinical implications of social scientific research. *JAMA, 252,* 2441-2446.

Walsh-Burke, K., & Marcusen, C. (1999). Self-advocacy training for cancer survivors. The Cancer Survival Toolbox. *Cancer Practice, 7*(6), 297-301.

Weissman, D. (2001, September). Fast Fact #21: Hope and truth telling. End-of-Life Physician Education Resource Center (EPERC). www.eperc.mcw.edu. Accessed August 28, 2001.

Weissman, D. E., Block, S. D., Blank, L., Cain, J., Cassem, N., Danoff, D., Foley, K., Meier, D., Schyve, P., Theige, D., & Wheeler H. B. (1999). Recommendations for incorporating palliative care education into the acute care hospital setting. *Academic Medicine, 74,* 871-877.

VI

PATIENT SKILLS, CONTROL, AND DECISION MAKING

20 | Cancer Patients as Active Participants in Their Care

Edward Krupat
Harvard Medical School

Julie T. Irish
The Health Institute
New England Medical Center

It is tremendously upsetting to learn that one has cancer, and coping with this disease requires a great deal of informational and emotional support. In addition to the role that family and friends can play, a growing literature has demonstrated that the skill with which clinicians and patients communicate with one another can make a great deal of difference (Arora, 2003; B. Butow & Baile, 2003; Kreps, Arora, & Nelson, 2003). Whether discussing a diagnosis, planning treatment, making decisions, or addressing palliative care, the relationship between the provider and the patient will be critical for helping the patient cope over a period of weeks, months, and years.

Despite the recognized importance of good communication, a wealth of empirical and anecdotal evidence exists to suggest that the communication process between patient and provider often breaks down. Providers limit the amount of information they give to patients and deliver it in jargon-laden terms. They fail to recognize the need for expressions of caring or have difficulty delivering emotional support to their patients. Decision making is often unilateral and patients are frustrated in their desires to be involved in their care.

To address this, clinicians, educators, and researchers have turned their attention to developing programs directed at the goal of improving patient–provider communication (Beckman & Frankel, 2003; L. Fallowfield, Lipkin, & Cockburn, 1998; V. Fallowfield et al., 2002). The vast majority of these programs involve communications skills training for medical students, residents, and practicing physicians, most often in primary care, but also in oncology and other specialties. These programs have demonstrated that improved outcomes can result from better communication on the part of the provider (Cegala, 2003; Cegala, Lenzmeier, & Broz, 2002; DiMatteo, 2003), but this focus only represents half of the equation. As noted by Hall (2003), the direction of influence is not unidirectional. Just as it is important for providers to learn to relate to and communicate well with their patients, it is equally important for patients to learn to communicate well with their providers, to ask questions, to make their needs and preferences known, to act assertively in times of conflict or uncertainty. Yet, although numerous programs have been developed and tested to train health professionals in communicating with their patients, Post, Cegala, and Miser (2002) were able to identify only 16 randomized controlled trials in the outpatient setting during the 25-year period from 1975 to 2000 in which patients were trained to communicate better with their providers. Of these 16 papers, only two focused on patients with cancer.

The relative scarcity of programs of "patient activation" in comparison to those on "provider education" can be explained in several ways. First, providers at all stages of their careers go through formal training in which communication can be made part of their curriculum; whereas no such formal opportunities exist for patients to learn how to communicate with those who care for them. Second, each physician trained has the capacity to impact thousands of patients over a career; whereas the training of patients has an impact that is obviously less broad, making such programs less cost-efficient. Although these two reasons might constitute sufficient explanation for the relatively small number of communication training programs for patients, it is believed that a more subtle "unconscious ideology" also underlies this. Despite all the rhetoric about practice that is patient-centered and the new found symmetry of power between patient and provider, an unstated assumption still seems to exist that, like ballroom dancers where one partner leads and the other follows, the physician still directs the flow of action, sets the tone, and ultimately determines whether the communication is successful or not. Therefore, the focus has been on training the "leaders" more than the "followers."

A growing body of evidence, however, suggests that a significant proportion of physician behavior is prompted by subtle signals as well as explicit requests conveyed by patients; in effect that the leaders take their cues from the followers and that the followers lead in ways that may not always be obvious (Street, 1992b; Street, Krupat, Bell, Kravitz, & Haidet, 2003). Therefore, the focus of this chapter is on communication from the patient's perspective. In the first part of this chapter we question what it is that patients want and examine how well they express their needs and preferences. In the second part, we discuss how patients can be taught to do a better job by reviewing the literature on patient patient-activation interventions, noting the directions they have taken, and the success they have had. We discuss research and programs of intervention within the arena of cancer care when they exist. However, because much of this work has been done in other health care contexts, we attempt to relate and apply these findings, to the extent relevant, to the care of patients with cancer. At the end of the chapter, we will propose directions that future programs of research and intervention might go in order to create better patient–provider communication, increased quality of life, and more positive health outcomes.

CLARIFYING TERMS

Much of the discussion of what patients want and how they might go about getting it suffers from a lack of conceptual clarity. In an exception to this, Kravitz (1996) presented a taxonomy of patient expectations. He noted noted that patient expectations may be thought of in terms of *expectancies* versus *values*. Patients' *expectancies* are expressed in the form of probabilities; beliefs that something will occur ("It is likely that I will be referred to the social worker to help me deal with my illness"). However, patients' values refer to what *ought to* or *should* happen rather than what *will* happen. Patient values can be expressed in the form of needs ("I am in need of a referral to a social worker"); desires, requests, or demands ("I want a referral to a social worker'); or entitlement ("I deserve a referral to a social worker"). As for content, patient's expectations can be specific (focused on a defined need in the course of a single visit) or general (dealing with overall goals in the course of treatment such a being treating as an equal). They may relate to structure (e.g., physical plant or organizational policies), process (what providers actually do in the course of treatment), or outcomes (end results that patients seek, whether physical or psychosocial).

Expectancies are often unspoken, but they serve as the baseline for judgments of satisfaction to the extent that large or small discrepancies exist between what was expected to happen and what actually occurred (e.g., patients are given more or less information than they had expected; patients are given the opportunity to be involved in selecting treatment options to the extent that they had anticipated). Broadly defined values determine the kinds of role relationships that patients believe should characterize their relationship to their providers; but specific values define the goals that patients have for treatment and determine the spoken and unspoken desires or demands that patients have during the course of a clinical encounter. If patients are to be effective communicators, they have to know (or be trained) how to participate in medical encounters in ways that generate processes and outcomes that meet their expectancies and fulfill their desires.

WHAT DO PATIENTS WANT?

Research within the context of primary care indicates that patients go into their doctors' offices with several kinds of expectancies, most principally that they will receive an explanation for their problem (Williams, Weinman, Dale, & Newman, 1995). According to Leventhal and Benyamini (1997), such explanations can be described in terms of five issues: identity (the name of the problem); timeline (its likely duration); cause; cure; and consequences (the extent to which it will interfere with everyday activities). During the course of a primary care visit, patients will not only ask questions of their providers, but also make explicit requests. In a study of 559 primary care patients who were seeing their physicians for a new or worsening problem, 23% requested a physical exam, 11% requested a new medication, 9% a refill, 8% some form of lab test, and 5% a referral to a specialist (Kravitz et al., 2003).

Within the context of cancer care, patients' specific expectancies and needs vary considerably. This is because there are so many different types of cancer affecting differing segments of the population; and the treatment process is complex, involving multiple providers over an extended period of time. In addition, patients' coping styles, their orientations toward their illness and their providers, and their desire to gain knowledge and be involved in decision making all differ greatly; and even these may change over time as a function of patients' perceived health and the stage of their disease (P. Butow et al., 1997).

The Desire for Information

Despite the many factors that affect cancer patients' needs, three themes emerge consistently. which These themes are, not surprisingly, almost perfectly parallel with the goals of the patient-centered provider. These are the exchange of information, the establishment of a good interpersonal relationship, and involvement of the patient in the process of decision making (Arora, 2003; Bakker, Fitch, Gray, Reed, & Bennett, 2001; P. Butow et al, 2002).

McWilliam, Brown, and Stewart (2000) described the characteristics of a positive working relationship between cancer patients and their providers (from which we may infer that such a relationship satisfies the patients' expectancies and meets their needs). Throughout the treatment process, but especially at the time of initial diagnosis, the prerequisite for any positive outcome between patient and physician is the sharing of information. Patients say that the news that they have breast cancer generates feelings of vulnerability and loss of control, and indicate that information from their providers is the key to mastering the experience of illness and restoring a sense of self-efficacy.

Lobb, Butow, Kenney, and Tattersall (1999) surveyed 100 women within 2 months of a breast cancer diagnosis and reported that the information that patients most wanted related to the probability of a cure, staging of their cancer, likelihood that the treatment would be successful, and 10-year survival figures with and without the use of adjuvant therapy. Jenkins, Fallowfield, and Saul (2001) surveyed more than 2,000 patients with various forms of cancer and found that 87% preferred to have as much information as they could about their disease, regardless of whether the news was good or bad. Of the sample, 54% felt that they "had an absolute need" for knowing all the possible treatments and for the chances of a cure; 60% wanted to know about all the possible side effects of the treatment; 45% questioned how the treatment works to treat the illness; and 39% wanted week-by-week progress during the course of treatment.

The fact that patients desire a good deal of information from their physicians stands in contrast to the finding that physicians typically underestimate the amount of information that patients want and overestimate the amount of information they have given (Kindelan & Kent, 1987; Waitzkin, 1984); and that those physicians who take a more paternalistic orientation toward their patients place a lower value on fully informing patients in the first place (Quill & Brody, 1996). In addition, the volume of information given hardly guarantees that the information was understood or seen as useful. When Lobb et al. (1999) questioned breast cancer patients after their visits, 73% did not understand the term *median* survival, 53% could not calculate risk reduction with adjuvant therapy relative to absolute risk, and the numerical equivalent of a "good" chance of survival varied greatly among patients. In addition, in a study of 115 pediatric visits, Street (1992a) found that the amount of information that the physician provided and the degree of physician informativeness as rated by the parents were not correlated.

The Desire To Be Involved in Decision Making

Although almost all cancer patients desire information of some sort, the extent to which they want to be involved in making decisions about their treatment and other matters relating to care varies widely. Degner et al (1997) surveyed more than 1000 breast cancer patients in Canada and found that 22% wanted to select their own treatment, 44% wanted to do so collaboratively with their physicians, and 34% preferred a more passive role, having their physicians make this decision for them. In Great Britain, Beaver, Luker, Owens, Leinster, and Degner (1996) reported a somewhat greater preference for passivity, with 20% of newly diagnosed breast cancer patients preferring the active role, 28% wanting shared responsibility, and 52% leaving the decisions to their providers. A third study in Sweden (Wallberg et al., 2000) showed even less desire for patient involvement among breast cancer patients, with 66% of these women preferring to leave decisions to their physicians. In another recent study, however, only 11% of a sample of breast cancer patients in Texas preferred the passive role (Bruera, Willey, Palmer, & Rosales, 2002).

Two studies of Canadian men with prostate cancer (Davison, Degner, & Morgan, 1995; Davison et al., 2002) show how decision decision-making preferences may vary not only by gender, type of cancer, and location of the study, but over time. In their 1995 paper, Davison and colleagues found that 58% of the men questioned wanted to leave decisions to their providers. However, in their more recent survey with a roughly equivalent sample of patients, the percentage of those preferring the passive role was only 7.5. Even comparing the same patients over time P. Butow et al. (1997), using a heterogeneous sample of cancer patients, reported that only 31% of the patients indicated the same preference for decision making from one visit to the next, usually only 3 to 6 months later. Those patients who were going for a routine follow-up generally preferred greater involvement; whereas those whose status had worsened generally preferred to remain in a more passive role.

These variations in the desire to be involved are underscored by several findings indicating that physicians have difficulty identifying the decision decision-making preferences of their patients, and that patients' desires for involvement are not typically matched by the actual amount of involvement that they achieve. Rothenbacher, Lutz, and Porzsolt (1997) asked the physicians of 145 patients whose cancers differed in both type and severity to estimate their patient's preferences for participation in decision making. They found that physicians overestimated their patients' preferred level of involvement in 28% of the cases, underestimated their preference in 36% of the cases, and identified their preferences correctly in 36% of the cases, which was not significantly greater than chance. Moreover, the ability to identify patients' preferences accurately did not differ as a function of duration of the patient–provider relationship nor the clinical experience of the physician. In a study of breast cancer patients, Bruera et al. (2002) reported a slightly higher agreement level of 42%.

Rather than focusing on whether physicians can identify their patients' preferences, other studies have investigated whether patients actually achieve the levels of involvement that they desire. Gattellari, Butow, and Tattersall (2001) reported that 33% of the patients studied achieved their preferred role in the course of treatment; whereas 29% were encouraged to take a more active role, and 37% were less active than they had wanted to be. Although only one third of the patient sample was able to contribute to decision making in a manner congruent with their preferences, those who achieved their desired level of involvement showed significantly greater reductions in post-visit anxiety compared with either of the other two groups. Degner et al. (1997) also reported significant mismatches of preferences and behavior, with a considerable asymmetry in the direction to which the mismatches occurred. Approximately 20% of those patients who preferred an active or shared role satisfied their desires. However, 80% of those who indicated that they "prefer to leave all decisions regarding treatment to my doctor" reported that their physicians had acted in a manner that was congruent with their preferences.

The Desire for Emotional Support

Rates of psychological distress among cancer patients have been estimated to range from 20 to 66% (Brietbart, 1995). Yet physicians are typically not attuned to looking for or are comfortable in addressing their patients' emotional issues (Ford, Fallowfield, & Lewis, 1994; Maguire, Faulkner, Booth, Elliot, & Hillier, 1996); and it has been estimated that less than 25% of those cancer patients who develop psychiatric symptoms disclose them to their physicians (Cormaroff & Maguire, 1981). Reasons cited for patient nondisclosure include the feeling that physicians are busy people and should not be burdened with their patients' worries; the fear that patients may be seen as weak, inadequate, or unreasonably concerned by their providers; and a feeling that patients' emotional responses are inevitable and therefore cannot be changed by their physicians (Maguire, 1985).

Patients may receive both information and support in one of two ways. They may do so directly, by asking direct questions ("What will be the side effects of my treatment?"); or indirectly by providing verbal *cues,* which are more subtle and defined as statements that signal a need for information or support (i.e., questions in nonquestion form). An example of a medically related cue might be: "So I guess I'll just have to start figuring out soon how much the side effects will limit me." An emotionally related cue might be: "I feel so upset when I think about what the disease is doing to my relations with my friends." Because each of the requests are subtlety masked, they require the provider to be attentive to the patient, and to be willing and able to switch gears and address the patient's perceived needs while the opportunity is at hand.

P. Butow et al. (2002) studied the ways in which patients with cancer use verbal cues to gain emotional and informational support, analyzing the transcripts of almost 300 visits of patients (who had differing forms of cancer) with five medical and four radiation oncologists. They found that patients asked a median of 11 questions (range 0–53) during their visits, but only about 8% of these addressed psychosocial issues and matters of social support, counseling, and stress management. Patients gave a median of two cues per visit (range 0–21), 32% of which focused on emotional as opposed to informational issues. The physicians' responses to their patients' cues were coded as to whether they were appropriate (i.e., offered information or showed empathy); or inappropriate (involving little empathy, ignoring or interrupting the cue, or postponing a response). Appropriate responses were given to informational cues 72% of the time; whereas only 28% of the emotional cues generated a helpful response on the part of the physician.

The finding that oncologists deal better with cues for information than for emotional support parallels those of Levinson, Gorawara-Bhat, and Lamb (2000) who studied primary care and surgical visits. Physicians responded positively with responses such as acknowledgement, encouragement, or praise to patients' emotional cues 38% of the time in surgery and

21% in primary care. However, in the majority of cases the physicians missed the window of opportunity or mishandled it, thereby failing to build a stronger relationship with the patient. Responses made by the physician included inappropriate humor ("You're getting so old . . . we're gonna have to shoot ya"), denial ("It's not that big a deal"), inadequate acknowledgment, or attempts at termination of the visit. The findings of these two studies suggest that patients are more likely to raise informational rather than emotional issues with their physicians; that when patients raise emotional issues they are likely to do so in indirect ways; and that this subtle approach to generating empathic and supportive responses from their physicians has a low probability of success.

Taken together, it would appear that a relatively clear gradient exists in which cancer patients have been found to have an impact on the three major areas of communication reviewed. When providers are not forthcoming with *information*, patients ask questions and provide cues that have a reasonable likelihood of being recognized and responded to positively. Information is not always given completely or in the form that patients can best digest, but patients can have an impact on having their informational needs met. Interventions to make patients better information generators and collectors have been the most common, and have generally been shown to have positive effects. Patients' *desires to be involved in care* are apparently harder for patient's to communicate and/or for providers to recognize. Nonetheless, some interventions to help patients indicate their preferred level of involvement and to encourage physicians to engage them in ways that fulfill their desires have been attempted, with varying levels of success. However, when patients have needs for *emotional support*, their physicians are not as likely to address them without some form of prompting; yet direct questions are uncommon and subtle prompts have not worked well. In this area involving communication about emotions, little if any direct intervention work has been attempted.

THE ASSERTIVE PATIENT

Depending on the practice style of the physician, it has been said that some patients are *allowed* or *invited* to participate in their treatment by their physicians, whereas others are not. However, verbs such as those just used imply that the patient's role is inherently passive. Do patients always have to wait for prompting from their physicians to participate, and what are the outcomes when patients act in ways that attempt to satisfy their needs without an invitation? That is, can assertive patient behavior make a difference in the care they receive? Two studies, the first involving cancer prevention and the second relating to diagnosis and treatment, suggest that assertive behaviors can have a significant impact.

M. Anderson and Urban (1997) surveyed almost 9,000 women in the state of Washington to determine if assertiveness was associated with whether they received mammograms as part of their health care. The women were characterized as assertive if they said that they asked their physicians to explain information if they didn't understand what was said; if they spoke up and repeated requests if they felt their doctors hadn't heard them; and if they reminded their doctors about screening tests if they weren't ordered every year or two. After controlling for age and other possible confounding variables, a strong association was found between assertiveness and receiving the service desired, in this case mammography.

Using an experimental approach, Krupat et al. (1999) showed 128 physicians videotaped interactions of women seeking care for breast cancer. The visits were all scripted and enacted by trained actors, however, they were extremely realistic. In half of the visits the patient was White and the other half African American, in half the patient was of lower socioeconomic class and the other half middle class, in half the patients had comorbidities and the other half did not. The content of all the visits was identical in every way with the exception that in half of the visits the patient made the following assertive statement: "Before we go any further, I have to say that I am very concerned about all this 'cancer' talk. I remember what my sister went through and if I really do have cancer I want to know what can be done about it. I want you to tell me what my options are because I'm willing to do whatever's needed to get this taken care of."

Following the viewing of this visit, the physicians were each asked to recommend treatment and evaluation plans. Although no main effect of patient assertiveness was found on the outcome measures, an interesting interaction emerged in which patients who came from "disadvantaged" groups (e.g., African American, comorbid, lower social class) were more likely to have full staging of their tumors ordered when they had made an assertive statement than when they had not. The findings of these two studies, very different in method from one another as well as from the majority of the previously discussed research, suggest the potential for programs that would facilitate assertive patient communication skills, increasing the probability that the squeaky wheel might get the grease.

REVIEW OF PATIENT COMMUNICATION INTERVENTIONS

A variety of approaches have been used in an attempt to educate and train patients to become more involved in their care, and the impact of these interventions has been examined using numerous outcome measures. As mentioned previously, in a recent review of patient communication interventions, Post et al. (2002) found only 16 clinical trials between 1975 and 2000 in which the interventions had been empirically evaluated. Based on the time, cost, and resources required to conduct the intervention, the authors categorized these into three groups representing varying levels of intensity—high, medium, and low. Although this is an important consideration assuming that patient educators may wish to implement these interventions in actual practice, we review the interventions according to the approach and content involved. The outcomes of interest have also varied considerably across the 16 studies, although the most common one measured has been patient satisfaction. Others include number of questions asked, knowledge of the disease, functional and health status, adherence, sense of control, anxiety, physician satisfaction, and length of visit. The differing intervention approaches and the varying outcome measures used make it difficult to draw generalizable conclusions about which methods are best, however, we attempt to note those areas that show promise for cancer patients, and offer recommendations for areas deserving further intervention and research.

Training in Question-Asking

There now exists ample evidence showing that patients who receive adequate information during the medical visit are more likely to adhere to recommendations and be active participants in their care. It is assumed that by asking more questions patients will acquire not only more information, but also more accurate information. Armed with this information, patients will leave the physician's office feeling more in control, better able to manage their health, and possibly better equipped in their ability to prevent future illness.

Encouraging or prompting patients to ask more questions of their health care provider is an approach that is often used because it requires relatively few resources and can be easily administered just prior to the medical visit. For these reasons, training patients to increase their question-asking behavior—even using simple formats—has been one of the more common approaches to help patients become more involved in their care.

In Post et al.'s review (2002) 10 of the 16 identified randomized controlled trials examined the effect of an intervention on patients' question-asking—perhaps underscoring an assumption that this behavior is an effective and easy strategy to empower patients and will lead to the provision of useful and appropriate information. Thompson, Nanni, and Schwankowsky (1990) conducted two studies using two different question-asking formats. In the first study, patients were given a handout that simply asked patients to think about questions they wanted to ask their doctor as a way to ensure a satisfactory visit. Results showed that patients who were given the opportunity to contemplate questions reported asking their doctor more questions and feeling less anxious, although they were no more satisfied with their visit than the control group. In the second study, the intervention was modified by either adding a checklist of information to the handout or informing patients that their physician was highly receptive to questions. As in the first study, the intervention groups asked more questions, although there was no impact on their recall of information. Both intervention groups also reported feeling more control in their treatment and were more satisfied, compared to the control group. The authors also found a positive relationship between asking more questions and the amount of information recalled, although this was not due to the intervention—suggesting that another mechanism may have produced these results.

A pilot study by McCann and Weinman (1996) demonstrated that a brief handout labeled "Speak for Yourself" had limited success in encouraging patients to increase their participation. The handout advised patients to identify concerns and questions for the doctor, and encouraged patients to write down this information prior to seeing the doctor as a way to increase the likelihood that their expectations were met. Based on audiotaped recordings, patients who received the handout tended to have longer visits and ask more condition-related questions. However, the intervention had no impact on patients' reported levels of satisfaction, nor did the results suggest that individual differences (such as levels of self-efficacy or locus of control) play a role in how well patients respond to the written intervention.

The goal of Frederikson and Bull's (1995) intervention study was to encourage patients to clearly state their reasons for coming to the doctor as well as to help them think about their expectations for the visit. As with the other question-asking intervention studies, this intervention was based on the assumption that activated patients will be more involved and better equipped to take care of their own health and have an improved sense of control. Patients were given a one-page handout outlined with the following instructions: "stop-think-tell-listen-remember," which emphasized the importance of telling the physician all pertinent facts and concerns because "the doctor is not a mind reader." The handout also included brief instruction as to how to carry out each action. However, unlike the majority of the intervention studies, the authors did not examine the impact of these instructions on patients' question-asking or satisfaction, but rather on how the study doctors evaluated their communication with each patient. Results showed that doctors gave a rating of "good" in

80% of the intervention patients, and only 57% of the control patients. Likewise, 35% of the control visits were rated "average" compared with only 18% of the intervention visits. Thus, an easily administered intervention was able to yield positive benefits—even from the physician' perspective.

In a study by Tabak (1988), family medicine patients were given a small booklet that encouraged information exchange and included 33 "modeling" questions for patients. The handout did not increase patient's question asking behavior nor did it increase their satisfaction. Yet, another study (Jacobson et al., 1999) that evaluated a brief patient handout demonstrated that this simple intervention was both effective in improving question-asking behavior and increasing the likelihood of patients receiving preventive care, even among those with low literacy. Inconsistencies such as these are not uncommon, and can be accounted for by a variety of factors that differ across studies, not only in the particulars of the approach taken, but in the sample used and the setting involved. For instance, patients in the former study had a mean age of 35 years, whereas the mean age of the patients in the latter study was 63 years.

In one of the few studies that examined patient communication interventions in the context of cancer care (P. Butow, Dunn, Tattersall, & Jones, 1994), cancer patients seeing an oncologist for the first time were reminded of the importance of having their concerns addressed, and given a list of the types of questions that cancer patients often ask their physicians "in order to help you make the most of your time with the doctor." These included questions about diagnosis (e.g., "What exactly is wrong with me?"), treatment (e.g., "Does the treatment have any side effects?"), and prognosis (e.g., "What will the outcome be, will I get better?"). Patients were encouraged to list the five questions that were most important to them, and to take the list, if they wanted, into the doctor's office to make sure that their concerns were addressed. Although there were no overall differences in the number of questions asked compared to those who received no handout, patients who were given the handout were more than twice as likely (35% vs. 16%) to ask questions related to their prognosis. The authors note that prognosis is probably the most emotion-laden and threatening issue that newly diagnosed cancer patients need to deal with, and suggest that the impact of the intervention may have been to encourage patients to ask the kind of questions that they might have otherwise avoided.

Brown, Butow, Dunn, and Tattersall (2001) conducted an intervention that replicated and extended the findings of P. Butow et al. (1994) using a larger sample of patients and oncologists. Half of the patients who were seeing their oncologists for the first time received a similar question prompt sheet. These prompted patients not only asked more questions about prognosis than controls, but they also received more prognostic information from their oncologists. However, the visits of the prompted patients also took longer, and patients' anxiety levels were significantly increased. The other half of the patients received the same prompt sheet, but their physicians were randomly assigned either to proactively address the question prompt sheet, actively endorsing it and systematically reviewing it; or to passively respond to it during the course of the visit. When the oncologists specifically addressed the prompt sheet, visits were shorter, anxiety levels were reduced, and patient recall of information was significantly improved.

Training Using Videos

A small number of studies have explored the value and effectiveness of showing training videos to patients prior to their medical visits. Based on the assumption that most patients would like to be more participatory in their medical visits, but lack the skills to achieve this, L. Anderson, DeVellis, and DeVellis (1987) used well-established modeling techniques to develop brief training videos for patients. Two experimental videos were developed in which a health educator presented various clinical and medical information to a patient who either displayed confusion by interrupting with many questions ("question-asking" model) or a patient who frequently interjected with comments about his condition ("disclosive" model). As hypothesized, the communication techniques shown in the videos led to more question asking and more self-disclosure of information. Specifically, patients who viewed modeling techniques to improve question-asking had an overall greater number of verbalizations— both in question and disclosure form. In contrast, patients who viewed disclosure modeling techniques made more disclosure statements, but did not ask more questions. Thus, knowing how to ask questions appears to generalize to overall participation to a greater extent than does knowing how to disclose information. However, despite the success in getting patients to participate and a positive relationship between participation and satisfaction, those patients who viewed the training videos were no more likely than the controls to retain the information they received from their doctor.

A similar study (Lewis, Pantell, & Sharp, 1991) was performed in a pediatric sample in which children, parents, and physicians each watched a videotape to build skills and motivation for the child's participation in the visit. The results showed that children who viewed the video were more activated, had better recall of medication information, and were more satisfied with the visit. Still, the video did not produce greater satisfaction on the part of the parents or the physicians.

Allowing patients to view effective communication techniques certainly creates the opportunity for patients to learn and model new skills they might not ordinarily develop. In addition, the video format is one that is likely to be more compelling than using written materials. Therefore, it is a methodology that deserves more attention and would benefit from a more critical and thorough evaluation in future studies.

Face to Face Training

Although patient handouts and training videos have the advantage of being relatively cost-efficient and easily administered, they lack the intensity and individualization that can be critical to the intervention process. In an early study by Roter (1977), an intervention in which patients were interviewed by a health educator prior to the visit was shown to have multiple effects, both positive and negative, on the doctor–patient interaction. Providing patients with the opportunity to identify and rehearse questions did indeed produce more patient question-asking, but it also produced more negative affect both in the patient and the physician, suggesting that the interview may have created heightened expectations on the part of the patient. Hoping for a more informative and interactive exchange with their physicians, patients may have displayed more anxiety and anger when these attempts proved unsuccessful. Yet because patients who received the training did show signs of increased adherence, as measured by future appointment-keeping, the greater patient involvement did yield positive effects.

In one of the most widely cited series of patient intervention studies (Greenfield, Kaplan, & Ware, 1985; Greenfield, Kaplan, Ware, Yano, & Frank, 1988; Kaplan & Greenfield, 1989), it was posited that specific aspects the doctor–patient communication are directly related to measurable health outcomes. This proposed causal relationship between patient involvement and medical outcomes is intuitively appealing because improved health is a major goal of almost all medical interactions. Ideally, giving patients the proper communication and negotiation tools allows them to more fully participate in the management and the control of their health, thereby resulting in better health status outcomes overall. In the first of three studies, the researchers compared a general previsit educational session to a highly personalized coaching session in which a health educator reviewed the patient's medical record and identified key medical decisions that were relevant to the visit. Various participatory behaviors, such as asking questions and negotiating medical decisions, were encouraged as well. Although there were no differences between the groups in the number of questions asked, patients in the experimental group did display other behaviors that clearly indicated more active participation. The most notable finding was that, compared to controls, these patients also reported a greater desire for increased involvement and better functional status (i.e., fewer limitations) (Greenfield et al., 1985). Using the same methodology, a similar pattern of results was shown in a sample of diabetic patients. In addition to reporting better functional status, patients receiving the intervention session also showed lower blood glucose levels and fewer diabetic-related problems (Greenfield et al., 1988).

In the last of the series of studies that examined the link between patient activation and health status, Kaplan, Greenfield, and Ware (1989) conducted four trials in which the impact of a communication intervention on various physiologic measures was assessed. As was found in the two earlier studies, compared to controls, patients who received individualized information about their condition prior to their visits and who were given strategies to improve their communication with doctors showed improved outcomes for three different chronic diseases as well as breast cancer (Kaplan et al., 1989). The exact mechanism that produced these results is not completely understood. Yet one of the more striking results of this study is the positive relationship found between expressed negative affect during the encounter and better health status—a pattern similar to that reported by Roter (1977). As the authors suggest, providing patients with the tools to become more participatory during the visit gives patients greater feelings of confidence and control and perhaps, on some level, a more intense feeling of commitment to the management of their condition. But at the same time that the patient is undergoing a renewed interest in his or her health care and a desire to be a more active participant in it, it is also possible that the physician and patient are experiencing some uneasiness due to a shift in perceived responsibility and control during their interaction.

The results of Greenfield and Ware's studies showing the significant link between patient activation and measurable health outcomes are often cited as clear evidence for further investigation in this area. However, to date, there has been little work that has either replicated or further tested the relationship between patient communication behaviors and functional health status. Because this pattern was evident in their sample of breast cancer patients, this training approach is one that might be considered particularly promising and worthy of follow-up in patients with many different types of cancer.

Multi-strategy Training

Although the interventions described here have each had varying levels of success in increasing patient involvement in the medical visit, few have approached the patient training as comprehensively as the recent work of Cegala and his colleagues. To increase the likelihood that both patients and doctors would have a successful communication exchange, Cegala, Marinelli, and Post (2000) developed patient workbooks designed to instruct patients on three distinct communication strategies: information provision, seeking, and verifying. Because patients often do not know how or what information to provide to their physicians, the initial step of the program helps patients to consider and verbalize all their medically relevant information. Next, patients are instructed on information seeking, a process similar to many of the earlier studies in which patients were given handouts to help them formulate questions they might want to ask their physician. Patients are also given sample questions to assist them in their preparation.

The purpose of the final, and perhaps most unique and important strategy, information verifying, was to train patients on how to clarify or confirm their understanding of the information given to them by their physician. Depending on the situation, patients can receive an enormous amount of information, often filled with clinical or technical terms that may be unfamiliar to them. Not knowing how to request a more simplified explanation or not realizing that they do not fully comprehend the information they are receiving is a common complaint of patients and can easily lead to misunderstandings, poor adherence, or even more serious outcomes, such as improper medication dosing or contra-indications. Cegala's work recognizes that the communication exchange between patient and provider is a more complicated process, and that multiple skills and strategies are required on the patient's part to assure that the end product of the exchange is shared meaning.

In addition to enhancing patient participation and increasing the number of important communication behaviors (Cegala et al., 2000; Cegala, Post, & McClure, 2001; Post, Cegala, & Marinelli, 2001) patients who received a training booklet 2 to 3 days prior to their appointment have been shown to have better compliance in terms of both behavioral recommendations and appointment keeping (Cegala et al., 2000). In a variation of the three-strategy approach, patients in another study received previsit instruction on these three skills, but no workbook preparation This resulted in more patient questions and better recall of information, but not more elicited information (Socha McGee, & Cegala, 1998).

Facilitating Patient Control

A range of patient-based approaches have been devised that involve medical decision making, although the majority of these are really directed at helping patients to make better decisions (i.e., focused on outcome) rather than at training patients about how to become more activated decision makers themselves (i.e., focused on process). For example, numerous decision aids have been developed to provide information on diseases and conditions, probabilities of outcomes, and clarify risks and personal values (Edwards, Evans, & Elwyn, 2003), however, these efforts, which are more outcome-based, are beyond the scope of this chapter.

With the goal of assisting men with newly diagnosed prostate cancer to become more involved in their own treatment decision making, Davison and Degner (1997) developed a self-efficacy intervention that contained several elements of the information-based efforts reviewed earlier. Patients received a written information package with discussion, a list of questions they could ask their doctors, and an audiotape of their visit, while control patients received the written package only. Men in the intervention group took a more active role in treatment decision making, and had lower state anxiety levels 6 weeks later.

A different approach makes use of the Control Preferences Scale (Degner, Sloan, & Venkatesh, 1997). This measure allows patients to identify their ideal role in treatment decision making by sorting cards that list different preferred roles. This has been converted recently into a touch-screen computer format that offers patients rapid feedback on their preferences for that particular visit. The developers of this scale believe that the act of completing the task makes active decision making roles more salient to patients, thereby encouraging them to initiate attempts to become more involved. An initial attempt at using the computer computer-based approach (Davison et al., 2002), however, generated limited results, as many of those who chose to complete the touch screen task were already among those preferring the most active roles. Although the exact use and timing of this method is yet to be fully refined, it stands as an innovative way of encouraging patients to become involved in at least thinking about how best to make decisions about their own care.

CONCLUSIONS AND FUTURE DIRECTIONS

Despite the relative scarcity of carefully controlled, published studies indicating which patient strategies work in clinical communications, there is apparently no scarcity of advice about how patients should communicate, as a recent Yahoo! search using the heading "how to talk to your doctor" generated 1,650,000 hits. Although movement toward consumerism of the overall health care arena is in full swing, the movement to improve health care through direct activation of patients on the part of researchers and providers is just in its infancy. The results of the studies reviewed have been generally positive, even those of relatively low intensity, yet few if any comparative studies have been done to evaluate the different interventional strategies. Also, with a few notable exceptions (e.g., Kahana & Kahana, 2003; Kreps, O'Hair, & Clowers, 1994), little conceptual work has been done in this area to identify the processes that mediate the relationship between patient activation and outcomes.

A number of interesting research questions call for investigation. For instance, why is it that objective measures such as amount of information given do not necessarily translate into subjective measures such as satisfaction? Why is it that patient activation can generate problems in process (e.g., negative affect), but also positive outcomes? More generally, to what extent is an active patient welcomed by some physicians at certain junctures in a relationship when discussing certain problems for some medical conditions?

As much as these research questions will allow us to understand the process, many practical questions call for immediate answers. What skills and strategies are most important to patients? What approaches to patient activation are most effective and/or most cost-effective? How does one determine trade-offs between the potential impact of such interventions versus their requirements in terms of time, staff, and cost? And how can the interventions be sustained over time, with outcomes studied longitudinally?

Recognizing that one size does not fit all, we need to ask which types of effort are most practical for different patient settings and patient types; and how much patient age, culture, education, condition, and preferences determine what the most appropriate intervention is. Considering when such interventions are best conducted, it would seem that patients would be most attentive and receptive to these when they are seriously ill and the stakes are greatest. Yet, during times of serious illness patients may be so emotionally focused on their medical problems that they may be less receptive, they may consider such attempts intrusive, and some patients may revert to dependence on the physician as the expert whom they feel they should rely on in times of threat and crisis.

Finally, there are many issues involved in patient activation that have barely been addressed at all. In the future, the care of cancer patients will likely be improved when the following are developed:

- Interventions that involve both sides of the equation, that train provider–patient pairs how to best utilize one another for the greatest benefit of all.
- Interventions that teach patients general skills of assertiveness and apply these to clinical communication.
- Interventions that move beyond information exchange and decision making to determine whether there are ways that patients can make their providers more attentive to their emotional needs.
- Interventions that train patients how to rely on different members of a care team for different kinds of information and support, and how to use the complementary knowledge and skills of the care team members to the patient's greatest benefit.
- Interventions that are personally and culturally sensitive, that offer skills to patients of differing races, ethnicities, and personal preferences in ways that are tailored to their individual needs and cultural values.

REFERENCES

Anderson, L. A., DeVellis, B. M., & DeVellis, R. F. (1987). Effects of modeling on patient communication, satisfaction, and knowledge. *Medical Care, 25,* 1044-1056.

Anderson, M., & Urban, N. (1997). Physician gender and screening: Do patient differences account for differences in mammography use? *Women & Health, 26,* 29-39.

Arora, N. K. (2003). Interacting with cancer patients: The significance of physicians' communication behavior. *Social Science & Medicine, 57,* 791-806.

Bakker, D. A., Fitch, M. I., Gray, R., Reed, E., & Bennett, J. (2001). Patient-health care provider communication during chemotherapy treatment: The perspectives of women with breast cancer. *Patient Education & Counseling, 43,* 61-71.

Beaver, K., Luker, K. A., Owens, R. G., Leinster, S. J., & Degner, L. F. (1996). Treatment decision making in women newly diagnosed with breast cancer. *Cancer Nursing, 19,* 8-19.

Beckman, H. B., & Frankel R. M. (2003). Training practitioners to communicate effectively in cancer care: It is the relationship that counts. *Patient Education & Counseling, 50,* 85-89.

Brietbart, W. (1995). Identifying patients at risk for, and treatment of major psychiatric complications of cancer. *Support and Cancer Care, 3,* 45-60.

Brown, R. F., Butow, P. N., Dunn, S. M., & Tattersall, M. H. (2001). Promoting patient participation and shortening cancer consultations: A randomized trial. *British Journal of Cancer, 85,* 1273-1279.

Bruera, E., Willey, J. S., Palmer, J. L., & Rosales, M. (2002). Treatment decision for breast carcinoma: Patient preferences and physician perceptions. *Cancer, 94,* 2076-2080.

Butow, B., & Baile, W. F. (2003). The importance of communication skills to effective cancer care and support. *Medical Encounter, 17,* 2-4.

Butow, P. N., Dunn, S. M., Tattersall, M. H., & Jones, Q. J. (1994). Patient participation in the cancer consultation: Evaluation of a question prompt sheet. *Annals of Oncology, 5,* 199-204.

Butow, P. N., Maclean, M., Dunn S. M., Tattersall, M. H. N., & Boyer, M. J. (1997). The dynamics of change: Cancer patients' preferences for information, involvement, and support. *Annals of Oncology, 8,* 857-863.

Butow, P. N., Brown, R. F., Cogar, S., Tattersall, M. H. N., & Dunn, S. M. (2002). Oncologists' reactions to cancer patients' verbal cues. *Psycho-Oncology, 11,* 47-58.

Cegala, D. J. (2003). Patient communication skills training: A review with implications for cancer patients. *Patient Education & Counseling, 50,* 91-94.

Cegala, D. J., & Lenzmeier Broz, S. (2002) Physician communication skills training: A review of theoretical backgrounds, objectives and skills. *Medical Education, 36,* 1004-1016.

Cegala, D. J., Marinelli, T., & Post, D. (2000). The effects of patient communication skills training on compliance. *Archives of Family. Medicine., 9,* 57-64.

Cegala, D. J., Post, D. M., & McClure, L. (2001). The effects of patient communication skills training on the discourse of older patients during a primary care interview. *Journal of the American Geriatic Society, 49,* 1505-1511.

Cormaroff, J., & Maguire, P. (1981). Ambiguity and the search for meaning: Childhood leukemia in the modern clinical context. *Social Science and Medicine, 15b,* 115-123.

Davison, B. J., & Degner, L. F. (1997). Empowerment of men newly diagnosed with prostate cancer. *Cancer Nursing, 20,* 187-196.

Davison, B. J., Degner, L. F., & Morgan, T. B. (1995). Prostate cancer: Information needs and treatment decision making. *Oncology Nursing Forum, 22,* 1401-1408.

Davison, B. J., Gleave, M. E., Goldenberg, S. L., Degner, L. F., Hoffart, D., & Berkowitz, J. (2002). Assessing information and decision preferences of men with prostate cancer and their partners. *Cancer Nursing, 25,* 42-49.

Degner, L. F., Kristjanson, L., Bowman, D., Sloan, J., O'Neil, J., Carriere, K. C., Bilodeau, B., & Mueller, B. (1997). Decisional preferences and information needs in women with breast cancer. *Journal of the American Medical Association, 277,* 1485-1492.

Degner, L. F., Sloan, J. A., & Venkatesh, P. (1997). The Control Preferences Scale. *Canadian Journal of Nursing Research, 29,* 21-42.

DiMatteo, M. R. (2003). Future directions in research on consumer-provider communication and adherence to cancer prevention and treatment. *Patient Education & Counseling, 50,* 23-26.

Edwards, A., Evans, R., & Elwyn, G. (2003). Manufactured but not imported: New directions for research in shared decision making support and skills. *Patient Education & Counseling, 50,* 33-38.

Fallowfield, L., Lipkin, M., & Cockburn, J. (1998). Teaching senior oncologists communication skills. *Journal of Clinical Oncology, 16,* 1961-1968.

Fallowfield, V., Jenkins, V., Farewell, V., Saul, J., Duffy, A., & Eves, R. (2002). Efficacy of a cancer research UK communication skills training model for oncologists: A randomised controlled trial. *Lancet, 359,* 650-656.

Ford, S., Fallowfield, L., & Lewis, S. (1994). Can oncologists detect distress in their outpatients and how satisfied are they with their performance during bad news consultations? *British Journal of Cancer, 70,* 767-770.

Frederikson, L. G., & Bull, P. E. (1995). Evaluation of a patient education leaflet designed to improve communication in medical consultations. *Patient Education & Counseling, 25,* 51-57.

Gattelleri, M., Butow, P. N., & Tattersall, M. H. N. (2001). Sharing decisions in cancer care. *Social Science & Medicine, 52,* 1865-1878

Greenfield, S., Kaplan, S., & Ware, J. E., Jr. (1985). Expanding patient involvement in care. Effects on patient outcomes. *Annals of Internal Medicine, 102,* 520-528.

Greenfield, S., Kaplan, S. H., Ware, J. E., Jr., Yano, E. M., & Frank, H. J. (1988). Patients' participation in medical care: Effects on blood sugar control and quality of life in diabetes. *Journal of General Internal Medicine, 3,* 448-457.

Hall, J. A. (2003). Some observations on provider-patient communication research. *Patient Education & Counseling, 50,* 9-12.

Jacobson, T. A., Thomas, D. M., Morton, F. J., Offutt, G., Shevlin, J., & Ray, S. (1999). Use of a low-literacy patient education tool to enhance pneumococcal vaccination rates. A randomized controlled trial. *Journal of the American Medical Association, 282,* 646-650.

Jenkins, V. , Fallowfield, L., & Saul, J. (2001). Information needs of patients with cancer: Results from a large study in UK cancer centers. *British Journal of Cancer, 84,* 48-51.

Kahana, E., & Kahana, B. (2003). Patient proactivity enhancing doctor-patient-family communication in cancer prevention and care among the aged. *Patient Education & Counseling, 50,* 67-73.

Kaplan, S. H., Greenfield, S., & Ware, J. E., Jr. (1989). Assessing the effects of physician-patient interactions on the outcomes of chronic disease. *Medical Care, 27,* S110-S127.

Kindelan, K., & Kent, G. (1987). Concordance between patients' information preferences and general practitioners' perceptions. *Psychology & Health, 1,* 399-409.

Kravitz, R. L. (1996). Patients' expectations for medical care: An expanded formulation based on review of the literature. *Medical Care Research and Review, 53,* 3-27.

Kravitz, R. L., Bell, R. A., Azari, R., Kelly-Reif, S., Krupat, E., & Thom, D. H. (2003). Direct observation of requests for clinical services in office practice. What do patients want and do they get it? *Archives of Internal Medicine, 163,* 1673-1681.

Kreps, G. L., Arora, N. K., & Nelson, D. E. (2003). Consumer/provider communication research: Directions for development. *Patient Education & Counseling, 50,* 3-4.

Kreps, G. L., O'Hair, D., & Clowers, M. (1994). The influences of human communication on health outcomes. *American Behavioral Scientist, 38,* 248-256.

Krupat, E., Irish, J. T., Kasten, L. E., Freund, K. M., Burns, R. B., Moskowitz, M. S., & McKinlay, J. B. (1999). Patient assertiveness and physician decision-making among older breast cancer patients. *Social Science & Medicine, 49,* 449-457.

Leventhal, H., & Benyamini, Y. (1997). Lay beliefs about health and illness In A. Baum, C. McManus, S. Newman, & R. West (Eds.), *Cambridge handbook of psychology, health, and medicine.* Cambridge, England: Cambridge University Press.

Levinson, W., Gorawara-Bhat, R., & Lamb, J. (2000). A study of patient clues and physician responses in primary care and surgical settings. *Journal of the American Medical Association, 284,* 1021-1027.

Lewis, C. C., Pantell, R. H., & Sharp, L. (1991). Increasing patient knowledge, satisfaction, and involvement: Randomized trial of a communication intervention. *Pediatrics, 88,* 351-358.

Lobb, E. A., Butow, P. N., Kenny, D. T., & Tattersall, M. H. N. (1999). Communicating prognosis in early breast cancer: Do women understand the language used? *Medical Journal of Australia, 171,* 290-294.

Maguire, P. (1985). Improving the detection of psychiatric symptoms in cancer patients. *Social Science & Medicine, 20,* 819-823.

Maguire, P., Faulkner, A., Booth, K., Elliot, C., & Hillier, V. (1996). Helping cancer patients disclose their concerns. *European Journal of Cancer, 32a,* 78-81.

McCann, S., & Weinman, J. (1996). Empowering the patient in the consultation: A pilot study. *Patient Education & Counseling, 27,* 227-234.

McWilliam, C. L., Brown, J. B., & Stewart, M. (2000). Breast cancer patients' experience of patient-doctor communication: A working relationship. *Patient Education & Counseling, 39,* 191-204.

Post, D. M., Cegala, D. J., & Marinelli, T. M. (2001). Teaching patients to communicate with physicians: The impact of race. *Journal of the National.Medical Association, 93,* 6-12.

Post, D. M., Cegala, D. J., & Miser, W. F. (2002). The other half of the whole: Teaching patients to communicate with physicians. *Family Medicine, 34,* 344-352.

Quill, T. E., & Brody, H. (1996). Physician recommendations and patient autonomy: Finding a balance between physician power and patient choice. *Annals of Internal Medicine, 125,* 763-769.

Roter, D. L. (1977). Patient participation in the patient-provider interaction: The effects of patient question asking on the quality of interaction, satisfaction and compliance. *Health Education Monographs, 5,* 281-315.

Rothenberger, D., Lutz, M. P., & Porzsolt, F. (1997). Treatment decisions in palliative cancer care: Patients' preferences for involvement and doctors' knowledge about it. *European Journal of Cancer, 33,* 1184-1189.

Socha McGee, D., & Cegala, D. J. (1998). Patient communication skills training for improved communication competence in primary care medical consultation. *Journal of Applied Communication Research, 26,* 412-430.

Street, R. L. (1992a). Analyzing communication in medical consultations: Do behavioral measures correspond to patients' perceptions? *Medical Care, 30,* 976-988.

Street, R. L. (1992b). Communicative styles and adaptations in physician-parent consultations. *Social Science & Medicine, 34,* 1155-1163.

Street, R. L., Krupat, E., Bell, R.A., Kravitz, R.L., & Haidet, P. (2003). Beliefs about control in the physician-patient relationship: Effect on communication in medical encounters. *Journal of General Internal Medicine, 18,* 609-616.

Tabak, E. R. (1988). Encouraging patient question-asking: A clinical trial. *Patient Education & Counseling, 12,* 37-49.

Thompson, S. C., Nanni, C., & Schwankowsky, L. (1990). Patient-oriented interventions to improve communication in a medical office visit. *Health Psychology, 9,* 390-404.

Waitzkin, H. (1984). Doctor-patient communication. *Journal of the American Medical Association, 252,* 2441-2446.

Wallberg, B., Michelson, H., Nystedt, M., Bolund, C., Degner, L.F., & Wilking, N. (2000). Information and preferences for participation in treatment decisions among Swedish breast cancer patients. *Acta Oncologica, 39,* 467-476.

Williams, S., Weinman, J., Dale, J., & Newman, S. (1995). Patient expectations: What do primary care patients want from the GP and how far does meeting expectations affect patient satisfaction? *Family Practice, 12,* 193-201.

Concordance and Communication in Cancer Management

Betty Chewning
University of Wisconsin

Carol J. Hermansen Kobulnicky
University of Wyoming

My oncologist sat down and said to me and my wife, "I work for you." That really struck a chord with us. I realized I wanted and needed to work together with my doctor in deciding what type of treatment I would have.

—Wiederholt and Wiederholt, *The WriteTrack* (2005, p. 6)

This chapter explores the concept of *concordance* and its potential for enhancing the communication between health care providers and individuals who have cancer. Concordance refers to the agreement between an individual and health care provider around a range of issues such as visit agendas, approaches to diagnosis and treatment, calibration of ongoing regimens, and even how actively an individual wishes to participate in a particular decision or visit. Across the full trajectory of visits and contacts with different health care providers, individuals with cancer face countless adjustments to people, health care procedures, and their physical status. The nature and quality of the communication process influences their quality of life (QOL) immeasurably.

We begin by exploring how the concept of concordance has been defined thus far and how it might be expanded. Second, we review cancer literature related to individuals' preference for involvement, their visit agendas, their symptom monitoring and pain management between visits, and patients' interactions with multiple providers related to pharmaceutical decisions regarding chemotherapy and palliative therapy. To help ground the discussion of possible approaches, we offer the experience of one individual with cancer who was a colleague of ours.

Joseph Wiederholt was a pharmacy school faculty member and former pharmacist. His wife, Peggy, is a nurse who directed clinical drug trials in cardiology and who now works with individuals who have cancer. During his 7 years with cancer we were privileged to have Joe relay his experiences with providers as he lived with cancer. A teacher to the end, one of the last things he said was, "Any more questions?"

Traditionally, the *concordance* term relates to whether the provider and patient agree on the initial prescribing decision with medications. We believe the concept can be applied much more broadly. Through Joe's experience, we hope to offer a wider view of what concordance can mean from the first meeting between a provider and individual when cancer is first diagnosed all the way through palliative care decisions.

RELEVANCE OF CONCORDANCE FOR CANCER

Concordance is especially applicable when a health condition is serious and the therapy options involve imperfect trade-offs with variable benefits and serious toxicities as well as damage over time, as in the case of cancer (Chewning et al., 2001). In the midst of great uncertainty and anxiety regarding their lives, individuals with cancer also have to cope with adverse effects and unknowns about how chemotherapy and possible palliative therapy will disrupt their lives. Chemotherapy and pain management side effects can add significantly to the burden of cancer related symptoms (Cleeland et al., 2000; Gunnars, Nygren, & Glimelius, 2001; Portenoy et al., 1994). In an extensive review of empirical literature on physicians' communication behavior, Arora (2003) noted that qualitative research confirms that cancer patients perceive more control when their physicians attempt to inform and involve them in decision making (Bakker, Fitch, Gray, Reed, & Bennett, 2001; McWilliam, Brown, & Stewart, 2000). Consistent with these findings, many have urged more collaborative relationships between patients and health care professionals (Blenkinsopp, 2001; Britten, 2003; Charles, Gafni, & Whelan, 1999; Chewning et al., 2001; Chewning & Wiederholt, 2003; Chewning & Sleath, 1996; Concordance Work Group, 1997; Golin, DiMatteo, & Gelberg, 1996; Stevenson, 2001; Wiederholt & Wiederholt 1997).

The Royal British Pharmaceutical Society has urged a concordance framework be widely implemented during patient–provider encounters with respect to their pharmaceutical regimens (Concordance Work Group, 1997). The Society's work group defined concordance as:

> . . . an agreement reached after negotiation between a patient and health care professional that respects the beliefs and wishes of the patient in determining whether, when and how medicines are to be taken. Although reciprocal, this is an alliance in which the health care professional recognizes the primacy of the patient's decisions about taking the recommended medications. (Concordance Work Group, 1997)

As Britten (2003) pointed out, concordance adds attention to the primacy of the individual's decision role. This view is based on the assumption that the individual and provider should negotiate and reach agreement on a regimen rather than have a patient passively receive medication and other therapy orders issued from a prescriber (Britten, 2003).

At its most basic level, concordance involves an exchange between the individual and the provider where each communicates his or her expertise and concerns in order to achieve an agreed on plan at the end of the visit. It requires the provider to assess how active the individual can and wants to be during this exchange. This process then shapes how visit agendas are established, what approaches are used for diagnosis and treatment, calibration of ongoing regimens, schedules and locations for treatment, side-effect management, self-care including complementary alternative medicines, how the individual can monitor and record symptoms between visits, and even how actively an individual wishes to participate in a particular decision or visit (See Fig. 21.1). The overall style of involvement and mutual respect sets the foundation for an effective partnership to achieve the optimal QOL for the individual. Each visit's interaction pattern influences the individual's role not only in the immediate visit but also with respect to the next visit. We are suggesting there is an iterative effect in the patient–provider interaction system across visits. Concordance lends itself to viewing partnership style across the trajectory of care, not simply at the initial diagnosis and therapy selection (Chewning & Wiederholt, 2003; Hermansen-Kobulnicky, Wiederholt, & Chewning, 2004). Both the individual's and the provider's expectations and behaviors at subsequent visits build on what happened earlier, as documented in an early observational study of clinic visits by Svarstad (1974) and others (Svarstad & Sitter, 2005).

Concordance depends on providers having strong interviewing skills to identify an individual's agenda, desire for information, and the degree to which the person wants to discuss his or her experience and preferences in the visit. This model depends not only on an individual being open and receptive to the provider's expertise, but equally important, concordance depends on the provider encouraging and welcoming involvement and the individual's potentially very different perspectives. From the concordance perspective, if the individual has unspoken reservations and concerns, the provider is at a terrible disadvantage when trying to achieve the best plan without feedback from the individual. Having strong processing skills is essential. As Fig. 21.1 suggests, the provider has a responsibility to clearly present his or her expertise, as well as to assess the individual's perspectives, be approachable and welcoming to the individual's questions and concerns, solicit and be responsive to input, and evaluate whether the individual agrees to the plan at the end of the visit. It is critical to gather feedback indirectly and/or directly throughout the encounter. Although at times this may seem overwhelming, perhaps it is easier to imagine if a multidisciplinary team can help respond to the varied concerns that may be identified in such an open interaction.

On the patient side, we assume that patients bring the best expertise they are capable of at that point in time to work with their provider. They are not blank slates. Consistent with the client centered model (Chewning & Sleath, 1996), we assume that individuals, better than any health care provider, understand their own: (a) personal goals and priorities for QOL as well as longevity; (b) preferred trade-offs of medication side effect/benefits for palliative as well as primary therapies; (c) preferences for how and when to receive chemotherapy (e.g., side-effect cycles may interfere with high-priority weekly activities, impersonal setting may be upsetting); (d) resources and constraints to handle toxicities, emotional issues, physical problems; (e) ability and interest to manage and evaluate a potentially complex regimen; and (f) plans for self-care (e.g., complementary alternative medicines). By integrating the provider's expertise with the patient's unique expertise about symptoms and priorities, the goal is to enhance concordance in regimen-related discourse, selection, and calibration over time as the person's needs and priorities change.

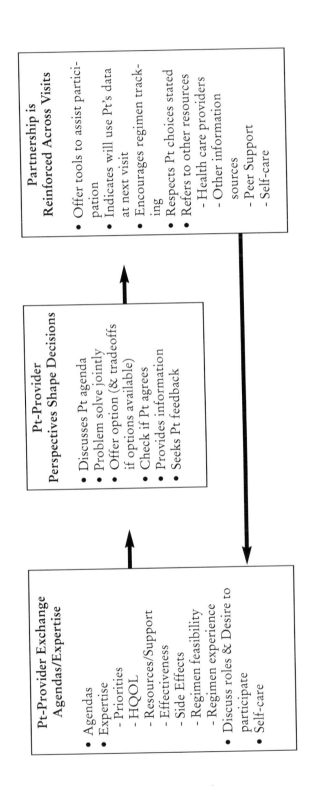

Pt-Provider Exchange Agendas/Expertise

- Agendas
- Expertise
  - Priorities
  - HQOL
  - Resources/Support
  - Effectiveness
  - Side Effects
  - Regimen feasibility
  - Regimen experience
- Discuss roles & Desire to participate
- Self-care

Pt-Provider Perspectives Shape Decisions

- Discusses Pt agenda
- Problem solve jointly
- Offer option (& tradeoffs if options available)
- Check if Pt agrees
- Provides information
- Seeks Pt feedback

Partnership is Reinforced Across Visits

- Offer tools to assist participation
- Indicates will use Pt's data at next visit
- Encourages regimen tracking
- Respects Pt choices stated
- Refers to other resources
  - Health care providers
  - Other information sources
  - Peer Support
  - Self-care

FIGURE 21.1. Concordance partnership across the trajectory of cancer care.

346

Given that individuals do vary in the degree of involvement they desire, it is interesting that so many studies have found that the majority of individuals with cancer prefer collaborative involvement in their cancer treatment decisions (Blanchard, LaBrecque, Ruckdeschel, & Blanchard, 1988; Bruera, Sweeney, Calder, Palmer, & Benishch-Tolley, 2001; Bruera, Willey, Palmer, & Rosales, 2002; Butow, Maclean, Dunn, Tattersall, & Boyer, 1997; Cassileth, Zupkis, Slutton-Smith, & March, 1980; Davison et al., 2002; Davison, Parker, & Goldenberg, 2004; Degner et al., 1997; Fielding & Hung, 1996; Gagnon & Recklitis, 2001; Hack, Degner, & Dyck, 1994; Helmes, Bowen, & Bengel, 2002; Hermansen-Kobulnicky & Chewning, 2002; Keating, Guadagnoli, Landrum, Borbas, & Weeks, 2002; Protiere et al., 2000; Rothenbacher, Lutz, & Porzsolt, 1997; Stewart et al., 2000). Even higher numbers of patients wish to be fully informed of options and outcomes (Barry & Henderson, 1996; Blanchard et al., 1988; Bruera et al., 2001; Butow et al., 1997; Cassileth et al., 1980; Degner et al., 1997; Fielding & Hung, 1996; Hack et al., 1994; Keating et al., 2002; Protiere et al., 2000; Rothenbacher et al., 1997; Stewart et al., 2000; Wallberg et al., 2000; Wong et al., 2000). A smaller number of studies found samples of patients, drawn largely from midwestern Canada and England, preferred a more passive role in their treatment decision (Beaver, Bogg, & Luker, 1999; Beaver et al., 1996; Bilodeau & Degner, 1996; Davison, Brundage, & Feldmann-Stewart, 1999; Degner & Sloan, 1992; Sutherland, Llewellyn-Thomas, Lockwood, Tritchler, & Till, 1989). Across several studies other than the few done in the United States and Australia, male, older, and less-educated patients often tend to prefer more passive roles than did younger, better educated, and female patients. Thus, demographic characteristics of study samples must be considered carefully. As well, there is evidence to suggest that providers may underestimate their patients' desire for involvement (Bruera et al., 2001, 2002; Keating et al., 2002; Rothenbacher et al., 1997). A significant portion of patients who report wanting an active or collaborative role indicate they did not participate as much as they would have liked (Barry & Henderson, 1996; Beaver et al., 1999; Bilodeau & Degner, 1996; Rothenbacher et al., 1997). It is important to note, however, that Keating et al. (2002) and others have documented a subset of individuals with cancer who report having had a more active role in the visit than they desired, reinforcing the importance of assessing patient preference for involvement in each visit.

One might ask if the desire for involvement is more a patient trait or a state. There is evidence that physicians may be able to increase participation in treatment decisions by using patient-centered behavior (Street, Voigt, Geyer, Manning, & Swanson, 1995). Similarly, in a randomized controlled intervention involving symptom monitoring, individuals with cancer who were given symptom diaries to use between visits reported that more shared decision making occurred in their subsequent visits than did the control group (Hermansen-Kobulnicky & Chewning, 2002; Kobulnicky, 2003). It appears that clear physician cues, approachability, and structures for involvement in the visit influence an individual's participation.

Taken together, this literature suggests that a considerable group of patients want to collaborate during their visit. Furthermore, there may be approaches and tools to assist this process. Another factor influencing the preferred decision role could be the individual's changing physical and emotional health status. Concordance offers a lens for framing the question of how, in the middle of all the changes a person with cancer goes through, the provider and individual can assess readiness to help calibrate care plans leading to an optimum QOL.

In the following sections, we discuss research literature related to communication and concordance with respect to patient visit agendas, symptom monitoring, pain management, and challenges in the multidisciplinary nature of care. Our goal is to contribute to improved QOL for individuals with cancer by exploring approaches and tools to establish and promote concordant patient–provider relationships through better communication. Taken together, although this research reinforces the importance of reciprocity between patient desire and an opportunity for input, it also points to how large our research gaps are. Therefore, we also comment on the need for further research throughout our discussion of these topics.

UNVOICED PATIENT AGENDAS

> At the first visit after I started chemo, the doctor went down a checklist of side effects and asked if I had had any of them. I rated each one. When he started to move on, I pulled out my list of the ones that had really bothered me a lot more and asked if he wanted to know about these other ones. He was really surprised. (Joe Wiederholt, personal communication)

A crucial step of concordance is identifying patient agendas for the patient–provider encounter. A second step is generating satisfactory plans to address them. Research on the visit agendas of patients with cancer suggests that physicians may not accurately perceive (a) the extent of patient concerns regarding treatment and physician-interaction issues (Goldberg, Guadagnoli, Silliman, & Glicksman, 1990); (b) physical symptoms not considered major by physicians (Newell, Sanson-Fisher, Girgis, & Bonaventura, 1998); and (c) psychosocial issues (Newell et al., 1998). This would be easier to correct if patients and providers had clear expectations as to who should take the lead in initiating discussions about patient agendas. However, work by Detmar, Aaronson, Wever, Muller, and Schornagel (2000) suggests that there are competing expectations between physicians and patients about who is to raise agenda items, particularly in the psychosocial area.

One recent observational study examined how patients' problems and concerns are communicated in 74 consultations with oncologists (Rogers & Todd, 2000). This study documented that doctor-initiated questions were the predominant communication pattern, both in initiating and directing talking by patients. More than 75% of doctor-initiated questions were closed-ended questions focusing on patient pain. The investigators of this study argued that doctors tightly controlled the agenda to focus narrowly on pain considered amenable to radiotherapy, chemotherapy, surgery, or hormone manipulation. In this context, it seems unlikely that patient agendas would be fully voiced and addressed.

Stromgren et al. (2001) investigated how completely symptoms experienced by advanced cancer patients were covered by the medical records. Consistent with other findings, there was consistent reporting of pain, but most other symptoms or problems reported by patients in three questionnaires were much less reported by physicians in the medical record as well. Fellowes, Fallowfield, Saunders, and Houghton (2001), similarly, found in interviews that patients reported more side effects from hormonal therapies for cancer than physicians reported in their medical notes. Examples of underreported side effects include fatigue, mood swings/changes, decreased sexual interest, achy joints, and weight gain. As Arora (2003) pointed out in his extensive literature review there is evidence that some cancer patients may think that depression, fatigue, pain, and other psychosocial problems are inevitable and therefore not report them to physicians. Likewise, a series of studies suggests that physicians do not discuss patients' psychosocial concerns as much as patient needs suggest they should be discussed (Detmar, Muller, Wever, Schornagel, & Aaronson, 2001; Fallowfield et al., 1998; McCool & Morris, 1999; Stead, Fallowfield, Brown, & Selby, 2001). Sadly, discussion of patient concerns could facilitate needed education, regimen adjustments, or problem solving of non-medication approaches to improve health quality of life.

Thus far, there has been little research on how patient roles in setting agendas and shared decision making change over time. One qualitative study, however, suggests important issues to study further. In one of the few longitudinal studies of terminally ill cancer patients' desire for shared decision making, 35 patients were interviewed during subsequent rehospitalizations. Across the study, patient desires to participate in decisions increased with the progress of the disease. Patients reported that over time they had come to know their own bodies and responses much better. Unfortunately, over time, they reported a greater discrepancy between their desired involvement in decisions versus the actual opportunity for involvement (Barry & Henderson, 1996). This suggests the need for tools and ongoing assessment of patient desire for involvement.

Interventions to address the problem have been proposed. Kahn, Houts, and Harding (1992) indicated a need to train medical students to conduct better patient history-taking. In their matched physician and patient surveys, physicians incorrectly estimated that older patients with cancer would experience more problems in four out of five QOL categories than young patients. The opposite was true according to their patients. A separate study focused instead on giving an intervention to patients. Butow, Dunn, Tattersall, and Jones (1994) randomized 142 patients with cancer to receive a question prompt sheet or a general sheet informing patients of services available. Consultations were audiotaped. The question prompt sheet increased discussion of prognosis; however, it did not increase the mean number of patient questions asked overall.

Both descriptive and intervention research is needed to identify (a) the nature of patient agendas, (b) whether and how they are voiced, (c) strategies to facilitate their expression during the visit, and (d) associated outcomes. Longitudinal work, in addition to the cross-sectional work done on other populations, is needed to track how patterns and interventions need to change over the trajectory from initial diagnosis and treatment selections up through palliative treatment in the end stage of care. Methodological work with observational tools are needed specifically to measure the actual patient and provider behaviors that are related to agenda setting and achieving concordance.

APPROACHES TO ASSIST SYMPTOM MONITORING

Being diagnosed with cancer made me feel like my life was spinning out of control. When I started chemotherapy, I kept a calendar and tracked how my body felt from one day to the next. I started to see certain trends. I could plan each day accordingly since I was able to predict my "good" days and "not-so-good" days. It also gave me a lot more information

to share with my doctor. This helped me stay with my treatment and it gave me a tremendous sense of control. (Wiederholt & Wiederholt, *The WriteTrack*, 2005, p. 24)

Leventhal and other researchers documented that patients naturally attempt to monitor and
understand symptoms (Baumann, Cameron, Zimmerman, & Leventhal, 1989; Baumann &
Leventhal, 1985; Baumann, Zimmerman, & Leventhal, 1989; Leventhal, Leventhal, &
Robitaille, 1998; Meyer, Leventhal, & Gutmann, 1985). According to Leventhal, people
develop schemas or theories about what makes their condition better or worse, its cause, and
what their symptoms signify. For example, one person may experience a side effect and feel
it reflects the chemotherapy is strong enough to be working. Another person could experience the same symptom and believe it is a sign that the therapy is reducing his or her strength
to fight the disease. We need much more research to identify how patients view their symptoms and how their attributions influence their perceptions, choices, and perhaps outcomes
with respect to their therapies.

As Joe Wiederholt noted in the quote given earlier, his ability to monitor and then anticipate good days when receiving chemotherapy enhanced his sense of control as well as an
improved QOL. Wiederholt and Wiederholt (1997) found the patient's ability to track
chemotherapy regimen side effects also provided the physician with important information
for subsequent concordant decisions at the follow-up visits. Symptom-tracking helped Joe
and his physician select the best schedule for Joe's chemotherapy during the week in light of
the teaching and family activities he considered highest priority. This same data facilitated
conversations about how Joe could titrate needed prescriptions or over-the-counter medications for associated side effects and cancer symptoms. It became the basis of changing the
anti-nausea prescription from a formulary approved drug to a much more effective nonfor-
mulary drug that Joe bought out of pocket. Aside from anecdotal evidence such as the above,
we know little about whether and how effectively providers discuss regimen refinements and
timing to improve symptom control. We know little about self-management decisions of people with cancer and how concordant these self-care decisions might be between patient and
provider, suggesting additional research agendas.

One promising approach being examined is the use of structured tools to assist patients
to write down and share their agendas and somatic data collected between visits. Jones et al.
(2002) gave cancer patients a paper prompt to list their questions 3 weeks before a hospital
doctor visit. About half of the patients subsequently attended the hospital visit with a written list. Physicians thought that 34% of the patients would not otherwise have asked the
questions, and physicians considered 91% of prompted discussions a worthwhile use of time.
In a review of interventions for cancer pain control, one of the most promising approaches
appeared to be patient pain diaries, in which patients systematically documented daily fluc-
tuations of pain levels followed by dose adjustment relatively quickly (Allard, Maunsell,
Labbe, & Dorval, 2001). Subsequent to this review, Schumacher et al. (2002) studied 155
patients with pain from bone metastases and 90 family caregivers using a daily pain management diary. Three quarters of the patients found the pain diary useful, with a large percent
reporting that the diary heightened awareness of pain and helped guide their self-management
of pain. Although much of the literature focuses on decisions during interactions with physicians, the diary opens the lens to include other health care providers and further reminds us
of the significant amount of decision making that patients and caretakers must make without
the benefit of a health care provider.

A similar diary approach was recently studied with patients systematically tracking side effects of chemotherapy. Recently, *The WriteTrack* (Wiederholt & Wiederholt, 2005) was made available to patients nationally by a pharmaceutical company. Its popularity with patients exhausted the supply within a year of its publication. A second paperback edition has been released. Patients use the diary to list their symptoms and side effects, coding each symptom daily on a 0–10 scale of severity. These diaries are taken to physician visits. A study at the *WriteTrack*, along with a smaller study of daily diary measures with patients in Phase I cancer drug trials, suggest that diaries are feasible for patients to use to assess coping, adjustment and symptoms for a large group of patients (Hermansen-Kobulnicky et al., 2004; Sherliker & Steptoe, 2000).

From a concordance perspective, the diary offers one strategy for a provider to prepare and reinforce a patient for a more active role in the next visit as he or she collects and brings the data to jointly evaluate and tailor the regimen to the individual's needs. This could become a basis for more concordant decisions. As noted earlier, diaries can help patients record and alert their providers about disruptive or disturbing side effects and symptoms unexpected by clinicians. QOL issues from the patient's perspective can be "on the table" regardless of whether the symptom is a threat to the patient's clinical status, often a more immediate concern to the provider. Given that physicians may tend to underestimate a patient's desire for involvement and information (Bruera et al., 2001, 2002; Keating et al., 2002; Rothenbacher et al., 1997), structured tools may offer an important cue to an individual that a provider wants the patient's input. In turn, a patient's responsiveness to this opportunity could provide an important cue to the provider about a patient's desire to be actively involved. As studied by Arora and McHorney (2000), patients vary in their desire to be actively involved. Although tools such as these diaries may not be desired by all patients, the general approach sets up the opportunity for discourse leading to concordant pharmaceutical regimen decisions and offers an interesting research opportunity to study intervention effects on the interaction and patient outcomes.

PAIN MANAGEMENT AND QUALITY OF LIFE

What I miss most is not sleeping with my wife. We did that for 30 years and now I can't. And also not being able to drive myself where I want to go. I can't do that either now that I'm on these pain meds. I really tried to keep the doses down so I could talk to people and think without being fuzzy, but the pain is just too bad to do that all the time. So now I've got myself on a schedule of taking my pills at 5 a.m. and again at 1:00 pm and at night before bed. That way I've got some good hours during the day when I can check in and call my students and colleagues and talk with my family. (Joe Wiederholt, personal communication 2001)

The cancer literature reinforces how challenging it is to manage symptoms and retain any semblance of normalcy in a patient's life (Emanuel, von Gunten, & Ferris, 2000). At times, palliative therapy can be equally if not more challenging than the condition. In one study of patients with cancer, in-patients averaged 12.5 symptoms, whereas outpatients averaged 9.7 symptoms (Portenoy et al., 1994). Sorting out which of these symptoms are due to the cancer and which to the treatment can be difficult for a patient. Provider expertise is needed to help interpret and then help identify possible options.

More than one third of patients undergoing therapy for cancer and 60% to 90% of those with advanced malignancy report significant pain (Foley, 2000). At the same time that opioid analgesic drugs are increasingly available, there is also evidence of significant nonadherence to prescribed pain control regimens with as much as nonadherence to opoid therapy 30% to 40% of the time (Ersak, Kraybill, & Pen, 1999; Ratka, 2002; Zeppetella, 1999). Patients report that side effects are an important factor for their nonadherence or discontinuation of pain therapy (Tarzian, Davidson, & Hoffmann, 2002; Zeppetella, 1999). As Ersak et al. (1999) indicated, cognitive reactions to opioids are a serious problem, especially among the terminally ill. The two goals of remaining alert and yet being free of pain are often in conflict. In her interviews with 21 adult patients with cancer, the most common side effect that prevented patients from taking some or all of the prescribed medication involved sedation and mental changes. In addition, there are numerous other problems such as constipation, sweating, and nausea/vomiting. Pellino and Ward (1998) added an interesting finding regarding patient satisfaction with pain management and their reported sense of control. Although individuals who report more severe pain are less satisfied with pain relief than are patients with less pain, their perception of control over the pain most related to satisfaction with pain relief. The question then is how best to support this sense of control.

In an excellent review article assessing the quality of life during chemotherapy, Gunnars and colleagues (2001) indicated that potential therapeutic gains must be weighed against the QOL costs of using the therapy. The same is true for palliative therapy. Does the toxicity and/or the inconvenience of the proposed treatment justify the expected gain? For recurring cancer, the decisions can be even more difficult. To make this judgment requires knowledge about an individual's values regarding QOL. Nothing can replace understanding a person's individual preferences. Unfortunately, commonly used QOL questionnaires often do not consider or weight ratings by individual preferences (Gunnars et al., 2001).

From a concordance perspective, the therapeutic alliance between patient and provider is never more obviously needed than when making these decisions about curative or palliative therapies. Yet, there appears to be little study of the patient's communication over time with their provider(s) and how it impacts on patients' QOL or survival. Nor do QOL instruments fill this gap. To the extent that patients and family members have established a pattern of voicing and agreeing on goals with their providers, an important foundation has been established for concordant end-stage care decisions. As reviewed by Arora (2003), several studies examine shared decision making in initial visits determining treatment of cancer. However, few studies address concordance issues in later stage care. In a literature review of information needs of families of cancer patients, Houts, Nezu, Nezy, and Bucher (1996) and Houts, Rusenas, Simmonds, and Hufford (1991) documented that caregivers wanted to know how to manage a variety of issues including side effects, to be listened to by health care professionals, to give as well as receive information, and to be involved in the treatment plan. In response to these needs, Houts developed a positive problem-solving model to be shared with caretakers. Both the caregivers' priorities and the problem-solving approach speak to the family members' active partnership with providers similar to those that the concordance framework posits for patients and their providers.

How to involve family members and yet maintain respectful attention on the individual in joint decisions deserves study. Patient and family members need to be prepared to make a myriad of decisions if optimum QOL can be achieved. Input from caretakers, with the individual's permission, may help identify better strategies to meet the individual's priorities across any 24-hour period throughout the week. We need observation tools to evaluate how concordant interactions are with caretakers as well as patients at end-stage care. Intervention studies may further help to determine if problem-solving programs, such as Houts proposed, can improve outcomes including QOL, sense of control, and satisfaction that pain can balanced with other priorities in the individual's life.

THE MULTIDISCIPLINARY TEAM

> It made such a difference to have people who knew me and treated me like a real human being. Sometimes I would see a nurse I knew and she would joke with me in the chemotherapy unit. I kept telling the younger nurses and staff to smile at patients and to touch us. That just meant so much, like I was known. Just like it hurt so much when people made me feel like it didn't matter what I wanted. Maybe it didn't seem important to them, but to me these things were very important. (Joe Wiederholt, personal communication)

Among the many challenges facing individuals with cancer is the sheer number of providers from different disciplines with whom they work over time. From anecdotal reports, we know that some staff respond warmly to new patients, whereas others do not. However, aside from these anecdotal reports, there is little empirical published literature on the multidisciplinary team's interaction with patients and with each other. The research literature focuses almost exclusively on physician–patient interactions in a single visit. There is limited observational research on the patient's interaction with any other providers. For example, we know of no published research on the individual's interaction with a pharmacist around cancer treatment and palliative care although there are articles promoting the use of pharmacists in cancer pain management (Ratka, 2002). There is little observational study of nurse–patient interaction, although there is substantial qualitative nursing research on patient self-management and symptom control.

An equally important gap in our empirical literature is the lack of research describing the degree of discontinuity between providers communicating with an individual about their needs and care over time. Anecdotally one hears from patients the extent to which they find diverging opinions and information overload at times from encounters with different specialists. We also have little research to identify factors that either lessen or enhance continuity of care between health care providers and disciplines within a single institution.

In the absence of research in this area, Joe and Peggy's experience is instructive. They estimated that they dealt with 30 to 40 health professionals including a surgeon, oncologist, radiologist, hospital pharmacist, community pharmacists, hospital nurses on several units, clinic nurses, nurses at the chemotherapy unit, social worker, hospice pharmacists, hospice nurses, and hospice physicians. They experienced both exquisitely sensitive care and communication, as well as the opposite. They reported an unfortunate silo effect within disciplines, with relatively few physician referrals to other health disciplines between visits for information or therapeutic help.

Joe and Peggy's health care expertise and preference for active involvement in decisions should have primed them for concordant partnerships with all their health providers. With each new contact and set of decisions, however, there was a negotiation of roles, rarely done explicitly. Feeling vulnerable to retain the goodwill of their providers, Joe and Peggy mostly tried to identify and get to those physicians with a reputation for a concordance interaction style. However, that was not possible with nursing staff. When Joe was able to work with nurses who had known him before the cancer or who had been supportive in his early care, it meant a great deal. The humor and the gift of being known almost seemed to buffer him from the vicious nature of the cancer and its treatment at times of chemotherapy or radiation. A specific example helps make the point of both the positive and negative impact a single person can have.

Joe's outpatient chemotherapy infusion unit was staffed by nurses. Many events occurred here that affected Joe's ability to stay positive. Joe arrived for his first day of infusion and realized that a mistake had been made. It appeared he would not be receiving his ondansetron 8 mg three times a day as prescribed by his physician to fight nausea. Instead, he would receive a lesser quantity of a less effective drug to control nausea. He asked the nurse on duty for help, and she refused to contact his physician. Desperate, Joe spoke to a colleague who was the hospital pharmacist for that area. The pharmacist intervened so that the nurse was given the authority to write the prescription with the doctor's permission. However, she wrote the dose for less than the physician had agreed to (i.e., only twice rather than three times daily) and refused to do anything further. When Joe reached his community pharmacy, he talked to his pharmacist (another friend) about the problem. The pharmacist filled the prescription and told Joe to take it three times a day while he arranged for a different prescription from the physician. Any average patient would have been stuck with a far less effective medication. It is easy to see how this might have an impact on an individual's QOL. It is also easy to see that a happy resolution occurred only because of Joe's expertise as a pharmacist as well as his colleagues' advocacy for him. What happens to those less well connected? Communication during the patient–physician encounter is only one aspect of communication that patients and families experience during the course of their care.

A broader agenda for research and definition of quality of cancer care is needed to encompass these additional environments and their impact on an individual struggling with cancer. There is little research on the climate of the chemotherapy rooms and the nature of the individual's interaction with staff. Joe reported that the tone and responsiveness of various nurses affected his ability to relax during the all important chemotherapy. The impact of time pressure on the nurse–patient interaction deserves to be studied. Efficiency and safe models offer only a piece of the puzzle for optimum organization of resources within these units. Evidence-based criteria for grading care that incorporates the perspective of the individual receiving chemotherapy is long overdue. We need much more research and attention to identifying how points of therapy for people with cancer can be structured, staffed, and offered in supportive ways.

A last example illustrates a significant success for multidisciplinary, cross-system coordination. As the end neared, Joe's pain caused by tumors in his spine made opioids necessary. Unfortunately, the mental side effects made him so "fuzzy" that he couldn't carry on the conversations he valued. This was key to retaining his humanity. As noted earlier, many patients are nonadherent with their opioid therapy. Joe and Peggy experimented with the schedule to dose Joe's opioids to balance his alertness and pain control for a predictable subset of hours each day. During those prized "cognitively clear" hours he called colleagues, talked with his family, and "watched the grass grow" as he sat outside on his backyard prayer bench. His physician and pharmacist offered information in response to his questions to support his pain-control strategies. He used his own agenda to select the best dose from the prescribed amount available to him. Thanks to the pharmacist, the physician knew both the over-the-counter and prescription drugs that numbered nearly 20 at the end of Joe's life. Joe double checked his dosing strategies with the pharmacist between visits and this prescriber during his visit. Far from worrying about adherence, the providers were a team that assisted with the goal of achieving Joe's priorities. This is what concordance is all about and points to the real difference between adherence models and concordance.

Although federally funded communication research has focused on the physician–patient encounter, the field of pharmacy has long voiced the goal of helping patients achieve the best trade-off of benefits against risk, costs, and side effects (Berger, 1993; Cipolle, Strand, & Morely, 1998; Hepler & Strand, 1990; Kozma, Reeder, & Schulz, 1993). Particularly given patients' apparent reliance on and attempt to interpret symptoms, at times related to medications, patient education by pharmacists about monitoring drug benefits and side effects could be a useful addition. Yet neither physicians nor nurses tend to refer patients to pharmacists for their medication-related questions. Thus, at this point, pharmacists' unique specialization in pharmaceutical knowledge appears to be underutilized. An additional research stream could examine what factors contributes to this underutilization or conversely what factors could facilitate better use of all non-physician providers.

While achieving patient–provider concordance in the patient's pursuit of improved QOL sounds fairly straightforward, several questions remain. How often does any professional, including physicians and pharmacists, examine a patient's total medication and self-care regimen with the patient? How often do any health professionals ask a patient what the person's priorities are to help balance side effects across the full trajectory of care for cancer? In many ways, it doesn't matter who helps the patient. However, if descriptive studies were to suggest that most patients have no one examining the entire picture, it would have important implications for the organization of the professions within our system of care.

IMPLICATIONS FOR PRACTICE AND HEALTH SERVICE ORGANIZATION

To move forward concordant communication between individuals who have cancer and their providers, it is useful to consider both the individual encounter and the health care system that supports and frames these encounters. Just as some things are encouraged within the current health care system, others are discouraged. It is important to consider how the system may unwittingly undercut the achievement of concordant encounters. To consider this possibility, first we discuss provider-level factors in practice followed by an exploration of health care system issues.

Practice

As sociologists have noted for half a century, physicians usually have far more power than do individuals in their encounter (Parsons, 1951). With this asymmetric power, physician cues and behavior strongly influence the likelihood an average person will express concerns and questions, let alone their opinions about a care plan. Concordance views the individual's encounter with a provider as an exchange. Thus, at the practice level there are key elements of physician behavior seen to influence whether agreement is achieved on the care plan at the end of the visit. Although both the individual and the provider have the potential to bring key knowledge and priorities to the table, physician behavior is critical for cuing the individual to share questions, information, preferences, agendas, and concerns.

Svarstad (1974), Roter and Hall (1992), and many others have identified the impact of several discrete elements of physician styles that seem to encourage achieving agreement with a patient. Svarstad's research documented for the first time how important it was to establish trust so that patient feedback could help steer care plans toward realistic and agreed on approaches. In Svarstad's observation of 220 visits, physician approachability was found to be a good predictor of both an individual's satisfaction and subsequent agreement with a regimen. Her index of physician approachability included several behaviors including the following: (a) solicits patient questions, (b) does not engage in clock-watching, (c) does not mumble or cut-off patient, (d) responds to patient's first question, (e) smiles or laughs. When a physician's approachability index was high, 46% of the patients asked three or more questions compared to 7% when approachability was low. Gathering feedback from the patient was key. Did the physician monitor the individual's regimen perception, symptom, and behavior? And if the individual indicated negative reactions about the regimen, did the provider move to nonjudgmental problem solving? If the provider simply offered a critical authoritarian response to a patient's negative reaction to the regimen, patients stopped disclosing negative experiences and reactions. So a basic question is not only how much the provider cues an individual that their questions and concerns are welcome, but also how successfully the provider then problem solves concerns in a nonjudgmental manner. Checking in by asking explicitly, "Are you Okay with this?" offers the minimal attempt to evaluate agreement. If the individual is not Okay with the plan, then concordance would suggest more exchange and problem solving is needed to achieve agreement.

Avis (1994) conducted an interesting exploratory study of whether patients in a day surgery unit in the United Kingdom realized they had the possibility of a participatory role. Their expectations of participation were found to be minimal. Patients had an instrumental model of involvement and considered themselves as the professional's "work object," which constrained the scope for any participation. This gets back to the extent to which providers and their institutions want and communicate that participation is valued. Patients may receive a message that they are a body, not a person, when their first contact at each visit is with a staff member whose primary role is to gather a history efficiently (and possibly mechanically). Thus, it is insufficient to analyze communication only on the physician, when either a medical assistant or nurse could set a tone by ignoring a patient concern or diary data. All too often overlooked is the stream of cues a patient receives from the time they check in and enter a health care setting.

Earlier in this chapter, literature on cancer patient preference for involvement was summarized. Clearly, we have not addressed sufficiently the findings that only a minority of patients report being involved at the level they preferred. One approach is to give a screening tool to each patient to identify their preferred level of involvement. Sweeney and Bruera (2002) suggested that the Degner and Sloan decision-making preference tool might be used for this purpose. Arora (2003) suggested that a new instrument is needed for this purpose. This is an important agenda for the future. Another approach is to give each individual a brief questionnaire and offer a summary printout both to the provider and patient at each visit to cue discussion of the individual's priority agendas. We are currently conducting longitudinal research using this latter approach.

Health Service Organization

Svarstad's (1974) early observational study documented that when physicians were pressured by time, their approachability index decreased. As physicians perceived their pressure and demands increasing, they became more task-oriented. Under the condition of low pressure, the physician was highly approachable in 61% of the cases. In comparison, physicians under a high amount of pressure were highly approachable in only 35% of the cases. These early findings are among the few that examine and document the association between time pressures and physician-interaction style related to encouraging patient involvement. Organizational factors within the health care system support or impede concordant approaches with patients. Thus, an additional research stream is necessary to look more broadly at our health care system's influence on concordant approaches. Do some of the same factors that promote efficient delivery of practice prevent rather than promote patient involvement and concordant decisions? Specifically, how are staffing and time constraints likely to discourage a provider from fully exploring an individual's agendas in the encounter? It seems likely that a hurried provider will feel less free to ask open-ended questions and explore an individual's perspective in a patient-centered assessment.

System resource allocations result in very concrete patient flow parameters, staffing ratios, and time allotted per visit. It is time to raise the question about bottom line not only in relation to safety but in relation to concordant encounters between an individual and provider. Going back to the example of Joe and his nurses at the time of chemotherapy, his insensitive infusion outpatient center nurses may have underattended to patient preferences and needs because of their staffing pressures. The average nurse may simply have been too busy to do anything other than address basic patient safety and efficient patient flow.

It appears we need better mechanisms and reward structures to promote cross-discipline collaboration and communication. System documentation and communication strategies need to be refined between departments, between in-patient and outpatient institutions, between disciplines of providers, and between providers and individuals with cancer. We lack studies on why there is such a series of silos within the health care system rather than a system designed for synergistic teams to facilitate nursing, pharmacist, dietician, physician referrals and collaborations with patients. The unique expertise each discipline offers could be described to patients openly so that individuals would take advantage of what the full team has to offer between as well as during physician visits. Oddly enough, even our reimbursement systems encourage a silo vision of care, with third-party reimbursement mechanisms heavily physician-oriented. Taken together, the organization and funding of health services for people with cancer may well be some of the most powerful influences on reducing the extent of concordant and multidisciplinary approaches to care.

An obvious point to examine is the education system for health professions. To what extent are multidisciplinary approaches to health sciences education of professions conceivable? It would be interesting to study whether and how health profession education (a) describes the unique expertise, training, and value of each of the other health professions; (b) encourages its trainees to openly refer patients to other health professions for expertise to complement their own, and (c) models how to work together effectively. As a slight indicator, to what extent do students hear a generic term such as "provider" when discussing patient care rather than only their own profession's title? If there were more interdisciplinary classes, it is possible that each profession could learn more about how and why team approaches are needed between encounters. If health profession education continues in a silo model, it is all the harder to overcome in practice.

CONCLUSION

This chapter used the concept of concordance as a lens to examine communication issues related to patient provider management of cancer. Ultimately, there is no magic answer but more than a set of questions has been generated. Our task is to have the tenacity to continue exploring these questions as we work toward improved communication and QOL for people with cancer and their caretakers.

Although there are more than 60 research studies of patient preferences for shared decisions and active involvement in oncology settings, there is a terrible absence of observational studies of cancer patient–provider encounters. We have very little evidence about the nature of patient and provider communication regarding pharmaceutical regimens from a concordance perspective.

A combination of cross-sectional studies at different stages of care as well as longitudinal studies are needed to track the evolving needs and adjustments in regimens, the symptoms and side effects experienced, the complexity of regimens that patients and families must manage over time and degree of concordant interactions and decisions around these issues.

In addition to descriptive studies, there is a need to identify interventions that can facilitate effective interactions between patients and providers. For example, how might we encourage a more complete identification of unvoiced patient agendas during patient–provider interactions? How might we encourage a more complete discourse of challenges to a patient's QOL at the same time curative or palliative treatment is being discussed? What are the means for encouraging patients to bring in specific observations regarding their symptoms and side effects to help promote an informed, concordant calibration of their regimens?

To accomplish either descriptive or intervention research agendas requires attention to measurement. Tools must carefully operationalize elements of concordance to detect if patient agendas have been addressed, if patient data regarding experiences and preferences with a regimen are solicited and used as input for regimen decisions. As Elwyn et al. (2001) suggested, we need measures devised specifically to detect the extent and nature of patient involvement in pharmaceutical and other regimen decision making and other aspects of shared decisions. Building on the review by Gunnars et al., (2001), QOL measures most frequently used need to take into account the priorities and preferences of patient respondents in addition to rating key dimensions. To know how patients weight the importance of different dimensions would add an important variable needed to interpret QOL ratings in outcome studies.

In closing, although research on the concordance perspective began in Great Britain, the review conducted by this chapter suggests that this country has the potential to make an important contribution. The qualitative work that has begun must be matched with quantitative studies. Theoretical frameworks, conspicuously absent, would enrich this line of work immensely were they generated from some of the qualitative research. We need research on the full array of regimen issues facing the individual, not simply the initial treatment selection. As long as we lack both a crystal ball and cures for many of our degenerative chronic conditions, patients and the full team of health providers need to bring their best knowledge together to achieve the best QOL outcomes for individuals with cancer.

ACKNOWLEDGMENT

We wish to dedicate this chapter to our mentor and colleague Joseph B. Wiederholt, who inspired our work in this area.

REFERENCES

Allard, P., Maunsell, E., Labbe, J., & Dorval, M. (2001). Educational interventions to improve cancer pain control: A systematic review. *Journal of Palliative Medicine, 4,* 191-203.

Arora, N. J. (2003). Interacting with cancer patients: The significance of physician's communication behaviors. *Social Science and Medicine, 57,* 791-806.

Arora, N. K., & McHorney, C. A. (2000). Patient preferences for medical decision making: Who really wants to participate? *Medical Care, 38,* 335-341.

Avis, M. (1994). Choice cuts. An exploratory study of patients' views about participation in decision-making in a day surgery unit. *International Journal of Nursing Studies, 31,* 88-98.

Bakker, D. A., Fitch, M. I., Gray, R., Reed, E., & Bennett J. (2001). Patient-health care provider communication during chemotherapy treatment: The perspectives of women with breast cancer. *Patient Education and Counseling, 43,* 61-71.

Barry, B., & Henderson, A. (1996). Nature of decision-making in the terminally ill patient. *Cancer Nursing, 19,* 384-391.

Baumann, L. J., Cameron, L. D., Zimmerman, R. S., & Leventhal, H. (1989). Illness representations and matching labels with symptoms. *Health Psychology, 8,* 449.

Baumann, L. J., & Leventhal, H. (1985). I can tell when my blood pressure is up: Can't I? *Health Psychology, 4,* 203.

Baumann, L. J., Zimmerman, R., & Leventhal, H. (1989). An experiment in common sense: Education at blood pressure screening. *Patient Education and Counseling, 12,* 53.

Beaver, K., Bogg, J., & Luker, K. A. (1999). Decision-making role preferences and information needs: A comparison of colorectal & breast cancer. *Health Expectations, 2,* 266-276.

Beaver, K., Luker, K. A., Owens, R. G., Seinster, S. J., Degner, L. F., & Sloan, J. A. (1996). Treatment decision making in women newly diagnosed with breast cancer. *Cancer Nursing, 19,* 8-19.

Berger, B. (1993). Building an effective therapeutic alliance: Competence, trustworthiness and caring. *American Journal of Hospital Pharmacy, 50,* 2399-2403.

Bilodeau, B. A., & Degner, L. F. (1996). Information needs, sources of information, and decisional roles in women with breast cancer. *Oncology Nursing Forum, 23,* 691-696.

Blanchard, C. G., LaBrecque, M. S., Ruckdeschel, J. C., & Blanchard, E. B. (1988). Information and decision-making preferences of hospitalized adult cancer patients. *Social Science and Medicine, 27,* 1139-1145.

Blenkinsopp, A. (2001). From compliance to concordance: How are we doing? *International Journal of Pharmacy Practice, 9,* 65-66.

Britten, N. (2003). Concordance and compliance. In R. Jones & N. Britten (Eds.), *Oxford textbook of primary medical care* (pp. 246-248). Oxford: Oxford University Press.

Bruera, E., Sweeney, C., Calder, K., Palmer, L., & Benishch-Tolley, S. (2001). Patient preferences versus physician perceptions of treatment decisions in cancer care. *Journal of Clinical Oncology, 19,* 2883-2885.

Bruera, E., Willey, J. S., Palmer, J. L., & Rosales, M. (2002). Treatment decisions for breast carcinoma: Patient preferences and physician perceptions. *American Cancer Society, 94,* 2076-2080.

Butow, P. N., Dunn, S. M., Tattersall, M. H. N., & Jones, Q. J. (1994). Patient participation in the cancer consultation: Evaluation of a question prompt sheet. *Annals of Oncology, 5,* 199-204.

Butow, P. H., Maclean, M., Dunn, S. M., Tattersall, M. H. N., & Boyer, M. J. (1997). The dynamics of change: Cancer patients' preferences for information, involvement and support. *Annals of Oncology, 8,* 857-863.

Cassileth, B. R., Zupkis, R. V., Slutton-Smith, K., & March, V. (1980). Information and participation preferences among cancer patients. *Annals of Internal Medicine, 92,* 832-836.

Charles, C., Gafni, A., & Whelan, T. (1999). Decision-making in the physician-patient encounter: Revising the shared treatment decision-making model. *Social Science and Medicine, 49,* 651-661.

Chewning, B., & Sleath, B. (1996). Medication decision-making and management: A client-centered model. *Social Science and Medicine, 42,* 389-398.

Chewning, B., & Wiederholt, J. B. (2003). Concordance in cancer medication management. *Patient Education and Counseling, 50,* 75-78.

Chewning, B., Wiederholt, J., Boh, L., Kreling, D., Van Koningsveld, R., Wilson, D., Bell, C., Boh, D., Nowlin, N., & Douglas, J. (2001). Does the concordance framework serve medicine management? *The International Journal of Pharmacy Practice, 9,* 71-79.

Cipolle, R. J., Strand, L. M., & Morely, P. C. (1998). *Pharmaceutical care practice.* New York: McGraw Hill.

Cleeland, C. S., Mendoza, T. R., Wang, X. S., Chou, C., Harle, M. T., Morrissey, M., & Engstrom, M. C. (2000). *Assessing symptom distress in cancer patients.* American Cancer Society.

Concordance Work Group. (1997). From compliance to concordance: Achieving shared goals in medicine taking. Report of the Royal Pharmaceutical Society Working Group. Available at http://www.medicines-partnership.org

Davison, B. J., Gleave, M. E., Goldenberg, S. L., Degner, L. F., Hoffart, D., & Berkowitz, J. (2002). Assessing information and decision preferences of men with prostate cancer and their partners. *Cancer Nursing, 25,* 42-49.

Davison, B. J., Parker, P. A., & Goldenberg, S. L. (2004). Patients' preferences for communicating a prostate cancer diagnosis and participating in medical decision-making. *British Journal of Urology International, 93,* 47-51.

Davison, J. R., Brundage, M. D., & Feldman-Stewart, D. (1999). Lung cancer treatment decisions: Patients' desires for participation and information. *Psycho-Oncology, 8,* 511-520.

Degner, L. F., Kristjanson, L. J., Bowman, D., Sloan, J. A., Carriere, K. C., O'Neill, J., Bilodeau, B., Watson, P., & Mueller, B. (1997). Information needs and decisional preferences in women with breast cancer. *JAMA, 277,* 1485-1492.

Degner, L. F., & Sloan, J. A. (1992). Decision making during serious illness: What role do patients really want to play? *Journal of Clinical Epidemiology, 45,* 941-950.

Detmar, S. B., Aaronson, N. K., Wever, L. D., Muller, M., & Schornagel, J. H. (2000). How are you feeling? Who wants to know? Patients' and oncologists' preferences for discussing health-related quality-of-life issues. *Journal of Clinical Oncology, 18,* 3295-3301.

Detmar, S. B., Muller, M. J., Wever, L. D., Schornagel, J. H., & Aaronson, N. K. (2001). The patient-physician relationship. Patient-physician communication during outpatient palliative treatment visits: An observational study. *JAMA, 285,* 1351-1357.

Elwyn, G., Edwards, A., Mowle, S., Wensing, M., Wilkinson, C., Kinnersley, P., & Grol, R. (2001). Measuring the involvement of patients in shared decision-making: A systematic review of instruments. *Patient Education and Counseling, 43,* 5-22.

Emanuel, L. L., von Gunten, C. F., & Ferris, F. D. (2000). Gaps in end-of-life care. *Archives of Family Medicine, 9,* 1176-1180.

Ersak, M., Kraybill, B. M., & Pen, A. D. (1999). Factors hindering patients' use of medications for cancer pain. *Cancer Practice, 7,* 226-232.

Fallowfield, L. J., Jenkins, V., Brennan, C., Sawtel, M., Moynihan, C., & Souhami, R. L. (1998). Attitudes of patients to randomized clinical trials of cancer therapy. *European Journal of Cancer, 34,* 1554-1559.

Fellowes, D., Fallowfield, L. J., Saunders, C. M., & Houghton, J. (2001). Tolerability of hormone therapies for breast cancer: How informative are documented symptom profiles in medical notes for 'well-tolerated' treatments? *Breast Cancer Research, 66,* 73-81.

Fielding, R., & Hung, J. (1996). Preferences for information and involvement in decisions during cancer care among a Hong Kong Chinese population. *Psycho-Oncology, 5,* 321-329.

Foley, K. M. (2000). Controlling cancer pain. *Hospital Practice, 10,* 36.

Gagnon, E. M., & Recklitis, C. J. (2001). Parents' decision-making preferences in pediatric oncology: The relationship to health care involvement and complementary therapy use. *Psycho-Oncology, 12,* 442-452.

Goldberg, R., Guadagnoli, E., Silliman, R. A., & Glicksman, A. (1990). Cancer patients' concerns: Congruence between patients and primary care physicians. *Journal of Cancer Education, 5,* 193-199.

Golin, C. E., DiMatteo, M. R., & Gelberg, L. (1996). The role of patient participation in the doctor visit. *Diabetes Care, 19,* 1153-1164.

Gunnars, B., Nygren, P., & Glimelius, B. (2001). Assessment of quality of life during chemotherapy. *Acta Oncologica, 40,* 175-184.

Hack, T. F., Degner, L. F., & Dyck, D. G. (1994). Relationship between preferences for decisional control and illness information among women with breast cancer: A quantitative and qualitative analysis. *Social Science and Medicine, 39,* 279-289.

Helmes, A. W., Bowen, D. J., & Bengel, J. (2002). Patient preferences of decision-making in the context of genetic testing for breast cancer risk. *Genetics in Medicine, 4,* 150-157.

Hepler, C., & Strand, L. (1990). Opportunities and responsibilities in pharmaceutical care. *American Journal of Hospital Pharmacy, 47,* 533-543.

Hermansen-Kobulnicky, C. J. (2003). *The behavioral impact of teaching patients to monitor side effects of chemotherapy: An intervention study.* Unpublished doctoral dissertation, University of Wisconsin, Madison.

Hermansen-Kobulnicky, C. J., & Chewning, B. (2002). *Teaching cancer patients to monitor side effects: An exploratory test to increase shared decision making.* Paper presentation, International Conference on Communication in Health Care, Warwick, England.

Hermansen-Kobulnicky, C. J., Wiederholt, J. B., & Chewning, B. (2004). Adverse effect monitoring: Opportunity for patient care and pharmacy practice. *Journal of the American Pharmacists Association, 44,* 75-88.

Houts, P. S., Nezu, A. M., Nezu, C. M., & Bucher, J. A. (1996). The prepared family caregiver: A problem-solving approach to family caregiver education. *Patient Education and Counseling, 27,* 63-73.

Houts, P. S., Rusenas, I., Simmonds, M. A., & Hufford, D. L. (1991). Information needs of families of cancer patients: A literature review and recommendations. *Journal Cancer Education, 6,* 255-261.

Jones, R., Pearson, J., McGregor, S., Barrett, A., Gilmour, W. H., Atkinson, J. M., Cawsey, A. J., & McEwen, J. (2002). Does writing a list help cancer patients ask relevant questions? *Patient Education and Counseling, 47,* 369-371.

Kahn, S. B., Houts, P. S., & Harding, S. P. (1992). Quality of life and patients with cancer: A comparative study of patient versus physician perceptions and its implications for cancer education. *Journal of Cancer Education, 7,* 241-249.

Keating, N. L., Guadagnoli, E., Landrum, M. B., Borbas, C., & Weeks, J. C. (2002). Treatment decision making in early-stage breast cancer: Should surgeons match patients' desired level of involvement? *Journal of Clinical Oncology, 20,* 1473-1479.

Kozma, C. M., Reeder, C. E., & Schulz, R. M. (1993). Economic, clinical, and humanistic outcomes: A planning model for pharmacoeconomic research. *Clinical Therapy, 15*, 1121-1132.

Leventhal, E., Leventhal, H., & Robitaille, C. (1998). Enhancing self-care research: Exploring the theoretical underpinnings of self-care. In M. Ory & G . DeFriese (Eds.), *Self care in later life: Research, program and policy issues* (pp. 118-141). New York: Springer.

McCool, J., & Morris, J. (1999). Focus of doctor-patient communication in follow-up consultations for patients treated surgically for colorectal cancer. *Journal of Management in Medicine, 13*, 169-177.

McWilliam, C. L., Brown, J. B., & Stewart, M. (2000). Breast cancer patients' experiences of patient-doctor communication: A working relationship. *Patient Education and Counseling, 39*, 191-204.

Meyer, D., Leventhal, H., & Gutmann, M. (1985). Commonsense models of illness: The example of hypertension. *Health Psychology, 4*, 115.

Newell, S., Sanson-Fisher, R. W., Girgis, A., & Bonaventura, A. (1998). How well do medical oncologists' perceptions reflect their patients' reported physical and psychosocial problems? Data from a survey of five oncologists. *Cancer, 83*, 1640-1650.

Parsons, T. (1951). *The social system.* Glencoe, IL: The Free Press.

Pellino, T. A., & Ward, S. E. (1998). Perceived control mediates the relationship between pain severity and patient satisfaction. *Journal of Pain and Symptom Management, 15*, 110-116.

Portenoy, R. K., Thaler, H. T., Kornblith, A. B., Lepore, J. M., Friedlander-Klar, H., Coyle, N., Smart-Curley, T., Kemey, N., Norton, L., & Hoskins, W. (1994). Symptom prevalence, characteristics and distress in a cancer population. *Quality Life Research, 3*, 183-189.

Protiere, C., Viens, P., Genre, D., Cowen, D., Camerlo, J., Gravis, G., Alzieu, C., Bertucci, F., Resbeut, M., Maraninchi, D., & Moatti, J. P. (2000). Patient participation in medical decision-making: A French study in adjuvant radio-chemotherapy for early breast cancer. *Annals of Oncology, 11*, 39-45.

Ratka, A. (2002). The role of a pharmacist in ambulatory cancer pain management. *Current Pain and Headache Reports, 6*, 191-196.

Rogers, M. S., & Todd, C. J. (2000). The "right kind" of pain: Talking about symptoms in outpatient oncology consultations. *Palliative Medicine, 14*, 299-307.

Roter, D. L., & Hall, J. A. (1992). *Doctors talking with patients, patients talking with doctors: Improving communication in medical visits.* Westport, CT: Auburn House.

Rothenbacher, D., Lutz, M. P., & Porzsolt, F. (1997). Treatment decisions in palliative cancer care: Patients' preferences for involvement and doctors' knowledge about it. *European Journal of Cancer, 33*, 1184-1189.

Schumacher, K. L., Doresawa, S., West, C., Dodd, M., Paul, S. M., Tripathy, D., Koo, P., & Miaskowski, C. (2002). The usefulness of a daily pain management diary for outpatients with cancer-related pain. *Oncology Nursing Forum, 29*, 1304-1313.

Sherliker, L., & Steptoe, A. (2000). Coping with new treatments for cancer: A feasibility study of daily diary measures. *Patient Education and Counseling, 40*, 11-19.

Stead, M. L., Fallowfield, L., Brown, J.M., & Selby, P. (2001). Communication about sexual problems and sexual concerns in ovarian cancer: Qualitative study. *British Medical Journal, 323*, 836-837.

Stevenson, F. A. (2001). Concordance: What is the relevance for pharmacists? *International Journal of Pharmacy Practice, 9*, 67-70.

Stewart, D. E., Wong, F., Cheung, A. M., Dancey, J., Meana, M., Cameron, J. I., McAndrews, M. P., Bunston, T., Murphy, J., & Rosen, B. (2000). Information needs and decisional preferences among women with ovarian cancer. *Gynecologic Oncology, 77*, 357-361.

Street, R. L., Voigt, B., Geyer, C., Manning, T., & Swanson, G. P. (1995). Increasing patient involvement in choosing treatment for early breast cancer. *Cancer, 78*, 2275-2285.

Stromgen, A. S., Groenvold, M., Pedersen, L., Olsen, A. K., Spile, M., & Sjogren, P. (2001). Does the medical record cover the symptoms experienced by cancer patients receiving palliative care? A comparison of the record and patient self-rating. *Journal of Pain and Symptom Management, 21*, 189-196.

Sutherland, H. J., Llewellyn-Thomas, H. A., Lockwood, G. A., Tritchler, D. L., & Till, J. E. (1989). Cancer patients: Their desire for information and participation in treatment decisions. *Journal of the Royal Society of Medicine, 82,* 260-263.

Svarstad, B. L. (1974). *The doctor-patient encounter: An observational study of communication and outcome.* Unpublished doctoral dissertation, University of Wisconsin, Madison.

Svarstad, B. L., & Sitter, D. C. (2005). The patient: Behavioral determinants. In A. R. Gennaro (Ed.), *Remington: The science and practice of pharmacy* (21st ed., pp. 382-389). Baltimore, MD: Lippincott, Williams, and Wilkins.

Sweeney, C., & Bruera, E. (2002). Communication in cancer care: Recent developments. *Journal of Palliative Care, 18,* 300-306.

Tarzian, A. J., Davidson, S. T., & Hoffmann, D. E. (2002). Management of cancer-related and non-cancer-related chronic pain in Connecticut: Successes and failures. *Connecticut Medicine, 66,* 683-689.

Wallberg, B., Michelson, H., Nystedt, M., Bolund, C., Degner, L. F., & Wilking, N. (2000). Information needs and preferences for participation in treatment decisions among Swedish breast cancer patients. *Acta Oncologica, 39,* 467-476.

Wiederholt, J., & Wiederholt, P. (1997). The patient: Our teacher and friend. *American Journal of Pharmaceutical Education, 61,* 415-423.

Wiederholt, J., & Wiederholt, P. (2005). *The WriteTrack personal health tracker for cancer patients.* Madison, WI: Wiederholt Group, Inc.

Wong, F., Stewart, D. E., Dancey, J., Meana, M., McAndrews, M. P., Bunston, T., & Cheung, A. M. (2000). Men with prostate cancer: Influence of psychological factors on informational needs and decision making. *Journal of Psychosomatic Research, 49,* 13-19.

Zeppetella, G. (1999). How do terminally ill patients at home take their medication? *Palliative Medicine, 13,* 469-475.

22 | Cancer Information On the Internet

Bernard J. Kerr, Jr.
Central Michigan University

The Internet is a wild frontier whose landscape changes frequently. It contains all sorts of health information—good and bad, true and false, complete and dangerously incomplete. Before you act on anything you learn online, we recommend that you make sure you check with your doctor.

—Consumer Reports

Studies conducted as part of the Pew Research Center's (2003) Internet and American Life Project reveal that 80% of adult Internet users, or about 93 million Americans, have searched for at least one of 16 major health topics online. This makes the act of looking for health or medical information one of the most popular activities online, after e-mail (93%) and researching a product or service before buying it (83%). In July 1999, *USA Today* published a special four-page cover story entitled "How the Internet is Changing Medicine." The story noted: "In ever-growing numbers, patients clutching Internet printouts are marching into doctors' offices nationwide, sometimes knowing more about their disease and ways to treat it than their physicians." Given the substantial growth of health-related Internet content, the parade of patients armed with Internet information must be quite a spectacle—and quite a challenge for today's health professionals. Hopefully, these patients and/or their family members are armed with quality, accurate information and the health professionals react favorably to the changing dynamic of caring for an Internet-informed population.

A search on the phrase "cancer information" using the Google search engine will produce about 2.7 million hits. How does one begin to differentiate the good sites from the not so good? Certainly, care should be taken in seeking and recommending health-related Web sites, given the importance and potential consequences of the information provided and how it is used in health care decision-making process. Recommending cancer-related Web sites presents a challenge and a responsibility. First, the person making the recommendation is suggesting a source of information that the user is likely to employ in making choices and decisions regarding their health care or that of a friend or relative. Second, the person making the recommendation may have little knowledge of why the inquiring party wants to know more about this particular health or medical issue. An emerging symptom, a recent diagnosis or simple curiosity emanating from something the individual read, saw, or heard may motivate him or her . No matter what the motivation, providing good guidance is important, as it is likely to be followed. Third, there is something of an expectation that the Web site suggested be a quality, reliable source.

The Harvard Center for Cancer Prevention (www.hsph.harvard.edu/cancer) suggests that when one surfs the Web to learn about cancer prevention, or any other health topic, one goes to reliable, well-known sources. Good starting points are governmental research institutions, such as the National Cancer Institute (www.cancer.gov) and the Centers for Disease Control and Prevention (www.cdc.gov); highly respected advocacy groups such as the American Cancer Society (www.cancer.org) and the American Lung Association (www.lungusa.org); and academic institutions. Two professionals who can help the users are a librarian and, more importantly, the individual's doctor. Information found on the Web cannot substitute for a physician's advice. If one has questions or is considering making a major lifestyle change, one should talk to his or her healthcare professional (The Source, 2002).

Because anyone can publish on the Internet and to a large extent information is unregulated, users should be aware of quality-of-information issues. Many sites offer high-quality information; however, there are reports of inaccurate and misleading information on the Internet. There are a number of groups proposing standards; however, because of the nature of the Internet these will be difficult to enforce (Quality, 2003). A search on the phrase "evaluating web resources" using the Google search engine will produce about 79,500 hits.

One solution is not to make cancer-related web site recommendations. Although this is an option, it does not represent the reply a friend, relative, or co-worker had hoped to hear. An alternative would be to recommend health-related Web sites that include cancer information and have been reviewed and recommended through some formal, structured evaluation process. One such process is the Utilization Review Accreditation Commission (URAC) Health Web Site Accreditation Program (URAC, 2003). Web sites that receive the URAC Health Web Site Accreditation Seal have been thoroughly evaluated against more than 50 URAC standards to ensure that they deliver quality health content and services. URAC's application process provides a third-party verification mechanism for compliance to facilitate the site maintaining its quality services over time.

Examples of URAC-accredited Web sites include the following:

- WebMD (www.webmd.com)
- healthAtoZ (www.healthatoz.com)
- Caremark (www.buildingbetterhealth.com)
- KidsHealth (www.kidshealth.org)

Indeed, there are many excellent health-related Web sites that have not undergone a formal evaluation and/or accreditation process. Therefore, when seeking and/or recommending such sites, the seven criteria developed by the Health Summit Working Group (1999), convened by the Health Information Technology Institute of Mitretek Systems, should be helpful. The criteria for Evaluating Internet Health Information are as follows:

- **Credibility:** includes the source, currency, relevance/utility, and editorial review process for the information.
- **Content:** must be accurate and complete, and an appropriate disclaimer provided.
- **Disclosure:** includes informing the user of the purpose of the site, as well as any profiling or collection of information associated with using the site.
- **Links:** evaluated according to selection, architecture, content, and back linkages.
- **Design:** encompasses accessibility, logical organization (navigability), and internal search capability.
- **Interactivity:** includes feedback mechanisms and means for exchange of information among users.
- **Caveats:** clarification of whether site function is to market products and services or is a primary information content provider.

The Health on the Net (HON) Foundation (2001) is widely recognized as a "Good Housekeeping seal of approval" for medical sites. HON (www.hon.ch) is an international not-for-profit foundation based in Geneva, Switzerland. Its council of medical informatics specialists developed minimum standards for health Web site content. Sites that display the seal meet or exceed HON standards for content. On HON sites, only health professionals give advice. If nonprofessionals provide advice, the site must reference where the information came from. HON is a voluntary system, so not all the sites that would qualify have been certified, but an increasing number of sites are coming on board (Bell, 1999). The HON site has a keyword search for retrieval of trustworthy medical documents. Examples of HON-participating cancer sites include the American Cancer Society (www.cancer.org), the University of Minnesota Cancer Center (www.cancer.umn.edu), the Prostate Cancer Institute (www.prostate-cancer-institute.org), Cancerpage.com (www.cancerpage.com), and the World Oncology Network (www.worldoncology.net).

The National Cancer Institute (NCI, 2003) points out that the growing popularity of the Internet has made it easier and faster to find health information. However, the Internet also allows rapid and widespread distribution of false and misleading information. It is important for people to carefully consider the source of information and to discuss the information they find with their health care provider. The NCI fact sheet, "How To Evaluate Health Information on the Internet: Questions and Answers," can help people decide whether the health information they find on the Internet or receive via e-mail from a Web site is likely to be reliable. A few among the many useful Internet sources of cancer information are the following:

- Guide to Internet Resources for Cancer, www.cancerindex.org/clinks1.htm
- Association of Cancer Online Resources, www.acor.org, provides access to disease-specific cancer listservs and allows a user to search or browse the archives of the lists.
- Cancer BACUP, www.cancerbacup.org.uk/, the United Kingdom's leading cancer information service. This site offers news and information on specific cancer types and topics, and includes an extensive and detailed question-and-answer section.
- Pediatric Oncology Resource Center, http://www.acor.org/ped-onc, focuses on psychosocial and medical issues and provides ways to connect with other parents of children with cancer. It is created and maintained by parents of children with childhood cancer.
- National Childhood Cancer Foundation, www.curesearch.org, features inspiring stories of children with cancer. This organization supports the Children's Cancer Group cooperative research organization.
- American Cancer Society, www.cancer.org, provides overviews of specific cancer types and topics such as nutrition, coping with side effects, support, and practical issues.
- National Cancer Institute, www.cancer.gov, contains Physician Data Query (PDQ) statements—peer-reviewed summaries on treatment of adult and pediatric cancer types, and various supportive care topics. Oncology specialists update the PDQ statements monthly. The site also contains a database of all cancer clinical trials (www.cancer.gov/clinicaltrials), and access to CancerLit (www.cancer.gov/cancerinfo/literature), an index of oncology peer-reviewed journal literature.
- Women's Cancer Network, www.wcn.org, was developed for women and their families by the Gynecologic Cancer Foundation (www.thegcf.org) and CancerSource (http://www.cancersource.com).
- Cancer Information Network, www.cancernetwork.com, provides extensive links to cancer organizations, cancer centers, and support groups.
- CenterWatch Clinical Trials Listing Service, www.centerwatch.com, provides clinical trials information for patients and health professionals, including industry-sponsored clinical trials that are actively recruiting patients.

There is an incredible amount of health information available on the Internet and, as is common with online publishing, there is a lot of opinion sold as fact, and users need to be aware of this when reading anything (Women's Health Information, 1997). The Federal Trade Commission (FTC, n.d.) is targeting false and unsubstantiated health claims on the Internet through Operation Cure.All—a law enforcement and consumer education campaign. The FTC's Operation Cure.All Web site (www.ftc.gov/cureall) offers information for consumers on how to recognize health fraud, guidance for businesses on how to market health products and services truthfully, and information about the FTC's initiatives. The Cleveland Clinic Information Center (2003) offers two important cautions along with tips for gathering cancer information on the Internet.

Caution 1: Misinformation is information that is incorrect, meaning there is no scientific evidence that the treatment does what it claims to do, even though many people say that it does. An example of this would be a treatment such as shark cartilage. In these cases, when people continue to repeat incorrect information, the conclusion becomes "understood." After all, how can so many people be wrong?

Caution 2: Another danger of information on the Internet is when the information is true but leads to misleading conclusions. Such is the case of a person who reviews a particular treatment or clinical trial on the Internet and concludes that this is the best treatment for him or her.

The following are tips for gathering cancer information on the Internet:

- Look for sites that are affiliated with known organizations or medical institutions.
- Use extreme caution when reviewing information. Look for facts, not opinions. If it sounds too good to be true, it probably is.
- Review the information with a health professional.
- Always let your doctor know if you are thinking of trying other therapies. Some can be dangerous.

Consumer WebWatch (www.consumerwebwatch.org) is a grant-funded project of Consumers Union, the nonprofit publisher of *Consumer Reports* magazine and *ConsumerReports.org,* supported by grants from The Pew Charitable Trusts, the John S. and James L. Knight Foundation, and the Open Society Institute. The organization's mission is to investigate; inform; and improve the credibility of information published on the World Wide Web. Consumer WebWatch (n.d.) cites "disclosure" as the most important principle underlying the promotion of Web credibility, indicating that many consumer concerns about the trustworthiness of Web sites can be addressed through consistent disclosure. Achieving better disclosure begins with a detailed "About Us" page, describing a Web site's mission, purpose, who owns it and how it is funded, where the staff offices and the site's content staff are based, how to reach the staff if there is a problem, how to alert the site to inaccurate information, and other such types of information. An example of a health care site identified by Consumer Web Watch as providing a relatively complete example of disclosure is Medscape (www.medscape.com), where the disclosure information is found in a "Privacy & Ethics" link.

The Internet is rapidly becoming a third party in the doctor–patient relationship, as the World Wide Web, e-mail, and discussion groups have dramatically increased the quantity of medical and health information available to patients (Pergament, Pergament, Wonderlick, & Fiddler, 1999). The availability of cancer information can have both positive and negative consequences. Providers of care may find that Internet-generated confusion and anxiety can make discussions with patients more difficult, but addressing Internet information may also represent an opportunity to clarify information and relieve anxiety, thus potentially strengthening rapport with patients (Helft, Hlubocky, & Daugherty, 2003).

Findings from the 2001 American Medical Association (AMA) Study on Physicians' Use of the World Wide Web found that the perception by physicians themselves of the Internet as a resource was increasingly positive. A team of AMA researchers interviewed 1,001 physicians in the United States between June and September 2000. They found that the percentage of physicians who actually used the Internet increased dramatically from 20% in 1997 to 70% in 2000. Importantly, the percentage of physicians who considered the Web to be a useful source for patient education has increased from 25% in 1997 to 39% in 2000. Similarly, 66% of doctors believed that Internet news and information has become an important component of patient care—up from 59% in 1997 (Willis-Knighton Cancer Center, 2001).

As evidenced by the AMA study and reflected in Table 22.1 (Lunenberg, 2000) there has been a remarkable growth in the use of the Internet by physicians. Medical professionals who reported regular use of the Internet felt that discussion of the results of patients' Internet searches was helpful in increasing patients' knowledge and improving communication between the medical professional and the patient. When physicians were asked which of three variables was the most important in seeking medical information on the Internet (Casebeer, Bennett, Kristofco, Carillo, & Centor, 2002), 41% felt that credibility of the source was most important, 35% felt that quick and 24-hour access to information was most important, and 24% felt that ease of searching was the most important.

As outlined in one health care system's strategy development document (Catholic Health East, 2003), "The Internet has the potential to erase one of the biggest handicaps of the health care industry—relay speed. It can slash the time it takes to make referrals, get test results, get paid, find patients for clinical trials, disseminate best practices and share cost information. It will quicken the pace for the adoption of new ideas, new therapies and new measurements." A study by the Boston Consulting Group (2003) revealed significant Internet usage by physicians and plans for growth in the use of online patient care tools as reflected in Fig. 22.1.

The increasing use of the Internet may effect physician–patient communication in that Internet resources are changing information access for patients and their providers. In a study of 102 patients (Ellis, Dimitry, Browman, Whelan, Nimmannit, & Brouwers, 2003) with breast, lung, genitourinary, or gastrointestinal cancer visiting a medical or radiation oncologist, the patients reported using the Internet to (a) gain a better understanding of medical terminology, (b) obtain more detailed information about treatment options, (c) clarify information given to them by a physician, and (d) find more detailed information about medications.

A survey (Chen & Siu, 2001) of 191 inpatients and 410 oncologists (including medical, radiation, and surgical oncologists) practicing throughout Canada published in the Journal of Clinical Oncology revealed the following:

- Almost 86% of patients wanted as much information as possible about their illness, but only 54% of those felt they received enough information from their doctors and other health care providers.

Table 22.1
Growth in Physician Use of the Internet

YEAR	ESTIMATED PERCENTAGE OF U.S. PHYSICIANS USING THE INTERNET
1995	3%
1996	15%
1997	32%
1998	60%
1999	80%
2000	80%

Does your practice use or plan to use any of the following online patient-care tools?

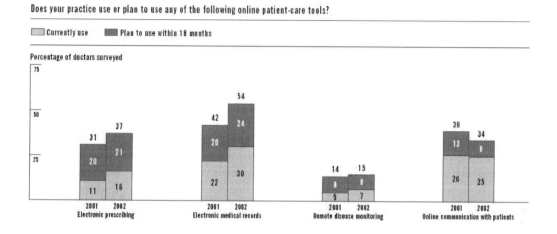

FIGURE 22.1. About One Third of Doctors Use/Plan To Use Online Patient Care Tools.

- Although 83% of patients relied on their doctors as their main source of information on their disease, 71% also searched for more—with the Internet as their most popular information source.
- About 88% of patients responded that their doctors were willing to discuss the Internet information they'd found with them—and 83% felt their doctors spent "a moderate" amount or "a lot" of time doing so.
- About 42% of patients felt Internet information helped them cope with their illness.
- Only 1% of patients felt Internet information had a negative impact on their ability to cope.
- Only 15% of oncologists surveyed thought Internet information helped their patients cope and 27% thought it interfered with their coping capabilities.
- Most patients and oncologists thought Internet usage had no impact on the quality of their relationship.
- Twenty-one percent of patients felt that Internet usage strengthened the doctor–patient relationship, compared with 8% of oncologists.
- Only 6% of patients and 9% of oncologists reported patient Internet usage had a negative impact on this relationship.

The Internet brings a new world of information to anyone with access. Patients and consumers are demanding more information about their health and illnesses and are increasingly eager to take a more active role in managing their well-being. This reinforces the merits of more extensive and higher quality Internet information for patients. Not only does strengthening Internet resource availability and quality make sense from the patient's perspective, it also makes sense from the health system perspective. Opportunities to conserve resources through Internet communication are emerging, outcomes of medication use can improve through Internet-based education and monitoring, and health budgets should benefit (Wold-

Olsen, 2001). For cancer health professionals, the availability of online continuing medical education (CME) helps make the maintenance of skills and credentials easier and cheaper than in the past. Sites such as the American Cancer Society's Online CME (http://cme.amcancersoc.org), CancerEducation.com, CancerNetwork.com, the Moffitt Cancer Center and Research Network (www.moffitt.usf.edu/education), The Oncologist CME Online (http://cme.alphamedpress.org), Baylor College of Medicine CME Online (www.baylorcme.org), and Meniscus Education and Communication for Health Professionals (www.meniscus.com) offer an array of CME opportunities.

The role of the Internet in cancer care communications is significant and growing. This vast information resource should be used by patients, families, and caregivers with both enthusiasm and caution. The World Wide Web has placed information at the fingertips of every connected consumer that the world's leading cancer researchers would have been envious of only a few years ago. The challenge is to sift through the myriad of available cancer information content and ferret out accurate and pertinent information specific to one's needs, without adding to the fear and anxiety that accompanies the cancer threat or diagnosis. The good news is there is a remarkable amount of quality information available.

REFERENCES

American Medical Association. (2001). Study on physician's use of the worldwide web. Accessed June 9, 2003, from www.ama-assn.org/ama/pub/article/1616-4692.html. .

Bell, H. (1999). Medicine online How useful is it? *Minnesota Medicine, 82*. Available at http://www.mnmed.org/publications/MnMed1999/April/Bell.cfm. Accessed June 10, 2003.

Boston Consulting Group. (2003). E-health in the United States. Available at http://www.bcg.com/publications/files/Vital_Signs_Rpt_Jan03.pdf. Accessed June 9, 2003.

Casebeer, L., Bennett, N., Kristofco, R., Carillo, A., & Centor, R. (2002). Physician Internet medical information seeking and on-line continuing education use patterns. *Journal of Continuing Education in the Health Professions, 22*, 33-42.

Catholic Health East. (2003). Healthcare strategic environmental scan—2003. Available at http://www.che.org/publications/pdf/Environmental-Scan-2003.pdf. Accessed June 11, 2003.

Chen, X., & Siu, L. (2001). Impact of the media and the internet on oncology: Survey of cancer patients and oncologists in Canada. *Journal of Clinical Oncology, 19*, 4291-4297.

Consumer WebWatch. (n.d.). Available at http://www.consumerwebwatch.org/. Accessed June 12, 2003.

Dillion, T. (1999). How the Internet is changing medicine. (1999, July 15). *USA Today*.

Ellis, P. M., Dimitry, S. J. D., Browman, G., Whelan, T. J., Nimmannit, A., Brouwers, M. (2003). American Society of Clinical Oncologists, Health Services Research Presentation, Oncologists, cancer patients and the Internet: Improving the clinical encounter and the quality of cancer care. *Proceedings of the American Society of Clinical Oncologists, 22*, 538. Available at http://www.asco.org/ac/1,1003,_12-002636-00_18-0023-00_19-00100958,00.asp. Accessed June 9, 2003.

Federal Trade Commission. (n.d.). Operation cure all: Introduction. Available at http://www.ftc.gov/bcp/conline/edcams/cureall/index.html. Accessed June 12, 2003.

Health on the Net Foundation. (n.d.). Available at www.hon.ch. Accessed June 15, 2003.

Health on the Net Foundation. (2001). Evolution of internet use for health purposes. Available at http://www.hon.ch/Survey/FebMar2001/survey.html. Accessed June 9, 2003.

Health Summit Working Group. (1999). Criteria for assessing the quality of health information on the internet—Policy Paper. Available at http://hitiweb.mitretek.org/docs/policy. html. Accessed June 12, 2003.

Helft, P., Hlubocky, F., & Daugherty, C. (2003). American oncologists' views of Internet use by cancer patients: A mail survey of American Society of Clinical Oncology members. *Journal of Clinical Oncology, 21*, 942-947.

Lunenberg, G. (2000). *Current trends in laboratory pathology*. Paper presented at the Clinical Laboratory Management Association Conference. Available at http:// www.ahcpub.com/ahc_root_html/hot/archive/diag082000.html. Accessed June 9, 2003.

National Cancer Institute. (2003). How to evaluate health information on the internet: Questions and answers. Available at http://cis.nci.nih.gov/fact/2_10.htm. Accessed June 13, 2003.

Pergament, D., Pergament, E., Wonderlick, A., & Fiddler, M. (1999). At the crossroads: The intersection of the Internet and clinical oncology. *Oncology, 4*, 577-83.

Pew Research Center. (2003). Internet health resources. Available at http://www.pewinternet.org/reports/toc.asp?Report=95. Accessed June 16, 2003.

Quality of medical information on the internet. (n.d.). Available at http://www.cancerindex.org/clinks18.htm. Accessed June 16, 2003.

The Cleveland Clinic. (n.d.). Cancer and the internet. Available at http://www.clevelandclinic.org/health/health-info/docs/2100/2156.asp?index=9054. Accessed June 15, 2003.

The Source. (2002). Harvard Center for Cancer Prevention Newsletter. Available at http://www.hsph.harvard.edu/cancer/publications/source/. Accessed June 10, 2003.

Utilization Review Accreditation Commission. (n.d.). URAC health web site accreditation program. Available at http://webapps.urac.org/websiteaccreditation/default.htm. Accessed June 10, 2003.

Willis-Knighton Cancer Center. (2001). Coping with internet information overload. Available at http://www.wkhs.com/cancerftr/CancerNews/052401.html. Accessed June 11, 2003.

Wold-Olsen, P. (2001). A holistic view of therapeutic advance, G10 Medicines Workshop on Information and Patients. Available at http://europa.eu.int/comm/health/ph_overview/Documents/contribution02_en.pdf. Accessed June 12, 2003.

Women's Health Information. (1997). Advice on the use of internet-acquired health information. Available at http://www.womens-health.co.uk/advice.htm. Accessed June 16, 2003.

23 | Patient Participation, Health Information, and Communication Skills Training

Implications for Cancer Patients*

Donald J. Cegala
The Ohio State University

Physician-patient communication has been seriously studied for about 30 years: however, most of this research has been conducted in a primary care setting (Roter & Hall, 1989; Thompson & Parrott, 2002). Although some aspects of the medical interview and associated communication principles generalize across medical contexts, there are also unique health and communication needs within various medical specialties. This is perhaps especially true for physician-patient communication about cancer. There are many types of cancer, each one presenting its own set of symptoms, risks, and stages of development. Additionally, cancer treatment often involves physicians from multiple disciplines, sometimes with different views and opinions about how cancer should be treated. Thus, cancer patients' concern, if not fear, about having a life-threatening illness is often further exacerbated by anxiety due to uncertainty about treatment options, their effectiveness, or related matters. These and other aspects of cancer result in unique communication needs for patients, physicians, and significant others within the patient's social network.

No single model or theory is likely to address adequately the entire complexity of communication needs associated with cancer. The focus of this chapter is on cancer patients' interactions with physicians. Although other communication contexts also influence patients'

An earlier version of this chapter was presented at the Kentucky Conference on Health Communication: Trends and Issues in Cancer Communication, Lexington, KY, April 18-20, 2002.

decisions about health matters, the physician plays a significant role in providing information and influencing decisions (Aspden & Katz, 2001; Pennbridge, Moya, & Rodrigues, 1999). A model, called The Integrated Patient Participation Model (IPPM), is presented that integrates health information with patient communication skills training. The basic premise of the model is that information alone about cancer is insufficient to prepare most patients to communicate effectively with physicians about their illness. It is suggested that the addition of communication skills training to information about cancer will enhance patients' use of information and promote more informed, adaptive decision making. The IPPM may be applied to several illnesses, including cancer; however, it is illustrated here with respect to prostate cancer.

HEALTH INFORMATION AND PATIENT PARTICIPATION

The traditional paternalistic model of the physician-patient relationship is being replaced with alternatives that in one way or another emphasize informed consent (Emanuel & Emanuel, 1992). In turn, this emphasis has led some scholars to advocate patient participation in medical decision making, such as that suggested in models of patient-centered interviewing, partnership, and shared decision making (Leopold, Cooper, & Clancy, 1996; Stewart et al., 1995; Towle & Godolphin, 1999). Although there are different views on what patient participation entails (Cahill, 1996), there is universal agreement that patients require health-related information in order for them to participate effectively in medical interviews. O'Connor et al. (1999) called this *informed choice*, whereas Kaplan and colleagues (Kaplan, Greenfield, Gandek, Rogers, & Ware, 1996) perhaps most succinctly capture the essence of patient participation as asking questions, eliciting treatment options, expressing opinions, and stating preferences. Studies in a primary care context support the value of patient participation with respect to enhanced health outcomes and related effects (Cegala, Marinelli, & Post, 2000; Greenfield, Kaplan, & Ware, 1985; Greenfield, Kaplan, Ware, Yano, & Frank, 1988; Kaplan, Greenfield, & Ware, 1989a). Research with cancer patients shows similar positive effects along the lines of less post-treatment anxiety, depression, and better overall adjustment (Davison & Degner, 1997; Johnson, Nail, Lauver, King, & Keys, 1988; Morris & Ingham, 1988; Morris & Royle, 1988; Rainey, 1985).

Although there is empirical support for the value of patient participation and agreement that health-related information is necessary for participation, the precise relationship between the two is less certain. Several studies within a primary care context have shown that patients often want detailed information about their illness, but that patients' desire for information and preference for participation are unrelated (Beisecker & Beisecker, 1990; Deber, Kraetschmer, & Irvine, 1996; Ende, Kazis, Ash, & Moskowitz, 1989; Strull, Lo, & Charles, 1984). Similar results have been reported with respect to cancer patients (Brandt, 1991; Cassileth, Zupkis, Sutton-Smith, & March, 1980; Davison & Degner, 1997). These studies suggest that patients' desire for health-related information is not predictive of their preference for participation in medical decision making. Thus, there is some reason to question whether providing health-related information alone is sufficient for enhancing patient participation. The IPPM assumes there are two significant issues relevant to the relationship between health information and patient participation: the manner in which information is presented to patients and training provided to patients for utilizing the information.

TAILORED HEALTH INFORMATION

One recent response to the matter of how best to present health-related information is the research on tailored messages (Kreuter, Farrell, Olevitch, & Brennan, 2000). Tailoring is sometimes confused with targeting, which involves designing a message to reach a specific subgroup, such as African Americans or women. Tailoring, on the other hand, involves designing a message(s) for a single individual (Kreuter, Strecher, & Glassman, 1999).

Overall, the first generation of research on tailored health information suggests that it is more effective than nontailored information in enhancing individuals' recall and perceptions of relevance and credibility of the information. Additionally, several studies report significant changes in intentions or health-related behavior due to tailored print communications (Skinner, Campbell, Rimer, Curry, & Prochaska, 1999).

Prevailing conceptualizations about the advantages of tailored information are based largely on the Elaboration Likelihood Model (ELM) (Petty & Cacioppo, 1981). Considerable research on the ELM supports the notion that individuals more actively and thoughtfully process information if it is perceived as personally relevant. Additionally, processing information in this way leads to greater recall and behavioral change than processing information in a less cognitively elaborated fashion. Thus, the effects of tailoring are thought to be due to the perceived personal relevance of the information, which, in turn, prompts attention, interest, and deeper cognitive processing.

There are two related aspects about the literature on tailoring that are especially relevant here. First, the majority of tailoring research has focused on cognitive effects, such as recall and perceptions of relevance. Although important, these effects do not clearly indicate *how* the tailored information is used or otherwise affects individuals' behavior. Second, many of the tailoring studies that do purport to assess behavioral effects in reality rely on self-reports of behavior change rather than more objective measures (Brug, Glanz, Van Assema, Kok, & van Breukelen, 1998; Campbell et al., 1994; Marcus et al., 1998; Skinner, Strecher, & Hospers, 1994; Strecher et al., 1994). Together, these observations suggest that at present it is not clear to what extent even tailored information enhances patients' health-related behavior. Additionally, as is argued later, there is a significant difference between using tailored information to promote preventive health behavior changes (e.g., weight loss, smoking cessation) and using it to facilitate complex decision making in an uncertain environment (e.g., where there are no clear treatment choices). Within the former context there is a clear correct choice (e.g., quit smoking and be healthier), whereas in the latter there is no clear right or wrong choice. In such uncertain decision-making environments, the amount and form of information (i.e., tailored or standardized) alone cannot guarantee quality decision making. As developed in the following section, effective communication may be a key factor in enhancing patients' use of health information, especially under uncertain conditions.

PATIENT COMMUNICATION SKILLS TRAINING

There is an enormous literature on physician-patient communication, of which only a small part is devoted to patients' communicative contributions to the medical interview (Anderson & Sharpe, 1991; Cegala & Lenzmeier Broz, 2003). Additionally, all of this work has been conducted in a primary care setting, with no reported evidence of transfer effects to other medical settings.

Nevertheless, the available results on patient communication skills training suggest that it is important for promoting individuals' participation in health care. For example, in comparison to their untrained counterparts, trained patients ask more questions, elicit more information from physicians, provide more detailed information about their illness, express greater preference for involvement and participation, are more compliant, and have better health outcomes (Cegala, Marinelli et al., 2000; Cegala, McClure, Marinelli, & Post, 2000; Cegala, Post, & McClure, 2001; Greenfield et al., 1985; Greenfield et al., 1988; Kaplan, Greenfield, & Ware, Jr., 1989b; Robinson & Whitfield, 1985; Rost, Flavin, Cole, & McGill, 1991; Roter, 1977).

The focus of communication training interventions has been on promoting patients' information exchange skills relevant to interactions with providers. Information-seeking skills in the form of question-asking have received the most emphasis, followed by information verifying and provision skills (Cegala & Lenzmeier Broz, 2003). Some research has applied communication skills training to patients with chronic illness (Greenfield et al., 1985; Greenfield et al., 1988; Kaplan et al., 1989b), but most of it has involved patients in a primary care setting regardless of the nature of their illness. To the author's knowledge, little or no research has examined the effects of communication skills training with cancer patients, although some work has explored ways to encourage cancer patients to ask more questions during the medical interview (Davison & Degner, 1997; Neufeld, Degner, & Dick, 1993).

The cancer environment provides an especially important and interesting context for studying the role of health-related information and the effects of patient communication skills training. The complexity of cancer demands that patients have baseline knowledge of their disease in order to communicate effectively with physicians about diagnosis and treatment choices. For example, a cancer patient seeking the physician's input about alternative treatments would likely ask more pertinent questions and make better assessments of the physician's response, if the patient already had some baseline information about options, possible side effects of treatment, and implications for quality of life. However, as suggested by the literature on desire for information and preference for participation, having an adequate baseline knowledge of one's cancer does not necessarily lead to effective, participatory decision making. Patients must have the desire to participate in decision making *and* the communicative skills to use the information they possess in furthering their understanding of choices and the implications of those options. In the case of prostate cancer, this integration of disease information and communication skills is even more essential for decision making due to the uncertain environment prostate cancer patients face in making treatment decisions. The Integrated Patient Participation Model provides a conceptual framework for integrating tailored health information and communication skills. Next is a brief explication of the prostate cancer environment, followed by an explanation of each component of the IPPM.

BACKGROUND AND SIGNIFICANCE OF PROSTATE CANCER

Prostate cancer is the second leading cause of cancer-related deaths among men in the United States. Approximately 198,000 men were expected to be diagnosed with prostate cancer in 2001, resulting in about 31,500 deaths (Greenlee, Hill-Harmon, Murray, & Thun, 2001). With the aging of America and projections of longer life expectancy (Beisecker, 1996; Beisecker & Beisecker, 1996), it is not unreasonable to anticipate the incidence of prostate cancer to increase over the next several years. From approximately 1987 until the mid 1990s prostate cancer diagnoses increased more than any other solid tumor. This is in large part due to the widespread application of PSA screening (Greenlee et al., 2001; Wingo, Landis, & Ries, 1997). The application of PSA screening has led to the detection of smaller tumors that have a lower risk of metastasis at diagnosis, thus more men are faced with decisions concerning which treatment is most appropriate for their specific situation. In fact, in the decade prior to 1992, the number of patients who underwent radical prostatectomy increased by 100%, whereas the number of patients presenting with advanced metastatic disease declined by 60% (Newcomer, Stanford, Blumenstein, & Brawer, 1997).

In this same period of time the choices for treatment of localized prostate cancer have increased. This has come about in part because technology has dramatically improved the ability of radiation therapy to increase the effective dose of irradiation to the prostate, while reducing collateral damage to adjacent tissues, such as the skin, colon, rectum, bladder, and the neurovascular tissues adjacent to the prostate. Dramatic advances in 3D confromal external beam irradiation and brachytherapy (seed implants) have made these modalities attractive for many men. The rapid adoption of the nerve-sparing radical prostatectomy by urologists, with its reputation for preserving sexual function and reducing incontinence, leads many men to choose surgery as an option. In the last two years, minimally invasive laparoscopic prostatectomy has emerged, with dramatically decreased hospitalization time and morbidity. The current direction of clinical research is to provide "risk-tailored" multimodality therapies that combine modalities with the goal of enhancing cure and survival, while limiting complications of treatment. The major obstacle to educating patients regarding treatment options is the lack of definitive data regarding outcomes, side effects, and quality of life.

The Ambiguities of Prostate Cancer Treatment

Prostate cancer presents comparatively unique problems and challenges for patients in processing information about treatment options and selecting a treatment. Although there are several treatment options, there are no long-term clinical trial data comparing the efficacy of these treatments (Albertsen, Hanley, Gleason, & Barry, 1998; Fleming, Wasson, Albertsen, Barry, & Wennberg, 1993; Millikan & Logothetis, 1997; Montie, 1994; Moore, O'Sullivan, & Tannock, 1988). Moreover, it is unlikely that such information will be available in the near future, if at all. The long natural history of the disease itself requires that trials of primary therapy may need to run 10 years (at great expense) in order to provide definitive data. To complicate matters further, providers often disagree on clinical endpoints to be used in evaluating the efficacy/safety of options, and there are personal biases among physicians of different disciplines (Moore et al., 1988). Expectations for the future of prostate cancer care suggest that treatment options are likely to increase in number and complexity, creating even more choices, but also more difficulty for patients' treatment decision making. Thus, the present and foreseeable future of prostate cancer treatment poses extremely complex information and choices for patients. Selecting a treatment under such conditions is often characterized by stress, uncertainty, and second guessing, which, in turn, can lead to distress and poor quality of life (Gotay & Muraoka, 1998; Gray, Fitch, Davis, & Phillips, 1997; Herr, 1997; Rainey, 1985). On the other hand, considerable research shows that the kind and quality of disease-related information and communication with health care professionals prior to medical treatments has beneficial effects on patients' recovery rate, level of post-treatment pain, and distress (Devine, 1992). There is, therefore, good reason to seek ways of facilitating prostate cancer patients' treatment decision making. The IPPM is intended to facilitate such decision making.

THE INTEGRATED PATIENT PARTICIPATION MODEL

The IPPM is displayed in Figure 23.1. The following is a brief description of the components and logic of the model.

Tailoring Antecedents

The tailoring antecedents are key group-level factors that are important for targeting information about prostate cancer. Due to the fact that prostate cancer onset is typically late in life and is slow growing, patients' age is a significant consideration in treatment decision making. For example, older patients (e.g., > 75) presenting with prostate cancer have a higher probability of experiencing significant trauma from invasive treatments and of dying from causes other than prostate cancer (Albertsen et al., 1998; Fleming et al., 1993). Similarly, considerable data indicate that ethnicity is significantly related to prostate cancer. African Americans, for example, tend to develop less differentiated and more aggressive malignancies than Caucasians, with no clear evidence of life-style or other factors to account for the difference (Fowler, Bigler, Bowman, & Kilambi, 2000; Hoffman et al., 2001; Jones, 2001). These antecedents, in part, are also likely to shape patients' values.

Values

O'Connor et al. (1999) noted that tailoring information on patients' values becomes essential in instances in which there is no clear cut evidence or consensus about treatment option efficacy. Values are personal factors that are important in assessing information about the benefits and risks of options. Because decisions based on values cannot be judged as right or wrong, the quality of such decisions is measured in terms of their consistency with personal values. The indicators of quality decisions include adequate knowledge, realistic expectations, clear values, low decisional conflict, decision implementation, and satisfaction with the decision and the decision-making process (O'Connor et al., 1998). Some of the associated outcomes of quality decisions include improved health quality of life, reduced distress, and decision regret. Tailoring information on the basis of patients' values requires patients to know what their values are, which are not always known or clear, particularly when value articulation is, in part, dependent on medical knowledge that the patient may not have or may not completely understand. A key aspect of decision aids is their ability to assist patients in identifying and focusing their values.

Although O'Connor's decision-support framework fits well with the logic and objectives of the IPPM, the fit is less precise within the context of prostate cancer. The matter of using

TAILORING ANTECEDENTS   PARTICIPATION INTERVENTION   OUTCOMES

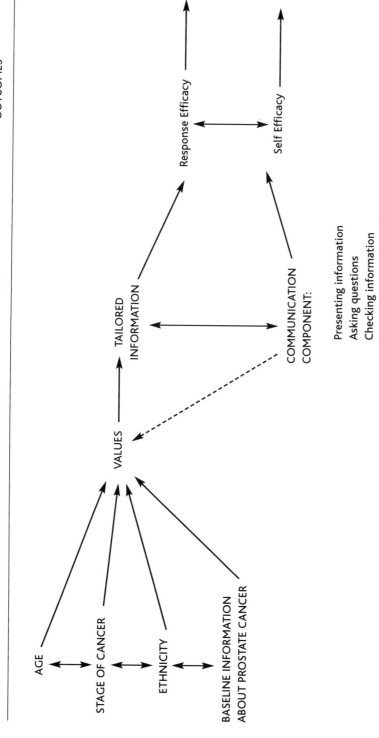

FIGURE 23.1. The integrated patient participation model.

one's values to weigh benefits and risks of prostate cancer treatment options assumes sufficient data to present benefits and risks of options that are tailored to individual patients. The problem with the prostate cancer environment is that there are insufficient data to provide patients with clear benefits and risks, even when information is tailored to individuals. Consequently, the application of the O'Connor et al. (1998) framework within a prostate cancer environment should emphasize the patient's attitudes toward risks, rather than desirability of benefits weighed against risks. In prostate cancer, such attitudes are defined in terms of the importance patients place on known treatment side effects (i.e., incontinence, impotence, rectal damage) and their understanding of what these side effects entail for matters of quality of life. In other words, enhancement of prostate cancer patients' adjustment to post-treatment life is most likely affected by pretreatment information and understanding of what to expect, should such side effects occur, and what options are available for mitigating their effects. In addition, prostate cancer patients selecting any treatment option other than watchful waiting, will experience basic changes in their experience of sex and, potentially, their definition of their own sexuality. Such information, though difficult to convey nonexperientially, is also important as an effective decision aid to incorporate as part of prostate cancer patients' decision making, particularly with respect to incorporating realistic expectations about post-treatment sexual life.

These relatively unique aspects of prostate cancer underscore the importance of the communication skills component of the IPPM. It is essential for prostate cancer patients to express their values and concerns about post-treatment life in discussions with physicians about treatment options and prognosis. By doing so, patients can gather additional information, refine or redefine their values (note the dotted line in the model from communication to values), and ultimately acquire more realistic expectations for post-treatment life. Such expectations are more likely to result in a better adjusted, higher quality of life post-treatment.

Tailored Information

Tailored information is perceived as more personally relevant, more deeply processed, and better recalled (Skinner et al., 1999). As such, tailored information is expected to promote response efficacy whereby information is believed to be effective in achieving a goal, such as solving a problem. Response efficacy has been shown to be an essential factor in persuading individuals to accept health-related recommendations (Witte, 1992; Witte & Allen, 2000). Response efficacy also should promote more confident decision making.

Communication Skills

The communication component of the model is based on previous research with the PACE System (Cegala, Marinelli et al., 2000; Cegala, McClure et al., 2000; Cegala et al., 2001). It currently consists of training in communication skills relevant to interacting with physicians in a primary care medical interview. To date, the PACE System has been presented to patients via a printed booklet and more recently as a Web site (http://patcom.jcomm.ohio-state.edu). Within the context of the IPPM, the PACE System is modified to communication about prostate cancer. Additionally, within the IPPM the PACE System is presented in an enhanced electronic form, with inclusion of video clips illustrating modeling of communication skills and integrated with tailored information about prostate cancer. The video models of the communication skills are expected to enhance patients' self efficacy, which has been shown to facilitate individuals' performance in a variety of behaviors, including health-related activity (Bandura, 1997). The communication skills component of the IPPM is expected to strengthen patients' self efficacy in their medical interview-related communication—that is, patients' belief in their ability to communicate effectively with health care providers about illness-related matters.

The integration of tailored information with communication skills training is the key feature of the IPPM. As patients are presented with tailored information about their illness, they are exposed to prompts and models of communication skills illustrating what they can do with the information during their appointment with a physician. This is consistent with Social Cognitive Theory, which specifies that modeling promotes self-efficacy and performance (Bandura, 1997). For example, as tailored information is presented about various prostate cancer treatment options, the patient is prompted to express his values relevant to treatment risks and side effects and is shown a model of a patient doing so. Later, as more detailed, tailored information is presented about a particular treatment option, the patient might be prompted to ask certain quality of life questions about the option, accompanied by another patient model doing so. In a similar way, as other information is presented, patients are reminded of the value of checking on their understanding of the information the physician gives them or the importance of expressing concerns, with appropriate models doing so.

Thus, with the IPPM, patients not only receive information that is tailored to their values and targeted on antecedent factors, but they are also provided with training prompts and models of communication skills that facilitate using the information while interacting with a physician. This integrated approach is expected to reinforce the connection between response and self-efficacy, thus enhancing patients' ability to make quality decisions about treatment selection and demonstrate better adaptation to any resulting impact on quality of life.

REFERENCES

Albertsen, P. C., Hanley, J. A., Gleason, D. F., & Barry, M. J. (1998). Competing risk analysis of men aged 55 to 74 years at diagnosis managed conservatively for clinically localized prostate cancer. *Journal of the American Medical Association, 280*(11), 975-980.

Anderson, L. A., & Sharpe, P. A. (1991). Improving patient and provider communication: A synthesis and review of communication interventions. *Patient Education and Counseling, 17*, 99-134.

Aspden, P., & Katz, J. E. (2001). Assessments of quality of health care information and referrals to physicians: A national survey. In R. E. Rice & J. E. Katz (Eds.), *The Internet and health communication: Experiences and expectations* (pp. 99-106). Thousand Oaks: Sage.

Bandura, A. (1997). *Self-efficacy: The exercise of control.* New York: Freeman.

Beisecker, A. E. (1996). Older persons' medical encounters and their outcomes. *Research on Aging, 18*, 9-31.

Beisecker, A. E., & Beisecker, T. D. (1990). Patient information-seeking behaviors when communicating with doctors. *Medical Care, 28*, 19-28.

Beisecker, A. E., & Beisecker, T. D. (1996). Research issues related to physician-elderly patient interactions. *Research on Aging, 18*, 3-8.

Brandt, B. (1991). Informational needs and selected variables in patients receiving brachytherapy. *Oncology Nursing Forum, 18*(7), 1221-1227; discussion 1227-1229.

Brug, J., Glanz, K., Van Assema, P., Kok, G., & van Breukelen, G. J. (1998). The impact of computer-tailored feedback and iterative feedback on fat, fruit, and vegetable intake. *Health Education Behavior, 25*(4), 517-531.

Cahill, J. (1996). Patient participation: A concept analysis. *Journal of Advanced Nursing, 24,* 561-571.

Campbell, M. K., DeVellis, B. M., Strecher, V. J., Ammerman, A. S., DeVellis, R. F., & Sandler, R. S. (1994). Improving dietary behavior: The effectiveness of tailored messages in primary care settings. *American Journal of Public Health, 84*(5), 783-787.

Cassileth, B. R., Zupkis, R. V., Sutton-Smith, K., & March, V. (1980). Information and participation preferences among cancer patients. *Annuals of Internal Medicine, 92*(6), 832-836.

Cegala, D. J., & Lenzmeier Broz, S. (2003). Provider and patient communication skills training. In A. D. T. Thompson, K. Miller, & R. Parrott (Ed.), *Handbook of health communication* (pp. 95-119). Mahwah, NJ: Erlbaum.

Cegala, D. J., Marinelli, T., & Post, D. M. (2000). The effect of patient communication skills training on treatment compliance in primary care. *Archives of Family Medicine, 9,* 57-64.

Cegala, D. J., McClure, L., Marinelli, T. M., & Post, D. M. (2000). The effects of communication skills training on patients' participation during medical interviews. *Patient Education and Counseling, 41,* 209-222.

Cegala, D. J., Post, D., & McClure, L. (2001). The effects of patient communication skills training on the discourse of elderly patients during a primary care interview. *Journal of the American Geriatrics Society, 49,* 1505-1511.

Davison, B. J., & Degner, L. F. (1997). Empowerment of men newly diagnosed with prostate cancer. *Cancer Nursing, 20*(3), 187-196.

Deber, R. B., Kraetschmer, N., & Irvine, J. (1996). What role do patients wish to play in treatment decision making? *Archives of Internal Medicine, 156*(13), 1414-1420.

Devine, E. C. (1992). Effects of psychoeducational care for adult surgical patients: A meta-analysis of 191 studies. *Patient Education & Counseling, 19,* 129-142.

Emanuel, E. J., & Emanuel, L. L. (1992). Four models of the physician-patient relationship. *Journal of the American Medical Association, 267,* 2221-2226.

Ende, J., Kazis, L., Ash, A., & Moskowitz, M. A. (1989). Measuring patients' desire for autonomy: Decision-making and information-seeking preferences among medical patients. *Journal of General Internal Medicine, 4,* 23-30.

Fleming, C., Wasson, J. H., Albertsen, P. C., Barry, M. J., & Wennberg, J. E. (1993). A decision analysis of alternative treatment strategies for clinically localized prostate cancer. Prostate Patient Outcomes Research Team. *Journal of the American Medical Association, 269*(20), 2650-2658.

Fowler, J. E., Jr., Bigler, S. A., Bowman, G., & Kilambi, N. K. (2000). Race and cause specific survival with prostate cancer: Influence of clinical stage, Gleason score, age and treatment. *Journal of Urology, 163*(1), 137-142.

Gotay, C. C., & Muraoka, M. Y. (1998). Quality of life in long-term survivors of adult-onset cancers. *Journal of the National Cancer Institute, 90,* 656-667.

Gray, R. E., Fitch, M., Davis, C., & Phillips, C. (1997). Interviews with men with prostate cancer about their self-help group experience. *Journal of Palliative Care, 13*(1), 15-21.

Greenfield, S., Kaplan, S., & Ware, J. E., Jr. (1985). Expanding patient involvement in care: Effects on patient outcomes. *Annals of Internal Medicine, 102*(4), 520-528.

Greenfield, S., Kaplan, S. H., Ware, J. E., Jr., Yano, E. M., & Frank, H. J. (1988). Patients' participation in medical care: Effects on blood sugar control and quality of life in diabetes. *Journal of General Internal Medicine, 3*(5), 448-457.

Greenlee, R. T., Hill-Harmon, M. B., Murray, T., & Thun, M. (2001). Cancer statistics, 2001. *CA Cancer Journal for Clinicians, 51*(1), 15-36.

Herr, H. W. (1997). Quality of life in prostate cancer patients. *CA Cancer Journal for Clinicians, 47*(4), 207-217.

Hoffman, R. M., Gilliland, F. D., Eley, J. W., Harlan, L. C., Stephenson, R. A., Stanford, J. L., Albertson, P. C., Hamilton, A. S., Hunt, W. C., & Potosky, A. L. (2001). Racial and ethnic differences in advanced-stage prostate cancer: The Prostate Cancer Outcomes Study. *Journal of The National Cancer Institute, 93*(5), 388-395.

Johnson, J. E., Nail, L. M., Lauver, D., King, K. B., & Keys, H. (1988). Reducing the negative impact of radiation therapy on functional status. *Cancer, 61*(1), 46-51.

Jones, J. (2001). African-Americans and prostate cancer: Why the discrepancies? *Journal of The National Cancer Institute, 93*(5), 342-344.

Kaplan, S. H., Greenfield, S., Gandek, B., Rogers, W. H., & Ware, J. E. (1996). Characteristics of physicians with participatory decision-making styles. *Annals of Internal Medicine, 124*, 497-504.

Kaplan, S. H., Greenfield, S., & Ware, J. E. (1989a). Impact of the doctor-patient relationship on the outcomes of chronic disease. In M. Stewart & D. Roter (Eds.), *Communicating with medical patients* (pp. 228-245). Newbury Park, CA: Sage.

Kaplan, S. H., Greenfield, S., & Ware, J. E., Jr. (1989b). Assessing the effects of physician-patient interactions on the outcomes of chronic disease. *Medical Care, 27*(3 Suppl), S110-127.

Kreuter, M., Farrell, D., Olevitch, L., & Brennan, L. (2000). *Tailoring health messages: Customizing communication with computer technology.* Mahwah, NJ: Erlbaum.

Kreuter, M. W., Strecher, V. J., & Glassman, B. (1999). One size does not fit all: The case for tailoring print materials. *Annals of Behavioral Medicine, 21*(4), 276-283.

Leopold, N., Cooper, J., & Clancy, C. (1996). Sustained partnership in primary care. *Journal of Family Practice, 42*, 129-137.

Marcus, B. H., Emmons, K. M., Simkin-Silverman, L. R., Linnan, L. A., Taylor, E. R., Bock, B. C., Roberts, M. B., Rossi, J. S., & Abrams, D. B. (1998). Evaluation of motivationally tailored vs. standard self-help physical activity interventions at the workplace. *American Journal of Health Promotion, 12*(4), 246-253.

Millikan, R., & Logothetis, C. (1997). Update of the NCCN guidelines for treatment of prostate cancer. *Oncology, 11*(11A), 180-193.

Montie, J. E. (1994). Counseling the patient with localized prostate cancer. *Urology, 43*(2 Suppl), 36-40.

Moore, M. J., O'Sullivan, B., & Tannock, I. F. (1988). How expert physicians would wish to be treated if they had genitourinary cancer. *Journal of Clinical Oncology, 6*(11), 1736-1745.

Morris, J., & Ingham, R. (1988). Choice of surgery for early breast cancer: Psychosocial considerations. *Social Science and Medicine, 27*(11), 1257-1262.

Morris, J., & Royle, G. T. (1988). Offering patients a choice of surgery for early breast cancer: A reduction in anxiety and depression in patients and their husbands. *Social Science and Medicine, 26*(6), 583-585.

Neufeld, K. R., Degner, L. F., & Dick, J. A. (1993). A nursing intervention strategy to foster patient involvement in treatment decisions. *Oncology Nursing Forum, 20*(4), 631-635.

Newcomer, L. M., Stanford, J. L., Blumenstein, B. A., & Brawer, M. K. (1997). Temporal trends in rates of prostate cancer: Declining incidence of advanced stage disease, 1974 to 1994. *Journal of Urology, 158*(4), 1427-1430.

O'Connor, A. M., Fiset, V., DeGrasse, C., Graham, I. D., Evans, W., Stacey, D., Laupacis, A., & Tugwell, P. (1999). Decision aids for patients considering options affecting cancer outcomes: Evidence of efficacy and policy implications. *Journal of The National Cancer Institute Monographs, 25*, 67-80.

O'Connor, A. M., Tugwell, P., Wells, G. A., Elmslie, T., Jolly, E., Hollingworth, G., McPherson, R., Bunn, H., Graham, I., & Drake, E. (1998). A decision aid for women considering hormone therapy after menopause: Decision support framework and evaluation. *Patient Education and Counseling, 33*(3), 267-279.

Pennbridge, J., Moya, R., & Rodrigues, L. (1999). Questionnaire survey of California consumers' use and rating of sources of health care information including the Internet. *Western Journal of Medicine, 171*(5-6), 302-305.

Petty, R. E., & Cacioppo, J. T. (1981). *Attitudes and persuasion: Classic and contemporary approaches.* Dubuque, IA: Brown.

Rainey, L. C. (1985). Effects of preparatory patient education for radiation oncology patients. *Cancer, 56*(5), 1056-1061.

Robinson, E. J., & Whitfield, M. J. (1985). Improving the efficiency of patients' comprehension monitoring: A way of increasing patients' participation in general practice consultations. *Social Science and Medicine, 21*(8), 915-919.

Rost, K. M., Flavin, K. S., Cole, K., & McGill, J. B. (1991). Change in metabolic control and functional status after hospitalization: Impact of patient activation intervention in diabetic patients. *Diabetes Care, 14*(10), 881-889.

Roter, D. L. (1977). Patient participation in the patient-provider interaction: The effects of patient question asking on the quality of interaction, satisfaction and compliance. *Health Education Monographs, 5*, 281-310.

Roter, D. L., & Hall, J. A. (1989). Studies of doctor-patient interaction. *Annual Review of Public Health, 10*, 163-180.

Skinner, C. S., Campbell, M. K., Rimer, B. K., Curry, S., & Prochaska, J. O. (1999). How effective is tailored print communication? *Annals of Behavioral Medicine, 21*(4), 290-298.

Skinner, C. S., Strecher, V. J., & Hospers, H. (1994). Physicians' recommendations for mammography: Do tailored messages make a difference? *American Journal of Public Health, 84*(1), 43-49.

Stewart, M., Brown, J. B., Weston, W. W., McWhinney, I. R., McWilliam, C. L., & Freeman, T. R. (1995). *Patient-centered medicine.* Thousand Oaks, CA: Sage.

Strecher, V. J., Kreuter, M., Den Boer, D. J., Kobrin, S., Hospers, H. J., & Skinner, C. S. (1994). The effects of computer-tailored smoking cessation messages in family practice settings. *Journal of Family Practice, 39*(3), 262-270.

Strull, W. M., Lo, B., & Charles, G. (1984). Do patients want to participate in medical decision-making? *Journal of the American Medical Association, 252*, 2990-2994.

Thompson, T. L., & Parrott, R. L. (2002). Interpersonal communication and health care. In M. L. Knapp & J. A. Daly (Eds.), *Handbook of interpersonal communication* (3rd ed., pp. 680-725). Thousand Oaks, CA: Sage.

Towle, A., & Godolphin, W. (1999). Framework for teaching and learning informed shared decision making. *British Medical Journal, 319*(7212), 766-771.

Wingo, P. A., Landis, S., & Ries, L. A. (1997). An adjustment to the 1997 estimate for new prostate cancer cases. *CA Cancer Journal for Clinicians, 47*(4), 239-242.

Witte, K. (1992). The role of threat and efficacy in AIDS prevention. *International Quarterly of Community Health Education, 12*, 225-249.

Witte, K., & Allen, M. (2000). A meta-analysis of fear appeals: Implications for effective public health campaigns. *Health Education Behavior, 27*(5), 591-615.

24 | Identifying Research Traditions Appropriate For Cancer Care and Communication

H. Dan O'Hair
University of Oklahoma

Identifying research traditions in the area of health communication is something of a paradoxical exercise for a short chapter in a book filled with many new exciting ideas about cancer care. On the one hand, it is relatively easy to list a number of the major research programs that constitute the corpus of studies focusing on patient-provider communication. On the other hand, it is impossible, in any narrative sense, to competently explicate the central issues involved in these important programs. Based on such challenges, I limit my discussion of research traditions to those in which I have the most experience. Specifically, I review research involving (a) relational control messages, (b) patient preferences and perception of quality, and (c) communication and health outcomes. For each of the sections, I briefly review important trends emanating from that research tradition and summarize each section with implications for future investigations. In the final section, I propose two promising directions of research for patient-provider communication.

RELATIONAL CONTROL MESSAGES[1]

The control dimension in the patient-provider relationship has been examined from both macro (strategic behavior) as well micro (specific message tactics) perspectives (O'Hair,

---

[1]Portions of this section were adapted from a previous article published by the author. O'Hair, D. (2003). Research traditions in provider-consumer interaction: Implications for cancer care. *Patient Education and Counseling, 50,* 5-8.

1988). Issues of paternalism and consumerism (Beisecker & Beisecker, 1993; Gadow, 1990) and participatory decision making (Gafni & Whelan, 1998; Kaplan, Greenfield, Gandek, Rogers, & Ware, 1996) are familiar standards in the control literature as are emerging models of shared control such as giving "voice" (Madson, 1999) and empowering patients (Gray, Doan, & Church, 1990; Wallerstein & Bernstein, 1999). These macro or strategic issues of control influence healthcare research in a number of important ways. Furthermore, "the currency with which they dot the landscape of psychosocial medical literature suggests that we will continue to view patient-provider communication from a control perspective for some time to come" (O'Hair, 2003, p. 5). A primary concern is investigations that discern how patients negotiate their roles within complex cancer delivery systems.

From a different perspective, relational control has been applied to message exchanges of dyads and triads in the healthcare delivery context. In this particular research paradigm, patients and providers define their relationships through the types of messages they exchange with their partners. Control is attempted by sending messages that define, direct, and dominate (Rogers & Farace, 1975; Millar & Rogers, 1987). Message control techniques include those that are confrontational, question authority, make assertions, disconfirm, change topics, initiate or terminate interactions, provide instruction, or possible answers to inquiries (McNeilis & Thompson, 1995; O'Hair, 1989; O'Hair, Allman, & Moore, 1996). Messages that allow control of the relationship (i.e., submission) consist of supporting messages, asking questions, providing approval, and offering confirmation (McNeilis, Thompson, & O'Hair, 1995; O'Hair, 1989; O'Hair et al., 1996). I would argue that cancer care is an especially appropriate context for studying relational control given the vast array of providers (oncologists, surgeons, radiologists, organ specific specialists, primary care providers, social workers, etc.) and the complex process of care associated with cancer delivery systems. Examining messages that identify relational control moves could be related to other patient and provider variables and certain types of outcomes from cancer treatment.

Observation and analysis of relational control is accomplished through relational coding techniques. The most widely used analysis system for this purpose is one designed by Rogers and Farace (1975) and validated by Rogers and colleagues (Millar & Rogers, 1987; Rogers, Courtright, & Millar, 1980; Rogers & Millar, 1982). This technique is touted as a genuinely relational system given that the emphasis of analysis is on interaction rather than simple utterances. By assigning a 3-digit code to an utterance, researchers can determine whether a message from one of the interactants is seeking control of the relationship (one-up message), relinquishing or offering control of the relationship (one-down message), or remaining uncommitted or neutral (one-across).

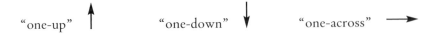

By pairing utterances from sequential interacts, a transaction sequence can be observed such as the following:

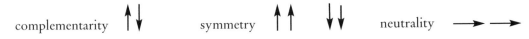

When examining entire interactions (e.g., clinical episode between patient and provider), a collection of transaction sequences could be observed offering cancer communication researchers opportunities to organize and analyze patterns of relational control for provider-patient relationships. The emergence of control patterns could be assessed through frequency counts and by determining the proportion of control or dominance attempted by each communicator. Over time, control patterns would reveal much about how patients perceive their communicative role in the therapeutic process.

The preponderance of relational control research on the patient-provider relationship demonstrates a dominant trend in which patients seldom attempt relational control with their providers (McNeilis & Thompson, 1995; McNeilis et al., 1995; O'Hair, 1989; Von Friederichs-Fitzwater, Callahan, Flynn, & Williams, 1991). In the main, when relational control is attempted or obtained, it is usually challenged by someone acting on behalf of the patient in the role of "advocate," such as with a child or parent (O'Hair, 1989; O'Hair & McNeilis, 1993). Cancer care is a disease causing family members to become involved with many aspects of care, and the role of advocate is likely to be observed among these advocates on behalf of the patient. In spite of the advocate's role, "most research involving relational control analysis empirically bears out what conventional wisdom and other studies suggests—physicians expect and exert control over their relationships with patients" (O'Hair, 2003, p. 6).

Limitations and Implications

Relational control analysis is often considered an appropriate method when transcripts of message exchange are available. Results from the analyses can have value for both researchers and practitioners who are interested in learning how providers and patients negotiate control over the relationship. Adding these data to patient training programs, such as the ones discussed in this volume, might be particularly illuminating for cancer patients. Alternatively, physician communication education programs could benefit similarly in facilitating a greater awareness of how messages can have undesirable control affects on patients. Critics of relational control analysis question the validity of the coding itself and find the necessity for multiple coders to ensure internal consistency to be impractical. Furthermore, the analysis requires a great deal of planning and execution, something that may not be appealing to some investigators and particularly practitioners. Relational control analysis seems to offer the most utility as a means of representing the relational control patterns of interactants over a period of time. Tracing relational control over time could serve to benchmark how surgeons, oncologists, or radiologists negotiate control in their relationships through the analysis of their messages and those of their cancer patients.

PATIENT PREFERENCES AND PERCEPTIONS OF QUALITY

Patient preferences for communication behavior and perceptions of communication quality have enjoyed a great deal of interest from health communication researchers in recent years. Although conceptually related, patient preferences and perceptions of quality serve different functions in research designs, occasionally alternating between independent and dependent variables. Although researchers point to previous research in general areas of medical care delivery, less is known about cancer specific preferences and perceptions of communication quality. For instance, patients may vary in their preferences depending on a number of disease-specific, therapeutic, and communication dimensions, and it stands to reason that cancer patients with more encouraging treatment diagnoses (e.g., breast, colorectal, prostate) will hold different communication preferences than cancer patients facing prognoses for treatments that are more pessimistic (e.g., pancreatic, brain, sarcoma).

Patient Preferences for Communication Styles

The research examining patients' preferences for physician communication behavior has been somewhat limited in its theoretical potential, although this line of research has demonstrated rather clearly what patients desire in provider communication patterns. Patients report that they prefer physicians who they perceive as interpersonally sensitive and willing to listen to patients' concerns (Ben-Sira, 1980; Buller & Buller, 1987; Cegala, McNeilis, McGee, & Jonas, 1995; Cline & McKenzie, 1998; DuPré, 1998; Frankel, 1984; O'Hair, 1986; O'Hair, Scannell, & Thompson, 2005; Street & Wiemann, 1987). Much of this work corroborates the notion that patients favor providers who are sensitive and caring. For example, Street and Wiemann (1987) discovered that patients desire physicians who exhibit involvement in the examination room and prefer a more expressive manner in their communication style. Research by Burgoon et al., (1987) observed that physicians who are attentive to their patients are more favorably rated. O'Hair (1986) examined the influence of patient anxiety on preferences for communication style. He found that patients with higher levels of receiver apprehension (low tolerance for high levels of information) preferred providers with a low affect/low information style. In the same study he discovered that patients with higher health beliefs (predisposition toward treatment compliance efforts) preferred physicians with a highly affective style (especially compared to low compliers). In a similar study, O'Hair, Behnke, and King (1983) found that younger and older patients preferred physicians who communicated less specific, detailed, and technical information. Patients preferring higher levels of information were middle-aged adults.

Communication preference studies focused specifically on cancer patients and oncologists have been reported with interesting results. The factors most likely to influence patient preferences for provider communication style include gender, age, education level, and physician perceptions of patient preferences (Blanchard, Labrecque, Ruckdeschel, & Blanchard, 1988; Bruera, Sweeney, Calder, Palmer, & Benisch-Tolley, 2001; Cassileth, Zupkis, Sutton-Smith, & March, 1980; Detmar, Aaronson, Wever, Muller, & Schornagel, 2000; Parker et al., 2001). Future research that would be especially meaningful should examine the connection between preferences and behaviors among cancer patients. The following questions would be especially pertinent: Does the realization of communication preferences translate into observable outcomes? How do providers determine and accommodate these preferences?

Communication Quality Perceptions

A widely used quality perception construct in the patient-provider context is satisfaction. Some research has suggested that satisfaction is only achieved through effective communication (Korsch & Negrete, 1981; Spiro & Heidrich, 1983). Another variable often used to index or gauge patient's perceptions of quality is treatment compliance. Burgoon et al. (1987) stated that a physician's influence used to achieve patient (treatment) compliance is one of the most important outcomes to medical interaction that communication researchers can investigate. Although patients' decisions to comply with prescribed regimen are dependent on many factors, undoubtedly a major component is the physician's communicative behaviors with the patient. Indeed, much of the research on provider-patient compliance focuses around the type of message strategy used (cf. Burgoon et al., 1987; Burgoon et al., 1990, O'Hair, 1986; O'Hair, O'Hair, Southward, & Krayer, 1987). It should be explicitly acknowledged that as an outcome variable, adherence to treatment regimen (compliance) has been questioned as a definitive outcome measure of provider-patient communication (Kaplan, Gandek, Greenfield, Rogers, & Ware, 1995). Patient compliance may have very little meaning for end-state cancer stages or surgery contexts, or may be difficult to measure in instances in which treatment is convoluted, especially those involving complementary and alternative therapies.

Recent research into the conceptualization of self-efficacy has special use for explaining communication quality perceptions. Self-efficacy is defined as one's ability to execute behaviors successfully in order to achieve specific goals (cf. Bandura, 1977; Woodruff & Cashman, 1993). Self-efficacy mediates the effect of situation difficulty and past experience on interpersonal communication. People who perceive themselves as interacting with minimal effort and attaining high success will possess a high degree of self-efficacy. One's communication with a physician is therefore affected by self-efficacy. Self-efficacy is a perception—almost an expectation of interaction. Previous literature has indicated a probable relationship between self-efficacy and satisfaction for general interpersonal relationships (c.f. Lopez & Lent, 1991; Rubin, Martin, Bruning, & Powers, 1993). It is worth noting that many medical communication researchers recognize that conceptions of self-efficacy are best conceived as a domain or behavior-specific construct. For example, self-efficacy perceptions have been specified for certain cancers (prostate, breast, etc.) and for certain cancer stages.

In a recent study, Moore, O'Hair, and Ledlow (2002) investigated the effects of patient self-efficacy on satisfaction and compliance. Results indicated that patients with higher degrees of self-efficacy generally reported a higher degree of satisfaction with the provider. In terms of compliance, those patients reporting a high degree of self-efficacy were more likely to comply with their caregiver, whereas those with lower degrees of self-efficacy were less likely to comply.

Other types of communication quality perceptions have captured the attention of researchers. In a study conducted by Ledlow, O'Hair, and Moore (2003), perceptions of quality (timeliness, accuracy, usefulness, and quantity of information) were investigated following communication among patients, nurses, and physicians in a nurse call center (triage) context. Nurse call centers involve integration of telephone triage, advice, and appointment systems as a means of demand management. The call centers serve as both gatekeeping and liaison functions between patients and physicians. As an intermediary to the care process, the nurse in the call center plays the vital role of communicator. Results from the Ledlow et al. (2003) study indicated that perceptions of communication quality (timeliness, accuracy, usefulness, and quantity) varied among both providers (physicians) and patients depending on a number of predictor variables. For example, distant providers (those practicing more than 30 miles from the nurse call center) perceived higher quality than local providers. Local providers expected more timely information. As provider age increased, so did perceptions of timeliness. Further research may find that older providers feel more comfortable with a slower pace of information flow or that older providers have lower timeliness expectations. Gender and health self-efficacy proved to be the best predictors for perceptions of timeliness for patients. Males perceived information to be significantly less timely than females. High health self-efficacy created greater levels of communication quality perceptions. Most patients perceived that the quantity of information was sufficient. Implications of these results for cancer patients negotiating treatment options with their managed care plans (especially those involving gatekeepers such as call centers) could be far reaching (O'Hair et al., 2003).

Limitations and Implications

One of the fundamental questions surrounding the utility of this line of research must address whether preferences and quality perceptions as cognitive states actually influence cancer patients' behavior and health outcomes. Granted, some of the communication preferences research articles are finding their way to practitioner-oriented journals (or citation of them), potentially influencing provider behavior. But how this research is directly affecting patient behavior is far from being understood. Additional research should extend previous work that reveals the association between preferences and interaction and post-interaction behavior of patients. Bringing to bear previous work on communication and relational expectations might offer some promising scenarios for future research in the area of patient preferences and perceptions of communication quality (Burgoon, Birk, & Hall, 1991; Klingle & Burgoon, 1995; O'Hair, Halone, Morris, & Ledlow, 1997). Research on patient preferences and quality perceptions might also benefit from complementary work investigating the influence of healthcare financial systems on patient perceptions. Although most of this work has focused on patient attitudes toward the system of delivery, some important work has considered how perceptions of the healthcare delivery system affect attitudes about providers (Greeneich, 1995; Moore, O'Hair, & Ledlow, 2002; Moore, Ledlow, & O'Hair, this volume; O'Connor, Hallberg, & Myles, 1998; Paletta, 1995). Importantly, it is not clear how and where cancer patients attribute quality perceptions when faced with treatment restrictions from managed care plans or obstacles faced when enrolling in clinical trials.

TRANSFORMATIONAL MODEL OF COMMUNICATION AND HEALTH OUTCOMES

In its original conception (Kreps, O'Hair, & Clowers, 1994), the Transformational Model of Communication and Health Outcomes (TMCHO) engaged general systems theory and Donabedian's (1980) model of health outcomes to reveal the dynamic forces involved in demonstrating the relationships among pre-existing conditions, communication behaviors, and health outcomes. Employing an input-process-output paradigm, the TMCHO, unlike other outcomes models, focuses exclusively on communication during the healthcare delivery process. Depicted below in Table 24.1, the three stages of the model are briefly described.

Table 24.1
Three States of the TMCHO Model.

ANTECEDENT CONDITIONS (INPUT)	COMMUNICATION (PROCESS)	OUTCOMES (OUTPUT)
Health problem/risk, provider/patient attitudes, beliefs, expectations	Provider/patient message strategies, language used, nonverbal cues, channels and media	Cognitive, behavioral, and physiological outcomes

The original TMCHO attempted to take full advantage of various elements of systems theory including equifinality, negative entropy, and interdependence. It also touted itself as applicable to any healthcare context and any level of communication (intrapersonal, dyadic, interdisciplinary healthcare teams, organization-wide, or community-based perspective).

What are the critical issues involved with an *outcomes-based* model? First, outcomes research is utilized by oncology researchers to sharpen their focus of inquiry, develop new questions for research, and compare benchmarked results with their own findings. Policymakers use outcomes research to profile the health status of the general public or particular groups and as a means for making arguments for funding priorities. Furthermore, in an age of rapidly evolving methods of paying for and delivering cancer care, it becomes essential to document the effectiveness, efficiency, and value of the treatment protocol. As a result, stakeholders at all levels (including patients and providers) have a vested interest in understanding the relationships among antecedent, process, and outcome variables. As a descriptive model then, the TMCHO offers a simplified view of the importance of communication in the healthcare delivery process. Where do we go from here?

Limitations and Implications

The most obvious limitation of TMCHO is a lack of explication for the component parts in the three stages. Explication should come in two forms. First, each of the components requires illumination in terms of their descriptive nature, but perhaps more importantly, in terms of how they become operationalized and then tested for their isomorphic qualities within each stage of the model. In addition, research should address how well these components predict or are influenced by other components in other stages of the model. Second, additional elements will no doubt find their place in each of the stages. Figure 24.1 depicts the three original categories composing the outcomes stage of the model along with a new category termed "philosophical." It seemed reasonable that the ethical treatment of cancer patients, the holistic consideration of a patient's needs, the heuristic potential of research, and patient privacy are outcomes that are difficult to ignore and certainly ones that are rich for study. Clearly, all of these variables are implicated by the communication process between cancer patients and providers. Additional elements for the original categories have also been added based on the emergence of new research focusing on patient-provider communication (identified with an asterisk in Figure 24.1).

COGNITIVE

Understanding/knowledge
Diagnostic information
Commitment to health
Adjustment of health beliefs
Confidence, satisfaction, and trust
Self-efficacy
Managed expectations, fears, and anxieties
*Adjusting to changes in self-identity
*Finding hope
*Emotions management

BEHAVIORAL

Compliance with regimen
Adoption of prevention/health promoting
  behaviors
Communication competence
Team/partnership building
Relational quality
Partner competence/satisfaction
Assertiveness/motivation
*Expanded social support network
*Empowered decision-making
*Accomplishing goals

PHYSIOLOGICAL

Disease prevention
Recovery and recuperation processes
Maintenance of desired health
Long-term survival
Quality of life
*Anxiety/depression management
*End of life management

*PHILOSOPHICAL

*Ethical treatment
*Holistic consideration of patient
*Heuristic potential
*Privacy

Revisions to Kreps, O'Hair, and Clowers (1994)

FIGURE 24.1 Health outcomes

Moreover, these new components are more reflective of a model that emphasizes communication between a provider and a patient within a cancer illness context. In addition, the previous discussion of relational control and communication preferences comes into play when considering outcomes. Empirical research could be directed toward predicting outcomes of cancer care based on consistent patterns of relational control attempts by patients and/or providers. Employing patients' preferences for communication styles could help to predict if patients are willing to follow through with participation in treatment regimens or clinical trials. From a prevention perspective, what effect do varying degrees of relational control have on patients receiving news that they carry a gene known to be expressive for a certain type of cancer? As a critical component of the cancer context, genetic counseling will become a more frequent element of the cancer care compendium, and understanding how relational messages and preferences for communication influence decisional outcomes regarding preventative behaviors will become critical.

Of course, a missing outcome variable that must become visible on the radar screen is costs. Few patients, and particularly cancer patients, can ignore the issue of cancer treatment (and palliative and hospice care) costs. I think it would be shortsighted for us to assume that cost is unrelated to communication processes between patients and providers. Furthermore, cost as an outcome variable could be considered in a macro sense (costs to society) and from a micro or personal perspective. The question at this point centers on where "cost" fits into an outcomes model similar to this one.

SUMMARY

As a means of offering some general conclusions to my thoughts on patient-physician communication research beyond those presented at the end of each section, I feel it necessary to share a couple of personal biases I hold regarding this type of research. First, I am finding it increasingly difficult to sort out the complexity of this relationship in isolation from its macroenvironment—in particular healthcare delivery systems. It might be argued that to introduce additional variables into an already multifarious research context would only complicate matters. I can agree with the basic assumptions (and advantages) for how experimental control offers substantial precision. However, I also side with Kreps (2001) who argues for a more ecologically valid effort from those of us who conduct health communication research. From my perspective that requires an inclusion (if not emphasis) on how the healthcare delivery system affects the patient-provider relationship. In the past decade, the communicative relationship between the provider and the patient has changed with the increasing complexity of health delivery systems (HDS) and insurance companies. At the patient level, patients are often confused with the allowances, policies, regulations, and procedures that are involved with their insurance plans, which is creating increased scrutiny by watchdog groups, federal regulators, and governmental officials. At a general level, research on patient-provider communication should be directed toward addressing the following issue: To what extent do cancer care delivery systems influence patterns of communication among patient and providers?

With the advent of the patient movement, the debate over "health care reform," and the highly visible marketing campaigns of the HDS industry, the traditional model of provider-patient communication has been called into question (Apker, 2001; Gillespie, 2001; Moore & O'Hair, 1997; O'Hair, Halone, Morris, & Ledlow, 1997). Because of the change in the provider-patient relationship, it is likely that individuals today feel like they have less control over communication with their healthcare providers. Providers report similar feelings—managed care systems have compromised their ability to relate to patients in traditional and meaningful ways (Apker, 2001; Gillespie, 2001; Miller & Ryan, 2001). As a result, empirical investigations must examine the control issues in this relationship: Relational control patterns among providers and patients involved in cancer care will be influenced by the effects of managed care policies and regulations.

A second bias that continues to influence (haunt) my thinking on patient-provider research, especially from a cancer context, involves *postdiagnostic* communication processes. The National Cancer Institute, along with other collateral cancer organizations do a wonderful job in providing patients with information about the etiology, symptomology, and support services associated with each type of cancer. This information is available for both patients and providers. What is missing is an extant body of research that addresses the difficult issues of patient-provider communication following the diagnosis of cancer. Most researchers in health communication have focused their talents on cancer prevention strategies, and it is hoped that they continue to enrich the scholarly literature with their efforts. However, theoretically driven, empirical research is desperately needed in the areas of survivorship, quality of life, palliative and hospice care, and loss, bereavement, and grief for those millions of patients who have been diagnosed with the second leading cause of death in our nation (see chapters in this volume). It is critical that focused study be directed toward these goals: What are the essential theoretical and practical attributes associated with explanatory models of postdiagnostic cancer care and communication among providers and patients.

Although elementary in its depiction, Figure 24.2 represents an initial model from which we can demonstrate essential relationships in the cancer communication process. Agency (see Richey & Brown, this volume; O'Hair et al., 2003; Villagran et al., this volume) becomes a key element in facilitating communication between cancer patients and critical players in the cancer care delivery system. Future research would do well in illuminating agency pathways for the cancer patients as they travel the postdiagnostic journey.

In sum, focusing on systemic effects and postdiagnostic care within a provider-consumer relational context is an ideal means of responding to the charge put forth by Health People 2010. That is, emphasizing communication within this unique context is a most cost effective approach for accomplishing essential goals for cancer care delivery. Funding sources, health communication researchers, and affected practitioners and patients are facing rich opportunities for moving cancer care to new levels of distinction. There has never been a better time for accomplishing those goals.

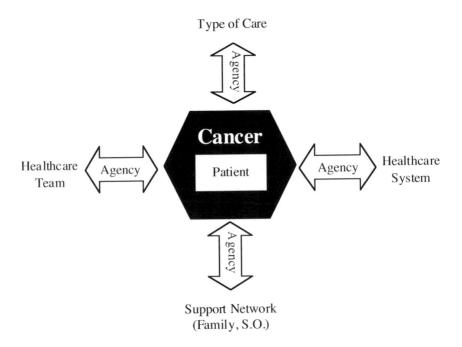

FIGURE 24.2. Cancer Care Process.

REFERENCES

Apker, J. (2001). Role development in the managed care era: A case of hospital-based nursing. *Journal of Applied Communication Research, 29,* 117-136.

Bandura, A. (1977). *Social learning theory.* Englewood Cliffs, NJ: Prentice-Hall.

Beisecker, A. E., & Beisecker, T. D. (1993). Using metaphors to characterize doctor-patient relationship: Paternalism versus patientism. *Health Communication, 5,* 41-58.

Ben-Sira, Z. (1980). Affective and instrumental components in the physician-patient relationship: An additional dimension of interaction theory. *Journal of Health and Social Behavior, 17,* 3-11.

Blanchard, C. G., Labrecque, M. S., Ruckdeschel, J. C., & Blanchard, E. B. (1988). Information and decision-making preferences of hospitalized adult cancer patients. *Social Science and Medicine, 27,* 1139-1145.

Bruera, E., Sweeney, C., Calder, K., Palmer, L., & Benisch-Tolley, S. (2001). Patient preferences versus physician perceptions of treatment decisions in cancer care. *Journal of Clinical Oncology, 19,* 2883-5.

Buller, M., & Buller, D. (1987). Physicians' communication style and patient satisfaction. *Journal of Health and Social Behavior, 28,* 375-388.

Burgoon, M., Birk, T. S., & Hall, J. R. (1991). Compliance and satisfaction with physician-patient communication: An expectancy theory interpretation of gender differences. *Human Communication Research, 18,* 177-208.

Burgoon, M., Parrott, R., Burgoon, J. K., Birk, T., Pfau, M., & Cocker, R. (1990). Primary care physicians' selection of verbal compliance-gaining strategies. *Health Communication, 2,* 13-27.

Burgoon, J. K., Pfau, M., Parrott, R., Birk, T., Cocker, R., & Burgoon, M. (1987). Relational communication, satisfaction, compliance-gaining strategies, and compliance in communication between physicians and patients. *Communication Monographs, 54,* 307-324.

Cassileth, B. R., Zupkis, R. V., Sutton-Smith, K., & March, V. (1980). Information and participation preferences among cancer patients. *Annals of Internal Medicine, 92,* 832-836.

Cegala, D. J., McNeilis, K. S., McGee, D. D., & Jonas, A. P. (1995). A study of doctors' and patients' perceptions of information processing and communication competence during the medical interview. *Health Communication, 7,* 179-203.

Cline, R., & McKenzie, N. (1998). The many cultures of health care: Difference, dominance, and distance in physician-patient communication. In L. Jackson & B. Duffy (Eds.), *Health communication research: A guide to developments and directions* (pp. 57-74). Westport, CT: Greenwood Press.

Detmar, S. B., Aaronson, N. K., Wever, L.D., Muller, M., & Schornagel, J. H. (2000). How are you feeling? Who wants to know? Patients' and oncologists' preferences for discussing health-related quality-of-life issues. *Journal of Clinical Oncology, 18,* 3295-3301.

Donabedian, A. (1980). *Explorations in quality assessment and monitoring, Volume 1. The definition of quality and approaches to its assessment.* Ann Arbor, MI: Health Administration Press.

duPré, A. (1998). *Humor and the healing arts.* Mahwah, NJ: Erlbaum.

Frankel, R. M. (1984). From sentence to sequence: Understanding the medical encounter through microinteractional analysis. *Discourse Processes, 7,* 135-170.

Gadow, S. (1990). Existential advocacy: Philosophical foundation of nursing. In S. Spicker & S. Gadow (Eds.), *Nursing: Images and ideas* (pp. 79-101). New York: Springer.

Gafni, A., & Whelan, T. (1998). The physician-patient encounter: The physician as a perfect agent for the patient versus the informed treatment decision-making model. *Social Science and Medicine, 47,* 347-354.

Gillespie, S. R. (2001) The politics of breathing: Asthma Medicaid patients under managed care. *Journal of Applied Communication Research, 29,* 97-116.

Gray, R. E., Doan, B. D., & Church, K. (1990). Empowerment and persons with cancer: Politics in cancer medicine. *Journal of Palliative Care, 6,* 33-45.

Greeneich, D. M. S. (1995). A model of patient satisfaction and behavioral intention in managed care (nurse practitioners) (University of San Diego; 0105). *Dissertation Abstracts International, 56*-05B, 2557.

Kaplan, S. H., Gandek, B., Greenfield, S., Rogers, W. H., & Ware, J. E. (1995). Patient and visit characteristics related to physicians' participatory decision-making style: Results from the Medical Outcomes Study. *Medical Care, 33,* 1176-1187.

Kaplan, S. H., Greenfield, S., Gandek, B., Rogers, W. H., & Ware, J. E. (1996). Characteristics of physicians with participatory decision-making styles. *Annals of Internal Medicine, 124.*

Klingle, R. S., & Burgoon, M. (1995). Patient compliance and satisfaction with physician influence attempts: A reinforcement expectancy approach to compliance-gaining over time. *Communication Research, 22,* 148-187.

Korsch, B. M., & Negrete, V. F. (1981). Doctor-patient communication. In G. Henderson (Ed.), *Physician-patient communication: Readings and recommendations* (pp. 29-65). Springfield, IL: Charles C. Thomas.

Kreps, G. (2001). Patient/provider communication research: A personal plea to address issues of ecological validity, relational development, message diversity, and situational constraints. *Journal of Health Psychology, 6(5), 597-601.*

Kreps, G., O'Hair, D., & Clowers, M. (1994). The influence of health communication on health outcomes. *American Behavioral Scientist, 38,* 248-256.

Ledlow, G. R., O'Hair, D., & Moore, S. D. (2003). Predictors of communication quality: The patient, provider and nurse call center triad. *Health Communication, 15,* 431-455.

Lopez, F. G., & Lent, R. W. (1991). Efficacy-based predictors of relationship adjustment and persistence among college students. *Journal of College Student Development, 32,* 223-229.

Madson, K. G. (1999). The voice of cancer. *Plastic Surgical Nursing, 19,* 127-129.

McNeilis, K. S., & Thompson, T. (1995). The impact of relational control on patient compliance in dentist-patient interactions. In G. Kreps & D. O'Hair (Eds.), *Communication and health outcomes* (pp. 57-72). Cresskill, NJ: Hampton Press.

McNeilis, K. S., Thompson, T., & O'Hair, D. (1995). Implications of relational communication for therapeutic discourse. In G. Morris & R. Chenail (Eds.), *The talk of the clinic* (pp. 291-313). Hillsdale, NJ: Erlbaum.

Millar, F. E., & Rogers, L. E. (1987). Relational dimensions of interpersonal dynamics. In M. Roloff & G. Miller (Eds.), *Explorations in interpersonal communication* (pp. 117-139). Beverly Hills: Sage.

Miller, K., & Ryan, D. (2001). Communication in the age of managed care: Introduction to the special issue. *Journal of Applied Communication Research, 29,* 91-96.

Moore, S. D., & O'Hair, H. D. (1997, February). *Patient expectations of communication within managed health care.* Paper presented to the Organizational Communication Interest Group of the Western States Communication Association, Monterey, CA.

Moore, S. D., O'Hair, D., & Ledlow, G. (2002). The effects of health delivery systems and self-efficacy on patient compliance and satisfaction. *Communication Research Reports, 19*(4) 362-371.

O'Connor, R. D., Hallberg, S., & Myles, R. (1998). Organizational communication and health care administration. In L. Jackson & B. Duffy (Eds.), *Health communication research: A guide to developments and directions* (pp. 103-124). Westport, CT: Greenwood Press.

O'Hair, D. (1986). Patient preferences for physician persuasion strategies. *Theoretical Medicine, 7,* 147-164.

O'Hair, D. (1988). Relational communication in applied contexts: Current status and future directions. *Southern Speech Communication Journal, 53,* 317-330.

O'Hair, D. (1989). Dimensions of relational communication and control during physician and patients interactions. *Health Communication, 1,* 97-116.

O'Hair, D. (2003). Research traditions in provider-consumer interaction: Implications for cancer care. *Patient Education and Counseling, 50,* 5-8.

O'Hair, D., Allman, J., & Moore, S. (1996). A cognitive-affective model of relational expectations in the provider-patient context. *Journal of Health Psychology, 1*, 307-322.

O'Hair, D., Behnke, R., & King, P. (1983). Age-related patient preferences for physician communication behavior. *Educational Gerontology, 9*, 147-158.

O'Hair, H. D., Halone, K., Morris, M., & Ledlow, L. G. (1997, February). *Extending the theoretical base of health communication research*. Paper presented to the Communication Theory and Research Interest Group of the Western States Communication Association, Monterey, CA.

O'Hair, D., & McNeilis, K. S. (1993). Advocates for the elderly patient: A case study of mutual influence. In E. B. Ray (Ed.), *Case studies in health communication* (pp. 61-73). Hillsdale, NJ: Erlbaum.

O'Hair, D., O'Hair, M., Southward, M., & Krayer, K. (1987). Patient compliance and physician communication. *Journal of Compliance in Health Care, 2*, 125-128.

O'Hair, D., Scannell, D., & Thompson, S. (2005). Agency through narrative: Patients managing cancer care in a challenging environment. In L. Harter, P. Japp, & C. Beck (Eds.), *Narratives, health, & healing* (pp. 413-432). Mahwah, NJ: Erlbaum.

O'Hair, D., Villagran, M., Wittenberg, E., Brown, K., Hall, T., Ferguson, M., & Doty, T. (2003). Cancer survivorship and agency model (CSAM): Implications for patient choice, decision making, and influence. *Health Communication, 15*, 193-202.

Paletta, J. H. (1995). Patients' perception of orthopaedic nursing competence (Columbia Teachers College; 0055). *Dissertation Abstracts International*, 56-07B, 3696.

Parker, P. A., Baile, W. F., de Moor, C., Lenzi, R., Kudelka, A. P., & Cohen, L. (2001). Breaking bad news about cancer: Patients' preferences for communication. *Journal of Clinical Oncology, 19*, 2049-2056.

Rogers, L. E., Courtright, J. A., & Millar, F. E. (1980). Message control intensity: Rationale and preliminary findings. *Communication Monographs, 47*, 201-219.

Rogers, L. E., & Farace, R. V. (1975). Analysis of relational communication in dyads: New measurement procedures. *Human Communication Research, 1*, 222-239.

Rogers, L. E., & Millar, F. E. (1982). The question of validity: A pragmatic answer. In M. Burgoon (Ed.), *Communication yearbook 5* (pp. 249-257). Beverly Hills, CA: Sage.

Rubin, R. B., Martin, M. M., Bruning, S. S., & Powers, D. E. (1993). Test of self-efficacy model of interpersonal communication competence. *Communication Quarterly, 41*, 210-220.

Spiro, D., & Heidrich, F. (1983). Lay understanding of medical terminology. *The Journal of Family Practice, 17*, 277-279.

Street, R., & Wiemann, J. (1987). Patient satisfaction with physicians' interpersonal involvement, expressiveness, and dominance. In M. L. McLaughlin (Ed.), *Communication yearbook* (Vol. 10, pp. 591-612). Newbury Park, CA: Sage.

Von Friederichs-Fitzwater, M. M., Callahan, E. J., Flynn, N., & Williams, J. (1991). Relational control in physician-patient encounters. *Health Communication, 3*, 17-36.

Wallerstein, N., & Bernstein, E. (1999). Empowerment education: Freire's ideas adapted to health education. *Health Education Quarterly, 15*, 379-394.

Woodruff, S. L., & Cashman, J. F. (1993). Task, domain, and general efficacy: A reexamination of the self-efficacy scale. *Psychological Reports, 72*, 423-432.

About the Contributors

Neeraj K. Arora is a social scientist in the Outcomes Research Branch of the Division of Cancer Control and Population Sciences at the National Cancer Institute, NIH. Dr. Arora received his PhD in Industrial Engineering with a major in Health Systems from the University of Wisconsin-Madison in 2000. Dr. Arora's research emphasizes the linkage and interrelationship among the areas of health communication, outcomes research, and cancer survivorship. Specifically, his work focuses on the measurement, determinants, and impact of physician–patient communication, patient participation in medical decision making, and cancer-related information seeking. Dr. Arora's research expertise also includes measurement and assessment of patient-reported outcomes including cancer patients' and survivors' experiences of and satisfaction with care, their information needs, and their health-related quality of life. At the NCI, Dr. Arora is conducting population-based studies that assess cancer survivors' perceptions of their follow-up care and their quality of life outcomes. He currently leads the NCI's efforts for planning a research initiative on patient-centered communication in cancer care.

Terri Babers holds a Master's of Professional Communication from the University of Alaska Fairbanks (2003), where her emphasis was Health Communication and Organizational Development. Her qualitative study of caregiver's communication experiences in triadic medical encounters stems from her experiences as the primary caregiver for her mother-in-law, who died from breast cancer in 1983; her ongoing work with people who have significant disabilities; and her work with the aging population in Fairbanks. Her personal and professional interest lies in facilitating human communication to help people connect from a perspective of their strengths. Terri lives near her three children in Fairbanks, where she is an independent communication consultant and coach. She is active in diverse community organizations such as the Alaska Geriatric Education Center, the Parent Academy, the Ballroom Dance Club of Fairbanks, Rotary International, and Fairbanks Paddler's Club.

Alexis D. Bakos is a health scientist administrator in the Office of Extramural Programs at the National Institute of Nursing Research, National Institutes of Health (NINR/NIH) in Bethesda, MD. She serves as a program director for scientific areas related to end-of-life and palliative care, ethics/research integrity, informal caregiving, and long-term care research. She also chairs the NIH-wide End-of-Life Scientific Interest Group. Prior to her appointment at NINR, she completed three years of postdoctoral training as a Cancer Prevention Fellow within the Division of Cancer Prevention at the National Cancer Institute, NIH. Previously, she worked as a staff member for the House of Representatives Select Committee on Aging as a specialist in health legislative affairs. Dr. Bakos is certified in gerontological nursing from the American Nurses' Association and is a member of Sigma Theta Tau International Nursing Honor Society.

Jozien M. Bensing is director of the Netherlands Institute for Health Services Research (NIVEL) and professor of Health Psychology at Utrecht University (the Netherlands). She is a member of several National Advisory Councils on the interface between the academic world and health care, such as the Dutch Health Council, the National Advisory Council for Science and Technology, the Social Research Council of the Dutch Royal Academy of Sciences, and the National Advisory Council on Health Research. She has published over 200 articles, books, and book chapters, mainly on communication in health care, but also on psychosomatic medicine (fatigue, pain, medically unexplained symptoms) and gender issues in health care. She has been active in the organization of several international conferences on communication in health care (Amsterdam, Oxford, Barcelona, Warwick, Chicago, and Basel), and is the co-founder and first president of the European Association for Communication in Health Care (EACH).

Jin Brown is the Chair of the department of communication at the University of Alaska Fairbanks, where he has served on the faculty since 1993. He received his MA and PhD degrees from the University of Oklahoma. Dr. Brown's research interests include secrecy in an organizational setting, assessment of public speaking (and how teaching, assessment, and accreditation can be a seamless process for the basic course in communication), narrative research (in health settings), and most recently, e-mail as supplement to face-to-face communication in romantic relationship formation. He is currently on sabbatical reading Simmel and thinking about the social construction of secrecy.

Kenneth M. Brown is a PhD candidate (University of Oklahoma) and an assistant professor of communication at Washburn University, Topeka, Kansas. Additionally, he is a seminary graduate, ordained minister, and was a pastor for 27 years. He and his wife Jean have 2 grown children and 2 grandchildren.

Donald J. Cegala, PhD, is a professor in the School of Communication and the Department of Family Medicine at The Ohio State University. He has been on the Ohio State faculty for over 30 years. Dr. Cegala is the former Chair of the Health Communication Division of the National Communication Association; he is a member of the OSU Institute for Primary Care

Research and the OSU Comprehensive Cancer Center. He has served as a consultant and grant reviewer for the National Cancer Institute, and has received federal funding for his own research. He has published over 30 articles in academic journals, and is known internationally for his research on physician–patient communication.

Betty Chewning, PhD, is an associate professor in the Division of Social Administrative Sciences and Director of the Sonderegger Research Center in the School of Pharmacy, University of Wisconsin-Madison. She teaches communication courses and studies methods to enhance and understand patient participation during their encounters with health care providers.

M. Robin DiMatteo, PhD (Harvard University, 1976), is Distinguished Professor of psychology at the University of California at Riverside. Her research involves the role of interpersonal and intrapersonal factors in the achievement of health, the utilization of medical care, and the adjustment to illness and disability. Her recent work on patient compliance/adherence to medical treatment focuses on the practitioner-patient relationship as a central component in bringing about patients' behavior change. She is using meta-analytic techniques for synthesizing the literature on adherence, and also examining the value of a multifactorial model in the determination of health-promoting versus health-compromising behavior. This model takes into account patients' beliefs and attitudes, social norms, commitment to action, rapport and effective communication with their practitioners, and the provision of supports for the removal of barriers to health action. She has been involved in research focused on enhancing both physician and patient use of preventive medical services and on adherence to pediatric regimens. She has conducted research in recent years on the psychosocial aspects of childbirth. She is interested in the sources and effects of stress on health professionals. Other research involves the study of the process of coping with illness, particularly the psychological and social consequences of chronic pain. Finally, Dr. DiMatteo is also interested in the development of curriculum materials in the field of health psychology.

Connie Dresser is the Program Director for the National Cancer Institute's Multimedia Technology Health Communication SBIR/STTR Grants in the Health Communication and Informatics Research Branch. The program promotes science-based, theory-driven, user-centered cancer communication research, and the development of products across the cancer continuum, from prevention to survivorship to end-of-life issues. Her program has produced four "Linking Science and Business SBIR Showcases" and an informative Web site for new and experienced applicants. She has accelerated ehealth research activities through her program as an NCI liaison to the Department of Health and Human Services' Science Panel on Interactive Communication and Health, and as a member of the Healthy People 2010 Health Communication Workgroup. Ms. Dresser has received four National Institutes of Health Merit Awards for these and other achievements. As a registered public health nutritionist, formally in clinical and private practice and a nutrition analyst for the CDC's National and Hispanic Health and Nutrition Examination Surveys, she brings her experiences in clinical and applied health communication, public health nutrition, epidemiology, and data collection and surveillance activities to her current role. She has written more than 30 peer-reviewed journal articles, book chapters, and Federal government publications.

Eileen S. Gilchrist (MA, University of Houston, 1997) is a third year doctoral student in the communication department of the University of Oklahoma (OU). Her primary research interest is health communication, with an emphasis in interpersonal, organizational, and risk communication within the aging, palliative care, and end-of-life populations. She has held a graduate teaching assistantship since 2003 and is currently the basic course director. The OU Department of Communication presented her with the 2005 Outstanding Graduate Student Award. Additionally, she was a participant in the 2005 NCA National Doctoral Honors Seminar. She also assisted NCA's 2005 1st Vice-president, Dan O'Hair, in planning the Boston NCA convention. During the 2004-2005 school year, she served her department and fellow students as co-president of the Communication Graduate Student Association. Since 2002, she has been an editorial and research assistant, under Jim Query's editorship, of *Communication Studies*. From 1994-2003, she taught in the University of Houston's Communication Department.

Lila J. Finney Rutten is a behavioral scientist for Scientific Applications International Corporation-Frederick, Inc. contracted to the Health Communication and Informatics Research Branch of the National Cancer Institute. She recently completed a post-doctoral fellowship in the National Cancer Institute's (NCI) Cancer Prevention Fellowship Program, during which she earned a Master's in public health from Harvard University. Prior to the fellowship, she earned her doctoral degree in psychology from Miami University of Ohio. Her research interests emphasize cancer prevention and control at the population-level with attention to the social contexts that influence cancer-relevant health behavior. Her program of research focuses on cancer relevant beliefs, information needs, and critical sources of cancer information among diverse populations. This work aims to provide an evidence base for delivering effective cancer prevention and control messages to the public, cancer patients, and patient advocates.

Lawrence R. Frey is a professor in the department of communication at the University of Colorado at Boulder. He teaches group interaction, applied communication, and quantitative and qualitative research methods courses. His research focuses on how participation in collective communicative practices makes a difference in people's individual, relational, and collective life. He is the author/editor of 14 books, 3 special journal issues, and more than 60 book chapters and journal articles. He has received 10 distinguished scholarship awards, including the 2000 Gerald M. Phillips Award for Distinguished Applied Communication Scholarship from the National Communication Association (NCA); the 2003 and 2000 Ernest Bormann Research Award from NCA's Group Communication Division for his edited texts, *New Directions in Group Communication* and *The Handbook of Group Communication Theory and Research*; and the 1998 National Jesuit Book Award and 1988 Distinguished Book Award from NCA's Applied Communication Division for his coauthored text, *The Fragile Community: Living Together With AIDS*. He is a past president of the Central States Communication Association and a recipient of the Outstanding Young Teacher Award from that organization, and the 2003 Master Teacher Award from the Communication and Instruction Interest Group of the Western States Communication Association.

Geoffrey H. Gordon is an associate professor of Medicine and Psychiatry at Oregon Health & Science University in Portland. Dr. Gordon followed his internal medicine residency with a fellowship in biopsychosocial medicine at the University of Rochester and has had a special interest in teaching clinical communication skills and the doctor-patient relationship. From 1997 to 2002 he served as Associate Director for Clinical Education with the Bayer Institute for Health Care Communication, where he developed interactive workshops on end-of-life communication. He currently directs the John Benson Program on Professionalism in the School of Medicine and serves as an Associate Director for the Center for Ethics in Health Care at OHSU. He has published over 40 articles and book chapters on communication skills and co-authored the popular *Field Guide to the Difficult Patient Interview*.

Linda M. Harris, PhD, is a Senior Health Communication Scientist in the Health Communication and Informatics Research Branch at the National Cancer Institute. She contributes to the Branch's efforts in information and communication technology research, focusing on coordinated cancer care. She came to the National Cancer Institute after spending five years in the private sector where she was involved in innovative uses of the Internet. Her previous public sector experience includes the exploration of family, community, and employer solutions to HIV while the Director of the Family Health Program at the Washington Business Group on Health; leading the development and evaluation of a community health and human services online network during her tenure as Chief of the Information Branch for the Office of Disease Prevention and Health Promotion, and Director of the National Health Information Center, HHS; and exploring translational health technology research as Senior Health Advisor to the Advanced Research Projects Agency, Department of Defense. Dr. Harris has written extensively about family communication and health communication technologies, including *Health and the New Media: Technologies Transforming Personal and Public Health*. She has advanced degrees in mass communication and interpersonal communication, and completed postdoctoral studies in family sociology.

Carol J. Hermansen Kobulnicky is an assistant professor in the School of Pharmacy at the University of Wyoming. She earned her PhD in Social and Administrative Pharmacy at the University of Wisconsin-Madison after working as a clinical pharmacist. Her research interests include studying interdisciplinary, collaborative, and patient self-care efforts to learn how to better involve the cancer patient in medication and symptom management across the course of care. Her teaching pursuits include preparing pharmacists in the area of practice management and communication with patients and other providers. She enjoys bringing her research into the classroom and serves as a member of the Wyoming Comprehensive Cancer Control Consortium.

Mary E. Husain is a lecturer in the Department of Communication and the Department of Mass Communication and Journalism at California State University, Fresno. She is a doctoral student in the California State University, Fresno/University of California, Davis, Joint Doctoral Program in Educational Leadership. Her research interests encompass two diverse areas: health communication/education and rhetorical criticism. She is co-author of a forthcoming article in the *National Women's Studies Journal*. She also serves as a member of the Board of Directors of University High School, on the California State University, Fresno campus.

Julie T. Irish is a research scientist at the Institute for Clinical Research and Health Policy Studies at Tufts-New England Medical Center and Assistant Professor of Medicine at Tufts

University School of Medicine. Her research interests include the psychosocial aspects of the medical interaction and quality care improvement. Dr. Irish's current research explores the linkages between physician–patient communication and racial disparities in diagnostic and treatment decisions. Prior to joining Tufts-New England Medical Center, Dr. Irish was a Research Scientist at The Picker Institute/Beth Israel Deaconess Medical Center, where she led survey development projects focusing on the assessment of nursing care for older adults with cognitive impairments and patients' and physician's satisfaction with telemedicine. Dr. Irish has also served as a consultant to the American Board of Internal Medicine.

Laura Jones Fox (MA, Texas State University-San Marcos, 2004) conducts research in the areas of health and organizational communication. She is especially interested in developing training and development materials to improve health communication among providers and older adult patients. Recently, she has been working as a communication consultant and teaching communication courses for the Dallas Community College District in Dallas, TX.

Boaz Kahana (PhD, University of Chicago, 1967) is a professor of psychology at Cleveland State University. Dr. Kahana joined the Department of Psychology in 1984 and served as chair from 1984-1987. He was director of the Center for Applied Gerontological Research from 1998-1997. Dr. Kahana has published extensively in the fields of mental health and clinical psychology of aging, trauma survivorship (focusing on both cancer survivors and Holocaust survivors), and on stress, coping, and health. His recent publications deal with planning for end-of-life care, successful aging among the chronically ill, the mental health of elderly cancer survivors, and late life adaptation of Holocaust survivors. Dr. Kahana served as President of the Ohio Network of Gerontological Consultants in Aging and has been honored with the Heller Award for excellence in Gerontological research. He has been a peer reviewer for the National Institute of Mental Health and the National Institute of Aging. He is a Fellow of the American Psychological Society and the Gerontological Society of America. He serves on the editorial board of the *Journal of Aging and Mental Health*.

Eva Kahana (PhD, University of Chicago, 1968) is the Pierce T. and Elizabeth D. Robson Professor of Humanities, Director of the Elderly Care Research Center, and Chair of the Department of Sociology at Case Western Reserve University. Throughout her career, she has pursued an applied program of research aimed at contributing to improved quality-of-life for older adults and focused on conceptualizing and operationalizing older people in a context— that is, how person–environment transactions explain late life well-being and quality of life. Her major research interests include social organization of health care institutions, late life sequelae of social stress, coping and adaptation among the elderly, environmental influences on aging individuals, institutionalization, migration, intergenerational family relationships, medical sociology, health care partnerships, and self-care. Dr. Kahana has received numerous awards for her scholarship including the John S. Diekhoff Distinguished Graduate Teaching Award, Case Western Reserve University, 2002; the Distinguished Scholar Lecturer, American Sociological Association, Section on Aging and the Life Course, 1998; the Distinguished Scholar from the American Sociological Association, Section on Aging and the Life Course, 1997; the Polisher Award for Creative Contributions to Applied Gerontology from the Gerontological Society of America, 1997; the Outstanding Gerontological Researcher in Ohio from the Ohio Research Council on Aging, 1993; and the Mary E. Switzer Distinguished Fellow from the National Institute of Disability and Rehabilitation, 1992-1993.

Bernard J. Kerr, Jr. is an associate professor with the Central Michigan University Doctor of Health Administration (DHA) Program. Immediately prior to joining the DHA faculty, Colonel Bernie Kerr was a United States Air Force Medical Service Corps professional health care administrator. He has nearly 30 years experience in the health care industry, including positions in public health, academia, and the military health system. His academic credentials include a bachelor's in health education and master's degrees in public health, health administration, business administration, and information management. He holds a doctor of education in curriculum and instruction and the instructional process and a graduate interdisciplinary certificate in gerontology. Dr. Kerr is a board certified health care executive and a Fellow in the American College of Healthcare Executives.

Paula Kim is known nationally and internationally for her work in research and patient advocacy and is becoming equally well-known for her efforts to bridge the gap between the research community and those with whom researchers must collaborate to achieve success in accelerating the science of research that benefits patients. Her efforts focus on accelerating the development of research and advocacy strategies that enhance the productivity of biomedical research. To further this goal, Ms. Kim has developed an innovative program, TRAC — Translating Research Across Communities[SM] — to identify and guide improvement opportunities in research collaboration, communication, outreach, funding, clinical trials, and public policy across all sectors of biomedical research. Ms Kim lost her father to pancreatic cancer just 75 days after his diagnosis in 1998. In 1999, she co-founded the Pancreatic Cancer Action Network (PanCAN), the first and only national patient advocacy organization for the pancreatic cancer community, serving as Board Chair, President, and CEO between 1999 and 2004. Prior to PanCAN, there was no national program providing key patient services; education and awareness of the disease; and engaging the research, government and industrial communities to ensure that pancreatic cancer research become a scientific priority on the national level. With a handful of volunteers and no paid staff, Ms. Kim and her co-founders immediately began providing vibrant national leadership in the battle against pancreatic cancer, the fourth leading cause of cancer death, where none previously existed. Under Ms. Kim's leadership, PanCAN public policy efforts resulted in an unprecedented increase of over 200% in federal government investments for pancreatic cancer research.

Gary L. Kreps (PhD, University of Southern California, 1979) is Professor and Chair of the Department of Communication at George Mason University (GMU) in Fairfax, VA, where he holds the Eileen and Steve Mandell Endowed Chair in Health Communication. Prior to his appointment at GMU, he served for five years as the founding Chief of the Health Communication and Informatics Research Branch at the National Cancer Institute (NCI), where he planned, developed, and coordinated major new national research and outreach initiatives concerning risk communication, health promotion, behavior change, technology development, and information dissemination to promote effective cancer prevention, screening, control, care, and survivorship. He has also served as the Founding Dean of the School of Communication at Hofstra University, Executive Director of the Greenspun School of Communication at UNLV, and in faculty and administrative roles at Northern Illinois, Rutgers, Indiana, and Purdue Universities. His areas of expertise include health communication and promotion, information dissemination, risk communication, organizational communication, information technology, multicultural relations, and applied research methods. He is an active scholar, whose published work currently includes more than 250 books, articles, chapters, and edited journal issues concerning the applications of communication knowledge in society. He has received many honors for his scholarship, including the 2005-2006 Pfizer Visiting Professorship of Clear Health Communication Award, the 2004 Robert Lewis Donohew Outstanding Health Communication Scholar Award, the 2002 Future of Health Technology Award, the 2002 Distinguished Achievement Award for Outstanding Contributions in Consumer Health Informatics and Online Health, the 2000 Outstanding Health Communication Scholar Award" from both the International Communication Association and the National Communication Association, and the 1998 Gerald M. Phillips Distinguished Applied Communication Scholarship Award from the National Communication Association.

Edward Krupat is the Director of Evaluation at Harvard Medical School and associate professor of psychology in the Department of Psychiatry at the Beth Israel Deaconess Medical Center. He holds a PhD in social psychology from the University of Michigan, and has taught previously as Rutgers University, Boston College, and the Massachusetts College of Pharmacy and Health Sciences. Dr. Krupat's interests revolve around the assessment of outcomes in medical education and research on doctor-patient communication. He has developed the Patient-Practitioner Orientation Scale, an instrument to assess the practice-related beliefs of patients and practitioners; and (with co-researchers Terry Stein and Richard Frankel) has developed the Four Habits Coding Scheme to measure patient-centeredness in the behaviors of physicians. He is currently involved in research and educational projects focusing on health disparities, and is actively engaged in the evaluation of several innovative programs to improve clinical teaching at Harvard Medical School.

Gerald (Jerry) Ledlow, PhD, MHA, CHE, is a board certified health care executive, bestowed by the American College of Healthcare Executives, and has earned a PhD from the University of Oklahoma, a Master's in Healthcare Administration from Baylor University, and a Bachelor's degree in Economics from the Virginia Military Institute. Dr. Ledlow has held academic positions as tenured faculty and director of the doctor of health administration program at Central Michigan University, executive positions with the Sisters of Mercy Health System, and the Department of Defense and has consulting experience in organizational development, leadership, planning, and communication with organizations such as the United Way, universities, charter schools, Department of Defense, and public health Agencies. Dr. Ledlow has published dozens of articles, several book chapters and served as an editor and contributing author for four books. He has been awarded the Regent's Award from the American College of Healthcare Executives in 1997 and 2003, and also the Federal Sector Managed Care Award in 1998. Currently, Dr. Ledlow is a Corporate Vice President for the Sisters of Mercy Health System.

Pamela McWherter is an associate professor and Graduate Program Coordinator of communication at University of Alaska Fairbanks. She holds bachelor's and master's degrees from Missouri State University and a doctoral degree from Southern Illinois University. A native of Arkansas, she has lived in Alaska since 1993. Her research and teaching interests include age-gap romantic relationships, the role of computer mediated communication in romantic relationships, and training assessment.

Scott D. Moore conducts research centered primarily in applied health communication, with an interest in organizational and interpersonal communication. Of particular focus is the perceived encroachment of outside agencies on provider-patient interaction. Recently, Dr. Moore has addressed the significance of environmental factors, and systemic and institutionalized influences on the delivery of healthcare. He has served as an Associate Editor for the *Journal of Applied Communication Research, Western Journal of Communication, Communication Research Reports,* and *Communication Studies,* and as Chair of the Health Communication Interest Groups for both the Eastern Communication Association and the Western States Communication Association. His most recent book, co edited with Kevin Wright, is titled *Applied Health Communication* (Hampton Press, 2007)

H. Dan O'Hair is a professor in the department of communication at the University of Oklahoma. His teaching and research interests include organizational communication, health systems, risk communication, and patient care communication processes. He has published over 70 research articles and scholarly book chapters in communication, health, management, and psychology journals and volumes, and has authored and edited 12 books in the areas of communication, business, and health. He is one of the founding directors of the Southwest Program for Pancreatic Cancer at the University of Oklahoma and was a co-chair of the Pancreatic Cancer Progress Group at the National Cancer Institute. He has served on the editorial boards of 18 research journals and is the immediate past editor of the *Journal of Applied Communication Research,* published by the National Communication Association. In 2006, Dr. O'Hair served as president of the National Communication Association.

Jim L. Query, Jr. (PhD, Ohio University, 1990) is an associate professor of communication at the University of Houston (UH), School of Communication. He holds a joint appointment with the University of Texas M. D. Anderson Cancer Center as an Adjunct Associate Professor of Neuro-Oncology. From 1991-1994, he served as the President of the Alzheimer's Association of Tulsa, Oklahoma. In addition to being a summer research fellow and consultant with the National Cancer Institute (NCI), he has worked and taught at the Indiana University School of Nursing, Indiana University Purdue University Indianapolis (IUPUI), the Ohio University College of Osteopathic Medicine, Ohio University, Ohio University East, University of Tulsa, and Loyola University Chicago (LUC). The bulk of his research examines the communication of social support during major life events such as retirement, caregiving during Alzheimer's, living with AIDS, and returning to higher education. His other research interests include communication among individuals with cancer and their caregivers, face-to-face and online support groups, health promotion interventions, multicultural health communication, Weick's model of organizing, and the Critical Incident Technique. Dr. Query is a Co-PI on a $25,000 grant from UH to establish the Center for Health and Crisis Communication (2005-2006). Dr. Query has authored or co-authored eight journal articles, sixteen book chapters, five book reviews, an encyclopedia entry, and a research methods instructor's resource manual. From 1998-2002, Dr. Query was a Contributing Editor for the *Journal of Health Communication: International Perspectives,* editing 21 book reviews. Dr. Query currently sits on two editorial boards and is the Editor of *Communication Studies* (*CS*) having recruited the largest editorial board in North America and Europe and currently featuring a 16% acceptance rate.

Sandra L. Ragan (PhD, University of Texas) is a professor in the department of communication at the University of Oklahoma. Her research in health communication began in the 1980s with an interest in women's health communication. This inquiry spawned a number of publications; it also helped to launch the careers of two health communication stars: Christina Beck and Athena duPre. In the last several years, Sandy has been writing in the area of palliative care communication and is currently working on a book on that topic. She is a passionate advocate for humane end-of-life care and patient-centered communication.

Amelie G. Ramirez, DrPH, Professor of Medicine at Baylor College of Medicine, is Director of the Office of Outreach and Health Disparities Research in Cancer at the Baylor Cancer Center and Deputy Director of the Chronic Disease Prevention and Control Research Center in the Department of Medicine. As a behavioral science and health communications investigator, she directs and participates in several research projects involving Latinos and such issues as breast cancer genetics, cancer risk factors, impact of breast cancer on families, breast cancer survivorship, and smoking prevention and cessation. Over the past 25 years, she has directed numerous state-, federal- and privately funded research programs focusing on human and organizational communication to reduce chronic disease and cancer health disparities affecting Latinos and other populations. She has authored over 60 peer-reviewed articles and is the recipient of state and national awards in the area of health disparities research and the advancement of Latinos in medicine, public health, and behavioral sciences professions across the United States. She is a recognized spokesperson for cancer disparities reduction and is a member of various national and regional advisory groups and coalitions. Her most recent appointments include membership on the National Cancer Advisory Board of the National Cancer Institute, the National Advisory Council of the National Heart, Lung and Blood Institute, Chair of the National Hispanic/Latino Advisory Council of the Susan G. Komen Breast Cancer Foundation, Board of Directors for the Lance Armstrong Foundation, and the Media and Counter Marketing Panel of the American Legacy Foundation.

Jean Richey is an assistant professor of communication at the University of Alaska Southeast in Juneau, Alaska. She is originally from Sacramento, California, but has lived and worked in Alaska since 1993. Jean's educational background includes a Bachelor of Arts in Psychology, 1998; Master of Arts in Professional Communication, 2001; and a PhD in Health Communication, 2003, University of Alaska Fairbanks. Prior to her academic pursuits, she had a 20-year career in public service with the State of California where she was a supervisor and trainer. Her research interests include ethical interpersonal communication and the construction of identity in co-cultural contexts.

Lisa Sparks (PhD, University of Oklahoma, 1998) is Professor of Communication Studies at Chapman University, Orange, CA. She is a highly regarded teacher-scholar whose published work spans more than 100 research articles and scholarly book chapters, and has authored and edited nine books in the areas of communication, health, and aging. Dr. Sparks' research and teaching interests include communication with, by, and about older adults, and how such communication relates to healthy and successful aging outcomes via theoretical frameworks such as lifespan development, social identity, communication accommodation, and intergroup behavior. Her research on intergroup (intergenerational, intercultural) communication and aging merges with research in health, risk, and crisis communication domains including provider-patient and family relationships and decision making, health organizations, communication about terrorism, and communicating relevant messages when information is uncertain during periods of health risk. She is currently Editor of *Communication Research Reports* and serves on several editorial boards including *Journal of Applied Communication Research* and *Communication Quarterly*.

Kiek Tates is a senior researcher at NIVEL, the Netherlands institute for health services research in Utrecht, the Netherlands. She has a background in linguistics (discourse studies) with a PhD in social sciences. Her areas of research interest include communication in health care and multiparty communication, with a focus on the participation of children in medical conversations. Before her current appointment at NIVEL, she conducted a social-oncological fellowship funded by the Dutch Cancer Society/KWF. The focus of her current research is on communication and role delineation in pediatric oncology, aiming to attain a multiperspective view on the policies, practices, and preferences regarding role delineation in information exchange and decision making within this setting.

A. M. (Sandra) van Dulmen studied clinical psychology. After graduation in 1997, she started working as a researcher in different fields of health care, first at the Department of Clinical Psychology, then, from 1988 till 1995, at the Department of General Practice at the University of Nijmegen, the Netherlands. She obtained her PhD in 1996 with the thesis titled "Exploring cognitions in irritable bowel syndrome: Implications for the role of the doctor," for which she received in 1996 the dissertation award from the Research Institute CaRe. From 1995 onward, she has worked at NIVEL (Netherlands Institute for Health Services Research), first as a researcher, and since 1999, as research coordinator of the research program Communication in Healthcare. In 2001 she co-founded and since then served as secretary of EACH (European Association for Communication in Healthcare). She has written a large number of scientific papers in the field of provider–patient communication (GPs, specialists, nurses), nonspecific/placebo factors, irritable bowel syndrome, psycho-oncology, and cognitive-behavioral interventions. She is a member of the Research Institute Psychology & Health, APS (American Psychosomatic Society), ESPCG (European Society for Primary Care Gastroenterology), and is a member of the editorial board of *Patient Education & Counseling*.

Melinda Morris Villagrán (PhD, University of Oklahoma, 2001) is an associate professor of communication at George Mason University. Her primary research program investigates messages in organizational and health care interactions to explore the intersections between organizational communication theory and health care practice in applied settings. Most recently, she has been conducting research on the role of communication and culture in health disparities among Latinos. Within this general framework, she has examined communication about cancer prevention and screening among low-income Latinos, misperceptions of the health care system, organizational and cultural barriers to cancer care, underutilization of mental health services among Latinos, effective prognosis communication, social identity and culture, and health care decision making. Dr. Villagrán currently serves on the editorial board for *Communication Research Reports*, and serves as reviewer for a number of peer-reviewed journals including *Health Communication, Journal of Applied Communication Research*, and *Public Understanding of Science*. Recent publications have appeared in *Communication Monographs, Health Communication, Communication Research Reports*, and *Case Studies for Organizational Communication*.

Elaine M. Wittenberg-Lyles is an assistant professor of communication at the University of Texas, San Antonio. Her research program entails a qualitative examination of the interpersonal processes occurring in the context of death and dying. She has examined the role of hospice volunteer-patient communication, the information-sharing strategies of hospice care managers in interdisciplinary team meetings, and communication apprehension with dying persons.

Kevin B. Wright (PhD, University of Oklahoma, 1999) is an assistant professor in the department of communication at the University of Oklahoma. The bulk of his research examines the relationship between the communication of social support and health outcomes in computer-mediated support group contexts among individuals dealing with health issues. His other research interests include communication among individuals with cancer and their caregivers, hospice and palliative care, provider-patient interaction, health promotion campaigns, aging and health, and face-face support groups for people facing health issues such as substance abuse, HIV, and eating disorders.

Author Index

Subject Index